Promoting the Emotional and Behavioral Success of Youths

Sergio V. Delgado • Ernest V. Pedapati
Jeffrey R. Strawn

Promoting the Emotional and Behavioral Success of Youths

A Practical Guide for Clinicians

Springer

Sergio V. Delgado
Cincinnati Children's Hospital and
Medical Center
Division of Child Psychiatry
Cincinnati, OH, USA

Ernest V. Pedapati
Cincinnati Children's Hospital and
Medical Center
Division of Child Psychiatry
Cincinnati, OH, USA

Jeffrey R. Strawn
University of Cincinnati
Psychiatry & Behavioral Neuroscience
Cincinnati, OH, USA

ISBN 978-3-030-88074-3 ISBN 978-3-030-88075-0 (eBook)
https://doi.org/10.1007/978-3-030-88075-0

This Springer imprint is published by the registered company Springer Nature Switzerland AG
The registered company address is: Gewerbestrasse 11, 6330 Cham, Switzerland

To my wife Erin and to my daughter Michelle
This is also dedicated to all the children and adolescents whose strengths and weaknesses provided the inspiration for this book.

—SVD

To Elliott Nicole and Rachel Marie

—JRS

To Carolyn, Noah, and Harrison, my beloved. To my parents and sister who taught me first the love of a family.

—EVP

Foreword

This work is an excellent exposition of a paradigm shift in the approach to the clinical understanding and therapeutic work with youths and their families. The authors offer an eminently useful and practical book grounded in their superb foundational work, *Contemporary Psychodynamic Psychotherapy for Children and Adolescents: Integrating Intersubjectivity and Neuroscience.* Central to this enlivening and dynamic model of practice are the four pillars of their Contemporary Diagnostic Interview. The first three pillars, temperament, cognition, and cognitive flexibility, form and ground the youth's personality, the interpersonal expression of the internal working model of attachment.

As noted by the authors, the four pillars are the synergy of innate and environmental processes that become the blueprint of how a child learns to develop and maintain self-regulation abilities to successfully interact with others. How this approach is applied, and the variables involved in the application, pave the way toward understanding how one arrives at accurate diagnostic formulations and how these are used in developing sequential treatment plans, tailored for each individual patient and his or her family, that have the best chance of a successful outcome. Useful tables, wise suggestions, and rich case vignettes give immediacy to the concepts, making them come alive for the reader.

The four pillars complement and work in concert, and no aspect of the youth's individual profile is overlooked or left out. This model of evaluation, diagnostic formulation, and treatment planning permits nimble clinicians to shift their center of attention, adjust aims, and deploy treatment interventions as the situation calls for, never stagnating, always building on blocks already laid.

The principles and concepts are saliently outlined in such a way that they become an implicit part of the clinician's memory and infuse an inherent mode of listening, evaluating, formulating, and applying the comprehensive understanding of the youth and important others. Flowing naturally out of this are practical and well-tailored treatment interventions that address areas of identified strengths and ongoing vulnerabilities. This was our experience as readers. The book is organized to flow in such a way that we were learning the material at an implicit level. Our recall had a clarity and substance that gave a conviction that we were ready to use these concepts without feeling the need to go back over things, re-read paragraphs, or laboriously memorize anything. Our reading experience was so attuned to the intentions of the authors that the material was entering into our implicit nondeclarative memory system. Extraordinary.

The importance of a disease-based model approach in understanding patients and the use of medication is not slighted. Rather, these aspects are given their proper place within the clinician's evaluation and treatment considerations. The youth is no longer a nail to be struck with the reflexively grasped, overused hammer in the clinician's toolbox. Clinical examples flesh out the important details to note and highlight. These examples are used to make the concepts vividly emerge from the background narrative through clear, easy-to-follow comparisons and contrasts.

The history obtained by utilizing the Contemporary Diagnostic Interview is clearly elucidated and, with practice, this approach becomes intuitive for both the skilled and newly minted clinician, who will experience the freedom of being unshackled from a solely *Diagnostic and Statistical Manual of Mental Disorders* (5th edition (DSM-5); American Psychiatric Association, 2013) interview style. In addition, the overall clinical view is broadened, and masterful clinical "pearls" become seamlessly part of the text, along with skillfully illustrated and interwoven informational tables and figures. These provide solid, succinct, and easily accessed reference sources for quick review.

The authors revitalize the concept of temperament and reframe its value for clinical acumen. Its importance as a genetically and biologically based innate behavioral style and its intimate relationship to the founding of personality is nicely illustrated. The relationship of temperament with regard to the youth's environment and his ability for emotional regulation is eloquently explained and rich examples are given. Importantly, the authors emphasize the bidirectional processes in all forms of interaction in how the emotional responses of others provide modeling and shape the youth's ability to self-regulate and develop distinctive personality patterns within the context of culturally determined aspects of the environment.

The authors work granularly, with attention paid to the multilayered aspects of development and its associated traits. The sediment of the initial presentation is put through a unique sieving process that refines the understanding into clear areas of demarcation and differentiation. As an example, what on the surface may appear equivalent, such as a full-scale IQ, appears so because of the overly simplistic lens utilized. Once one considers the subtest indices and places these in perspective, one is using multiple lenses in a more refined approach. The use of comparison tables rightly divides the primary diagnostic sediment into clinically useful layers.

The various subtest indices are clearly described, and the comparison case presentations make the concepts come alive. The various discrete and ingrained patterns, in each of the subtests, are provided with telling and clever monikers for characteristic profiles. As an example, for processing speed, "The Clerk" and "The Brave Turtle" are illustrated. For verbal comprehension, "The Librarian" and "The Imposter" are profiles delineated. These creative descriptors serve as memory hooks for the practitioner. This is just one example of the many skilled means used by the authors aimed at cementing the concepts into the implicit memory of the treatment specialist.

The area of cognitive flexibility, or theory of mind as noted by the authors, includes executive functioning, attention, working memory, and regulation of emotion. Cognitive flexibility provides the capacity for viewing situations from another person's perspective. The complement and contrast to the concept of mentalization is noted and takes into account the relationship of social context and the malleability of reflective function. How this important area is assessed, formulated, and applied is nicely expanded upon. The foundations of personality are explored and attachment theory explained, along with clear definitions of attachment styles. The commonly used testing instruments and evaluative procedures are outlined. Cognitive profiles are again a useful part of the narrative, and disorders of personality are described within the context of the overarching system.

The identification of strengths and weaknesses, particularly as they relate to the various components of the four pillars—and how parents and families can incorporate this understanding to positively impact their modes of relating—are powerfully illuminated for the reader. Nontraditional and nonintuitive parenting approaches are described in a practical manner, with innovative and skillful interventions. Interestingly, this unique encompassing approach gives a new spin and perspective on concepts from the field of positive psychiatry and associated work regarding character strengths and virtues.

The authors of this foreword are graduates of the Karl Menninger School of Psychiatry Child and Adolescent Psychiatry Training Program where the senior author, Sergio V. Delgado, MD, was a highly valued teacher and supervisor. His openness and accessibility, his clinical skill and grace, and his rare teaching abilities have served us well over the years. Here we again find ourselves being rewarded by his work and trailblazing ideas. We are in the process of incorporating the fresh paradigm developed by Sergio and his colleagues in our work with children, adolescents, families, and schools. We see the striking depth and wide scope of these readily applicable ideas and concepts. This superb book is an invaluable resource and guide for this endeavor.

Topeka, KS, USA Kirby Pope
Topeka, KS, USA Charles Millhuff

Preface

The seeds for this book were sown over many years of practicing and teaching in both the traditional *Diagnostic and Statistical Manual of Mental Disorders* (5th edition (DSM-5); American Psychiatric Association, 2013) disease-based model and the four pillars multidimensional approaches. We recognized that the traditional models of conceptualizing the psychological difficulties of children and adolescents was limiting. Colleague mental health clinicians spoke with us about cases with limited improvement with standard care: psychotherapy and medications. They often described these cases as "difficult to treat" or "treatment-resistant." The prevailing narrow explanations of why these patients were difficult to treat or treatment-resistant were severe forms of a disease-based model diagnosis. The goal was to search for the "right" form of therapy, medication, a combination of medications, or medical intervention (electroconvulsive therapy (ECT), transcranial magnetic stimulation (TMS), etc.) to treat the patients' "symptoms." Although, at times, this approach was successful, often it fell short. As such, we became disenchanted by the *DSM–5* disease-based model approach. It did not account for the patients' (and their parents') four pillars strengths and weaknesses—information necessary to develop a contemporary diagnostic formulation of their difficulties (e.g., understanding temperament, cognition, cognitive flexibility, and attachment). Over the last decade, we came to understand that the root of the patients' "symptoms" was often due to innate cognitive weaknesses, which would improve with psychosocial interventions tailored to their needs. We concluded that there was an urgent need for a practical and clinically relevant approach to help mental health clinicians elucidate their patients' cognitive strengths and weaknesses to help tailor truly individualized treatment interventions. This is particularly relevant in the current era, in which mental health clinicians now evaluate and treat more psychologically ill patients and increasingly struggle to find the right treatment modality or medication.

Moreover, now more than ever, we treat children who need help learning how to survive and grow in disruptive and unpredictable environments. Thus, the decision to write this book began with multiple discussions among us, and took advantage of our generational differences in incorporating the four pillars into diagnostic formulations and treatment plans. We became increasingly aware of the limited teaching and supervision opportunities in the contemporary four pillars model approach of many mental health specialties. This dyssynchrony occurred in the context of the traditional *DSM–5* disease-based model, wherein the relevant and practical concepts from the four pillars are neither taught nor integrated into clinical practice. Importantly, this is perpetuated by a shortage of user-friendly material in the standard psychiatric texts and journals frequented by psychiatrists, advanced practice nurses, psychologists, and social workers, thus limiting its dissemination.

Further, the insights learned from four pillar diagnostic assessments, as well as tailored treatment interventions, are not easily accessible to mental health clinicians to share with the patient's parents, who are desperate for parenting models that "best fit" their youth's strengths and weakness. Additionally, we also noted the dyssynchrony in mental health clinicians, who often want to know more about the patient needs but hesitate to work collaboratively with our psychology colleagues to understand and use clinically the results of the psychological assessments of our patients to improve the development of practical treatment plans beyond careful attention to the diagnostic rating scales the psychologist may use. However, rating scales do not account for the patients' or their parents' ability to understand the questions asked, nor do they ask balancing questions that may elucidate what the patient is succeeding in. Ultimately, this book aims to provide clinicians with contemporary assessments and treatment interventions that have day-to-day clinical relevance to the practicing mental health clinician. To accomplish this, there is an urgent need to have a user-friendly multidimensional approach that integrates varied clinical perspectives to provide a bio-psycho-social diagnostic formulation that helps understand the distressed patient and family. In short, we must learn to create what psychoanalyst and pediatrician Donald Winnicott, MD, termed a secure "holding environment" to promote the success of youths. Therefore, after many conversations, we concluded that we needed to write a book about how we use the four pillars approach diagnostically. Clinically, this approach has been well received when we teach it, and clinicians and parents want our approach available to them in written form.

We are happy to say that what started as a collection of ideas has become a reality. We are pleased and relieved to say that we completed our book with the hope that it will become a go-to resource for mental health clinicians who may have never been exposed to the four pillars diagnostic approach, and may wish to learn about the rewarding Contemporary Diagnostic Interview and use of psychological assessments to elucidate the strengths and weakness of youths' and parents' four pillars. Our destination has been the same: to share with our colleagues what we have learned and what has shaped us. We further hope that clinicians will share pertinent sections of this book to help parents make use, at home, of the tailored treatment interventions provided. We hope this book persuades clinicians to use the many references we offer or contact us directly to expand their knowledge about youths' four pillars to improve their clinical work. As we state throughout our book, a one-size-fits-all diagnostic approach can lead to ineffective treatment interventions, with risk of poor outcomes.

Importantly, we wrote this book through many virtual meetings during the COVID-19 pandemic. This led us to miss the many curbside and lively in-person discussions among ourselves and with our friends and colleagues, which would have further enriched the content of these chapters. Clearly, the pandemic affected people in different ways, and we were not excluded.

The Authors' Journeys

Sergio V. Delgado

My personal and professional experiences shaped me and contributed to making my mission to help youths with unrecognized cognitive difficulties that often led to their emotional and behavioral problems. After years of clinical experience with youths with cognitive weaknesses at the root of their problems, I developed the concept of the four pillars, which helps clinicians understand these children, adolescents, and their parents' cognitive strengths and weaknesses, which come in different profiles. This understanding will help clinicians develop unique, individualized treatment interventions necessary for the success of youths. Furthermore, I am honored that my co-authors were hooked on the value of using the four pillars in our care of patients, and have joined me in teaching and writing about the four pillars concept in more depth and with more clinical application.

Personal Journey

As an immigrant from Mexico 35 years ago, although bilingual, I experienced first-hand difficulties with some of the nuances of the English language. The most vivid example that remains a standing joke with my family and friends is that when I drop them off at various locations, I often say, "We're here. You can get down now," which is received with polite, disapproving looks, although it would be correct if said in Spanish. Now I *mostly* say, "We're here. You can get out now." Of course, this is not my only difficult phrase in English, as my co-authors can happily attest. Additionally, my wife continues to laugh about grocery-store trips in which I bring home limes, although she assures me she asked for lemons. In Spanish, the word *limes* ("limones") is used for both limes and lemons, and my wife assumes I will remember that lemons are "yellow limes"; hence, I always bring home green limes. Happily, we put the extraneous "green limes" to good use by making ceviche or margaritas.

Having learned to monitor how I say certain phrases has led me to develop a so-called thick skin. This helps me tolerate the disapproving looks or comments made in jest and has made me sensitive to youths who have difficulties communicating or being understood in their native language. Further, having family members and close friends who struggled in high school and college because of cognitive weaknesses and who, as a consequence of these weaknesses, had emotional and behavioral problems encouraged me to learn how to help these people work around their weaknesses and not hit a wall trying to change what is hardwired.

Most of these family members and close friends are now successful in music, photography, advertising, art, and animal care. This has helped me understand that effective communication in relationships is mostly contextual. When youths are in the right context, they can excel; in the wrong context, they can become overwhelmed managing affect-laden situations, quickly displaying emotional and behavioral problems. I have had many clinical encounters in which youths have difficulties describing basic concepts, identifying emotions, feeling misunderstood, etc., and receive disapproving looks from their parents, which has a profound and negative effect on their self-esteem. My empathy for these youths has encouraged me to look deeply at how their cognitive weaknesses led to their emotional and behavioral problems and to find practical solutions based on their weaknesses, as a one-size-fits-all proved to be detrimental to them.

Professional Journey

I was fortunate to train in child and adolescent psychiatry and become a faculty member at the Menninger Clinic in Topeka, Kansas, more than 30 years ago. The Menninger Clinic's rich tradition in the bio-psycho-social model helped me become thoroughly immersed in this model when evaluating patients' and families' frailties in managing their life. Working beside many psychologist colleagues, I learned the value in using information obtained from psychological tests to help corroborate and expand upon the information gathered from clinical diagnostic interviews. Further, I was in close clinical collaboration with social workers, school psychologists, and special education teachers, who unknowingly contributed to the formulation of this book.

While at the Menninger Clinic, I served as a school consultant to special education classrooms with at-risk youths and collaborated with many school psychologists and educational specialists, who, at the time, understood that youths' emotional and behavioral problems could be best understood if attention were given to their cognitive abilities and weaknesses. I developed an emerging awareness about the importance of attending to youths' cognitive abilities in understanding their behavior beyond the classroom. I was asked by Dr. Michele Berg, Director of the Center for Learning Disabilities at Menninger, and her colleagues, to help develop a comprehensive plan to help children with learning difficulties and attention-deficit/hyperactivity disorder that we took to many schools across the state of Kansas. This experience was inspirational, as we met teachers, special education teachers, and school psychologists who demonstrated a genuine wish to help youths with cognitive weaknesses succeed in new ways at school and in their home lives. I am also grateful to continue to work closely with my Menninger colleagues and friends, psychologists Carleen Franz and Anthony (Tony) Bram, in very difficult cases, and educational specialist Trudy Olde. They are masterful at integrating findings from their excellent psychological and psychoeducational evaluations into clinically practical approaches for complex young patients.

In 2001, I moved to Cincinnati and joined the department of child psychiatry at the Cincinnati Children's Hospital Medical Center, which proved to be a wise decision. I was fortunate to work in both inpatient and outpatient settings to care for the emotional needs of children and adolescents. My inpatient teams have been composed of wonderful colleagues. We made one of our priorities to request that our patients have intelligence testing to better understand their innate strengths and weaknesses through their WISC-V subtest indices score. This information proved to be very helpful when assessing which of our patients' day-to-day emotional and behavioral difficulties were attributable to their cognitive weaknesses and which were due to their disease-based diagnoses. We corroborated our clinical impression of the patient's weakness with additional evaluations: speech and language and occupational therapy. As an inpatient team, we participated in several grand rounds demonstrating how the four-pillars approach augmented the traditional *DSM–5* approach and helped develop optimal treatment plans for outpatients.

My work in the outpatient setting allowed me to meet young patients and their parents, who are the true contributors to this book. They taught me to give importance to why certain emotional and behavioral problems occur in some contexts and not in others. I discovered that the context variability was related to problems with temperament, cognition, cognitive flexibility, and personality styles. Parents were surprised learning about the impact their child or adolescent's cognitive weaknesses, nonverbal learning disorder, or dyslexia had on him or her emotionally outside of the classroom. This understanding of children and adolescents allowed me to explain the four pillars to parents and develop tailored interventions for the weaknesses in each pillar. After years giving real-life trials of these interventions, I learned, from parents, which interventions have been most successful for their youths.

Jeffrey R. Strawn

After completing my general psychiatry residency at the University of Cincinnati and a fellowship in child and adolescent psychiatry at Cincinnati Children's Hospital, I embarked on a career as a clinician-scientist, conducting clinical trials and treating patients. My training had strong foundations in traditional psychotherapeutic and disease-based approaches and my early work with patients and their families reflected this. However, I began to notice that my formulations "fell short" and that the standard, evidence-based, disease-based approaches failed a number of my patients. As I worked closely with my friend and colleague, Sergio Delgado, and as I became a father, I increasingly appreciated the way in which the pillars could—independent of psychopathology—drive behaviors, influence interactions, and sculpt emotional reactions.

Over the years, my approach with patients and their families shifted. I no longer used the same pharmacologic or psychotherapeutic strategies. I saw my patients' interactions with their families, teachers, case managers, and other clinicians through a different lens. As I worked with clinicians who also exposed this approach, my patients' outcomes improved. They and their families were happier, and I was more professionally satiated and more able to enjoy my daily clinical work.

When presented the opportunity to contribute, as a co-author, to this book, I immediately said "yes." Moreover, as I worked with my co-authors to draft this book, some of the more nebulous aspects of this approach, which had implicitly been part of our writing and daily work, became clearer. As I worked with my co-authors, the concepts crystalized, often as a result of our enthusiastic discussions in which we challenged each other's application of the model and interventions and from my co-authors' understanding of my own relative visuospatial processing weaknesses as we drafted this book. From these discussions, our approach became clearer, and nuances were included in the text and powerful visual images were incorporated into the book which you are about to enjoy.

Ernest V. Pedapati

In my final year of medical school at the University of Massachusetts, I still could not decide between the body and the mind. Instead, I embraced my ambivalence and pursued the Triple Board Residency at the University of Cincinnati and Cincinnati Children's Hospital Medical Center. Unlike conventional child psychiatry training, the Triple Board emphasizes pediatric medicine with later specialization in psychiatry and child psychiatry. Rather than distance myself from mental health, my training in pediatrics inspired a curiosity for childhood development and gave me a new lens through which to view pediatric psychopathology. I struggled with understanding why a child ravaged with bone cancer struggled so vigorously to live or why a child caught in the depths of depression would so earnestly wish for death. Although my early supervisors helped me understand children psychologically through a traditional one-person lens, over time I found common ground with my pediatric training as I began to deepen my understanding of attachment theory, neuroscience, and social cognition. I am grateful for the lead author's invitation to collaborate in writing this book, which will enhance my colleagues' psychotherapeutic experience.

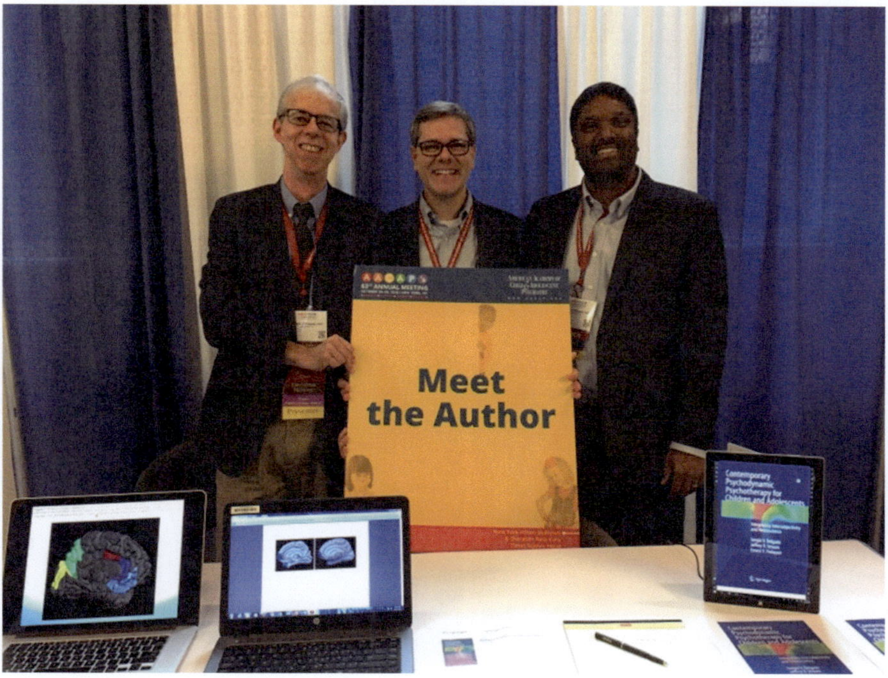

Cincinnati, OH, USA — Sergio V. Delgado
Cincinnati, OH, USA — Ernest V. Pedapati
Cincinnati, OH, USA — Jeffrey R. Strawn

Acknowledgments

We would like to express our heartfelt gratitude to our young patients and their parents, who unknowingly contributed to this book in remarkable ways. They provided the clinical material through their subjectivities in here-and-now moments with us as clinicians. We are in great debt to the many parents, colleague psychiatrists and residents, advanced practice nurses, and social workers, who often said, "Please write a book about the four pillars. It's very important, although it can be overwhelming. We need a how-to guide to understand how to use the four pillars diagnostically and practically."

Additionally, we are indebted to our colleagues and students, who helped us appreciate the pressures of trying to "fit in" learning about the evolution of four pillar psychology, due to the prevailing pressures by the traditional *DSM-5* disease-based model and those loyal to mainly psychopharmacological interventions. Our colleagues and students were pivotal in encouraging us to provide rich case examples, and we discussed them from both a traditional *DSM-5* disease-based model and a four-pillar multidimensional diagnostic approach, which we realized was very much needed.

We thank Kirby Pope, MD, who read the early drafts of this manuscript, as well as subsequent revisions, and was gentle in sharing comments that helped shape the flow of the content of this book. We want to express our warm thanks to members of the clinical medicine Springer Publishing team, who were instrumental in the acceptance of our book proposal and shepherding us through the completion of this book. Also, we give a heartfelt thank you to Becky Adnot-Haynes for her masterful and sensitive editorial assistance, with her attention to detail and careful work to make clearer our sometimes-muddled sentiments with skillful use of the written word and grammatical prowess. We thank Becky for bringing greater coherence to our concepts and significant improvement to our original work.

We are also indebted to Andre Delgado (CEO of Grupo Cinco in Monterrey, Mexico), whose expertise in advertising inspired and helped our co-author and magician in graphic design, Ernest Pedapati, to create the jovial four pillar cartoon figures, which bring to life our concepts and profiles.

Further, we are thankful to colleagues who took the time to read selected chapters and generously provide constructive criticism. They were kind enough to point out what was not clear, what was confusing, what required further elaboration, and what we had omitted. Among these colleagues are Steve Hoersting, Kelly Bunker, Sam Vaughn, Charles Millhuff, Patricia Smith, and Megan Eastman.

We thank the many inpatient colleagues that contributed to the importance of the four pillars: Jennifer Creedon, Amanda Jones, Hannah D'Souza, Adam Diggs, Catherine Stine, April Nelson, Chad Duncan, Laurie Mack, Allison Carter, and Barb Velarius. We were honored when Susan Franer, lead advance practice nurse, asked us to share with her team the importance in using the four pillars approach in outpatient work, which led to many fruitful curbside conversations about youths' maladaptive behaviors as a result of their cognitive weaknesses.

We also can't thank enough our friend and lead outpatient intake department coordinator, Ryan Jennings, who kindly kept his ears open for families requesting help for their youths with behavioral problems who were also struggling in school. He knew we would gladly accept them into our busy schedules. We also express our gratitude to Michael Sorter, MD, who encouraged and supported us in making our work a reality.

We apologize to the many other wonderful people that we are sure we have left out.

To all, we say thank you!

The Authors' Acknowledgments

Sergio V. Delgado

I would have never thought I had the knowledge and energy to work on a book of this length, especially during a pandemic. I want to thank my friends and coauthors Jeff and Ernie, who believed this was possible and were instrumental in the depth and quality of this book. The task felt daunting, but their ability to provide me a "holding environment" helped me write the first draft of this book. Our close friendship helped us decide what needed more in-depth work or expansion, and what we had to delete. Most of all, I thank them for tolerating my "Mexican" written-sentence structure and for their gracious comments when providing the editing needed. Today we continue to teach about the four pillars.

Finally, I am indebted to Erin, my true better half, who provided the warmth that kept me from giving up; provided the useful, unedited critiques needed to improve the readability of this book; and was instrumental in helping me keep my eye on the project as there were plenty of times I would have preferred to quit. She provided the energy behind these pages and believed in us and supported this project by taking over many of my home duties, which I dread, as they await me.

—SVD

Jeffrey R. Strawn

This work would not have been possible without the loving support of my wife, Lara, who from the beginning helped me to balance our life with the writing of this book, although she may still not agree that we reached equilibrium. Also, I thank my daughters, Elliott Nicole and Rachel Marie, for their daily lessons in intersubjectivity and attachment theory. My regular reminders of implicit relational knowing and development ultimately made the writing of this book possible. Finally, I thank my friends and co-authors, Sergio and Ernie, whose encouragement and always-present enthusiasm were the driving force for this work.

—JRS

Ernest V. Pedapati

Apologies are not meant to change the past, but rather the future. My contributions to this book are inspired by my own shortcomings and desire to be a better father, husband, and clinician. More than anything, the message of this book is to investigate, recognize, and cherish the great diversity found in parents and children. Our field is lurching toward a new paradigm in which people are not simply placed in categories but thought of across multiple dimensions, both within the self and the network of people that surround them. I am thankful for my own two growing and ambitious sons, Noah Francis and Harrison Paul, and my loving wife, Carolyn, who often must endure the multiple "pillars" found within the household. As we conclude this most recent work, I am even more impressed with the tenacity and creativity of my colleagues, Sergio and Jeff, who began as mentors, then as partners, and now as friends.

—EVP

Contents

About the Authors

Sergio V. Delgado, MD is Professor of Psychiatry, Pediatrics, and Psychoanalysis at Cincinnati Children's Hospital Medical Center and the University of Cincinnati. Dr. Delgado is a graduate of the School of Medicine of the University of Nuevo Leon, and the psychiatry and child psychiatry programs of the Karl Menninger School of Psychiatry and Mental Health Sciences. He also completed training as a supervising and training analyst in adult and child psychoanalysis at the Topeka Institute for Psychoanalysis. He also served as a Child and Adolescent Psychiatry Oral Board Examiner for the American Board of Psychiatry and Neurology. Currently, Dr. Delgado is an adult and child supervising and training analyst at the Cincinnati Psychoanalytic Institute. He currently is the medical director of the Compliance and Information Services in the Department of Psychiatry at Cincinnati Children's Hospital Medical Center. Dr. Delgado is the co-chair of the Psychotherapy Committee to the American Academy of Child & Adolescent Psychiatry. He is the president of the Cincinnati-Dayton Regional Council of the American Academy of Child & Adolescent Psychiatry.

Dr. Delgado actively teaches in the adult and child psychiatry training programs. He is a frequent recipient of numerous teaching awards for his helpful and pragmatic teaching and supervising style. Dr. Delgado is frequently sought for supervision and consultation involving difficult psychiatric cases. He is a strong advocate for the integration of the multidimensional four pillars approach to best provide practical and individualized treatment interventions. He is a strong proponent for the integration of individual psychotherapy, family psychotherapy, and pharmacologic interventions in the treatment of patients. Dr. Delgado has authored multiple journal articles and book chapters on the integration of psychopharmacologic and psychotherapeutic treatments in youth, on the assessment and treatment of learning disorders, and on psychological development and intersubjectivity-based interventions in adolescents. Dr. Delgado is the founder and director of the relational advanced psychotherapy program (RAPP) in Cincinnati.

Jeffrey R. Strawn, MD received his bachelor's degree in biology from the University of Kentucky and then completed his residency training in general psychiatry at the University of Cincinnati. Following his general psychiatry training, he completed a fellowship in child and adolescent psychiatry at Cincinnati Children's Hospital.

Currently, Dr. Strawn's is Professor of Psychiatry and Pediatrics at the University of Cincinnati and Cincinnati Children's Hospital Medical Center and is the director of the Pediatric Anxiety Disorders Clinic at the University of Cincinnati. His clinical work focuses on the treatment of anxiety and related disorders in children and adolescents and his research program focuses on elucidating the underlying brain circuitry of these conditions, using functional magnetic resonance imaging. Additionally, he is actively involved in the testing of innovative treatments for youth with mood and anxiety disorders. Dr. Strawn has published nearly 200 papers and book chapters and his research has been acknowledged by numerous organizations, including the American Psychiatric Association and the American Academy of Child & Adolescent Psychiatry.

He enjoys teaching and is actively involved in the teaching of psychotherapy with adolescents and the treatment of adult and pediatric anxiety disorders to medical students, general psychiatry residents, and child and adolescent psychiatry fellows at the University of Cincinnati and Cincinnati Children's Hospital Medical Center

Ernest V. Pedapati, MD is an Associate Professor of Psychiatry (affiliate) at the University of Cincinnati and maintains a joint appointment in the Division of Psychiatry and Neurology at Cincinnati Children's Hospital Medical Center. He completed medical school at the University of Massachusetts. He completed his Triple Board Program at Cincinnati Children's Hospital Medical Center which is a combined residency in Pediatrics, Adult Psychiatry, and Child and Adolescent Psychiatry. He is Board Certified in Pediatrics, General Psychiatry, and Addiction Medicine.

Dr. Pedapati is extensively involved in clinical and research work involving autism, learning disorders, and developmental disabilities. He is currently a child psychiatry consultant to the Division of Developmental and Behavioral Pediatrics at Cincinnati Children's Hospital Medical Center. Dr. Pedapati is a member of the Autism Research Group at Cincinnati Children's Hospital Medical Center and conducts clinical trials and basic psychological research in children with social impairments and repetitive behaviors. In addition, he is a part of an interdisciplinary research team which studies the neurophysiology of neuropsychiatric illness through transcranial magnetic stimulation. Dr. Pedapati federally funded research program in Fragile X Syndrome focuses on detecting differences in brain activity using electroencephalography. He continues to have a great interest in the promotion of healthy families including maintaining a psychotherapy and family coaching clinic.

Chapter 1
Introduction: Biological, Emotional, and Social Development

With the new day comes new strength and new thoughts.
— Eleanor Roosevelt (1884–1962)

The successful development of a child's emotional, social, behavioral, and academic skills is essential for a bright future. In guiding their child's development, parents often lean on their own personal history, plus advice from family, peers, pediatricians, and parenting manuals, in deciding how to best assure their child's emotional and social well-being. However, there persists a misconception that all children can be "fixed" emotionally, socially, and behaviorally—if only we apply the correct parenting strategy.

For decades, mental health clinicians have wrongly relied on authoritarian behavioral plans undergirded by clear limit-setting that allowed—supposedly—a child or adolescent to learn through a structure that rewarded good behavior and enacted consequences for poor decision-making. Additionally, many clinicians and parents believe that a child or adolescent's maladaptive behaviors represent a mental health disorder requiring psychotherapeutic and often pharmacological interventions. As such, there has been limited attention given to the many possible causes of emotional, social, and behavioral problems in children and adolescents beyond the school of thought of clinicians. This book provides a neurodevelopmental view of children and adolescents, as well as their parents. In this way, we provide tailored interventions to help children, adolescents, and parents develop the skills needed for stable and healthy relationships. To do this, we encourage clinicians to consider the strengths and weaknesses of both the child and parent in four areas:

- Temperament.
- Cognition.
- Cognitive flexibility.
- Personality style.

S. V. Delgado et al., *Promoting the Emotional and Behavioral Success of Youths*,
https://doi.org/10.1007/978-3-030-88075-0_1

This will allow a multidimensional understanding of the root of their problems and improve the success rate of interventions. We define these four pillars as those that provide the foundation of a person's unique personality. The four pillars are the convergence of biological and environmental processes that become the blueprint of how a child learns to develop and maintain self-regulatory abilities and unique implicit relational patterns to successfully interact with others. The first three pillars—temperament, cognition, and cognitive flexibility—form the foundation of the fourth pillar, personality, the interpersonal expression of the internal working model of attachment (IWMA). By understanding the contribution from each of the pillars, the clinician will have a true biopsychosocial understanding of the specific needs of both the patient and the parent [9].

Of note, this book was written during the 2019–2020 coronavirus pandemic, when many countries faced multiple challenges: systemic and individual healthcare stress, social distancing, feelings of isolation, high unemployment, remote learning, and racial divide, which led to uncertain and difficult times. We address these issues throughout the book and provide suggestions for the clinician to adopt in order to help parents in areas in which their child's innate weaknesses, or challenges, may have been further exacerbated by this difficult period.

Biological Development

Neuroscientists recognize that the psychological phenomena of thought, planning, and emotion are complex biological processes that are poorly understood. Furthermore, researchers believe that understanding psychological processes might not be possible without study of the underlying biology [19]. It is accepted that there are significant underlying neurobiological factors influencing the emotional and social development in children and adolescents. In recent epigenetic (DNA modifications that do not change the DNA sequence but switch on and off gene activity) and molecular biology research, individual differences in intellectual and emotional abilities were recognized to be strongly influenced by the interactions of nature (epigenetic and genetic) and nurture (environment). The epigenetic and molecular underpinnings are apparent in children with cancer, cystic fibrosis, autism, learning disabilities, etc., when other family members are not affected by these conditions. Additionally, recent findings from genomic research remind us of the limitations of knowing which person may be more apt to be positively or negatively affected by their environment.

While biology has always been an important factor in medicine, the field of psychiatry has been striving, for the last several decades, to make use of clinically relevant discoveries from molecular, epigenetic, genetic, and neuroscientific research. However, although promising scientific advances have occurred in understanding certain disorders—PANDAS and autoimmune encephalopathy, for example—the advances have been of limited clinical use in the understanding of most common mental health disorders in children and adolescents. Neuroscientists emphasize neuroplasticity in the expression of a neuron's genome, with continual changes influenced by complex environmental factors. This concept lays to rest the misconception of a linear pathway linking mental health disorders (e.g., schizophrenia, depression, bipolar disorder, anxiety, etc.) directly to specific gene sequences. Rather, there is limited scientific information supporting the notion that mental health conditions have distinguishing familial genetic predispositions. To date, genes identified by the human genome project only explain 1–5% of the variance between groups for psychological traits of all kinds, including temperament, intelligence, and cognitive flexibility [11]. For example, innate DNA polygenic codes remain elusive in elucidating the origins of mental health disease based–model disorders, e.g., schizophrenia, depression, and anxiety. Furthermore, these codes are independent of race or culture, although these factors may influence the expression without changing the code. Research of human development estimates that there are over 70 trillion potential human genotypes, and each of them may be coupled across a person's life with an even larger number of physical and social contexts and interpersonal relationships and experiences [17]. Therefore, the diversity of development in each person's lifetime trajectory is unique, and people become more different from each other with age [3].

Additionally, culturally mediated measures of intelligence are strongly predicted by genetics [20]. Loughnan et al. add "a note of caution: it [interpreting the genome-wide polygenic score of intelligence] should not simply be thought of as a proxy for genetics or 'nature.' Each individual in this study inherited half of their genome from each parent and so these genetic effects can also have indirect influences on their cognitive performance through the cognitively enriching environments that parents provide." Furthermore, in addition to DNA sequence, epigenetic effects at a molecular level (e.g., chromatin and histone modifications, DNA methylation) are also biological factors that have been shown to impact cognition [7].

As such, the vast body of neuroscience research has not provided mainstream psychiatry and mental health journals the answers that were hoped for, which has led some practitioners of child and adolescent psychiatry to take a reductionist approach. Instead of drawing on potentially valuable neuroscience research in diagnosing patients, clinicians more commonly perform brief, one-hour diagnostic evaluations, using diagnostic scales to support a disease-based model diagnosis, followed by the use of algorithms to decide which medications are indicated. This approach gives limited attention to important cognitive, family, and social factors that may influence the presentation of signs and symptoms in children and adolescents. Furthermore, clinical research in youth has focused on the treatment of disease-based model psychiatric disorders as opposed to prevention of these disorders. This focus is largely due to the relative lack of information of the precursors regarding early emerging symptoms and later disorders in youth [18]. A multidimensional approach helps understand the many hardwired precursors of the most common "symptoms" youth present to the clinician which do not neatly fit a *Diagnostic and Statistical Manual of Mental Disorders* (5th edition (DSM-5); American Psychiatric Association, 2013) [1] diagnostic disease-based model formulation.

Furthermore, biological psychiatry has mostly limited its attention to the pharmacodynamics and pharmacogenetics of psychotropic medications used for disease-based model conditions. This knowledge has given somewhat limited results due to the complex interactions of proteins in DNA and mRNA at the cellular level of neurons and inter-neurons, which make predicting response to medication unclear. For example, up to 50% of children and adolescents respond to the first antidepressant used for depression while 40–60% also respond to placebo [5]. High placebo response rate in adolescent depression is poorly understood. Consequently, mixed results from psychopharmacological interventions have brought to light the limitations of accurate diagnosis of children and adolescents with mental health problems with poorly defined diseases. There has been limited attention given to developmental factors that can be expressed with signs and symptoms that can mimic a mental health disorder. Accordingly, poor treatment outcomes have led to high rates of nonadherence with pharmacological recommendations: Youth patients and their families are not adhering to their prescribed treatment plans because of side effects or a lack of efficacy [8].

As Appelbaum and Benston [2] aptly state,

> Translation of research findings into clinically useful genetic tests, however, has been limited by the some of the inherent characteristics of psychiatric disorders themselves. Findings by the Schizophrenia Working Group of the Psychiatric Genomics Consortium [23] on the genetics of schizophrenia indicate that—with the exception of uncommon conditions related to copy number variations (CNVs), such as DiGeorge syndrome—variants in a large number of genes are implicated in its etiology.

They further remind us that the variance in most mental health disorders is likely due to polygenic mechanisms involved in their etiology. Thus, although pharmacogenomic tests are being actively marketed to mental health providers, the database supporting their use is weak.

Furthermore, limitations in research regarding mental processes are made evident by the extant literature about the origin of love, sexual orientation, altruism, and hate in individuals, which, although important, remain poorly understood.

Gender is also likely to affect the impact of the family context on children's self-regulatory abilities. Studies indicate that the development of self-regulatory abilities differ by gender. Girls are typically better self-regulators than boys, which may be due to innate differences in reactivity levels [21].

Lesbian, gay, bisexual, transgender, and queer (LGBTQ) people possess a complex set of sexual orientations and behaviors whose origins are poorly understood. Some understand sexual orientations as a result of environmental factors, which could range from hormone exposure in the womb to social influences later in life. Others believe that sexual orientation is explained by genetics, although recent research shows that only 8–25% of nonheterosexual behavior can be explained by genes [15]. Moreover, LGBTQ youth are more susceptible to mental illness due to factors, such as family disapproval and stigmatization, particularly in conservative regions. As with other traits, such as personality, there is no single "gene" that can explain same-sex attraction and other forms of sexual behavior.

Emotional Development

In the last decade, there has been renewed interest in identifying people's temperamental traits to develop tailored psychosocial interventions to help with emotional regulation and social interactions. Child temperament, neurophysiology, and cognitive development play important roles in youth's development of emotional regulatory skills [16]. It is important for parents to model emotional regulation of different affective states for their children—a skill that children and adolescents must develop to handle intense affect and anxiety. Occasionally, children and adolescents are temperamentally better able to regulate emotions than their parents. Emotional regulation is an essential component of mental health, and problems with it are a hallmark characteristic of a variety of disorders, particularly anxiety disorders. For children, adolescents, and adults, the anxiety created by the pandemic will be hard to define.

Clinicians treating children and adolescents are in a unique position to integrate information about innate temperamental patterns and cognitive abilities to gain a better understanding of the root of children and adolescents' emotional, social, and behavioral maladaptive patterns and provide effective treatment recommendations and practical parental advice. While many clinicians view cognitive weaknesses as impairments in specific academic skills (e.g., reading, language, mathematics), up to 40% of children and adolescents with varied cognitive weaknesses experience maladaptive behaviors and poor self-esteem [10] with significant short- and long-term effects on their emotional, social, and educational development. These impairments vary from child to child, and it is crucial to understand cognitive abilities to develop practical interventions for parents to employ to help their children improve self-esteem, intellectual abilities, and emotional success. Children and adolescents with better emotional regulation will have better problem-solving and conflict-resolution strategies. Studies of resilience in children and adolescents discovered that those with at least one stable and nurturing adult were able to adapt better to adversity than those exposed to dysfunctional environments—family conflict, food shortage, violence, substance use, limited academic access—without a consistent adult to provide support. Regardless of their family environment, all children and adolescents require sound cognitive abilities in order to develop internal relational schemas for emotional regulation, which will allow them to achieve resilience and, accordingly, positive outcomes. Early onset of child mental health problems (before the age of 10 years) is associated with chronically poor social adjustment, as well as psychological and physical health disorders, which makes early intervention even more crucial [6].

Furthermore, mainstream psychiatric texts base most treatment recommendations in biological and pharmacological terms and often do not address interventions based on a child's cognitive abilities, which are often the precursors to their maladaptive behaviors. Furthermore, the clinician may find herself feeling frustrated when a youth's emotional and behavioral problems do not improve with traditional forms of psychotherapies and medication. She may consider the failure of response to be from intentional resistance to treatment or due to dysfunctional family systems. This is further complicated by pressure from parents who request, or demand, quick fixes. It is essential to understand children and adolescents' strengths and weaknesses in cognitive abilities to best understand their maladaptive behaviors and provide useful steps for a successful scaffolding of the practical interventions needed to help them acquire the necessary developmental skills.

Social Development

In recent years, neurodevelopmentally informed research has extended the works by psychology/psychiatry pioneers John Bowlby, Mary Ainsworth, and Mary Main in expanding the understanding of biological, emotional, and social development in children and adolescents. Bowlby hypothesized that a child's temperament influences how the child is experienced by their parents and significantly shapes how the parents interact with the child [4]. Thomas et al. [25] aptly stated that "some children with severe psychological problems had a family upbringing that did not differ essentially from the environment of other children who developed no severe problems," and later added that "domineering authoritarian handling by the parents might make one youngster anxious and submissive and another defiant and antagonistic." Thus, "theory and practice of psychiatry must take into full account the individual and his uniqueness" [25]. Phrases such as "the apple doesn't fall far from the tree" are pejorative and no longer helpful. Social development in children and adolescents can be influenced by parents although children will develop skills to communicate with other people and process their emotions in ways that may not be like their parents' methods.

Additionally, there are some biological mechanisms that can be altered by one's environment and accordingly influence the development of a person's brain structure and cognitive functioning dynamically throughout life. A person's interactions with other people are markedly influenced by early relational experiences, innate temperamental patterns, cognitive schemas, attachment patterns, and, most importantly, his or her cultural background [13]. Today, most scientific researchers don't consider personality to be a static process.

The search for environmental conditions that differentiate the common childhood mental health disorders has yielded little fruit. That is, the major environmental risk factors identified for mental health disorders—family disruption, child abuse, substance use, and poverty—appear to be largely nonspecific rather than unique to particular disorders [12]. Therefore, an integrative view of the four pillars is essential to have a multidimensional understanding of the complexities of the development of personality and mental health issues (Fig. 1.1).

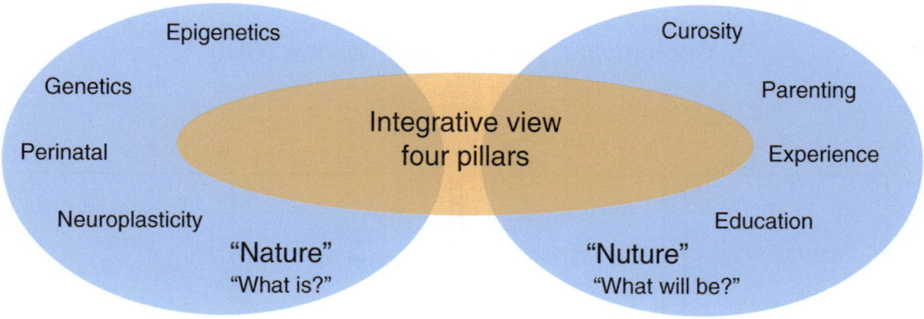

Fig. 1.1 Integrative view of the four pillars

How to Use this Book

This book is written with several audiences and several goals in mind. First, we want to expand the body of psychiatric literature aimed at treating children and adolescents and to present an effective, collaborative method of working with complex or difficult clinical cases. Second, we seek to integrate the four pillars in psychiatric interviews and diagnostic formulations. Third, we aim to guide experienced clinicians, advanced psychiatric nurses, psychologists, psychiatric residents, and clinical fellows, toward using a multidimensional friendly diagnostic tool to develop tailored and practical treatment interventions in complex psychiatric cases (Fig. 1.2).

The goal of our book is to help clinicians and child and adolescent psychiatrists learn how to integrate in useful clinical ways the four pillars in order to: (1) determine which maladaptive behaviors are a result of cognitive weaknesses and not "symptoms" of a disease-based model psychiatric disorder, (2) develop "best fit" practical interventions to help parents of children and adolescents with varied cognitive abilities, (3) develop realistic emotional, social, and academic goals, (4) improve self-esteem and promote adaptive behaviors, and (5) decrease conflict in day-to-day interactions between children and adolescents and their parents and friends.

Furthermore, we provide relevant cases that allow the reader to be on the shoulder of the clinician, and we include tables to give readers an efficient, at-a-glance picture of how to apply these methods for efficient review of relevant information from a contemporary diagnostic interview and psychological assessments clinically. This will allow clinicians to tailor treatment interventions as needed, and encourages collaboration with psychologists to help children, adolescents, and their parents. The clinical cases examples described are from a diverse race and ethnic group. We have omitted to identify race and ethnicity to highlight the context of the four pillars.

Of note, we will use the term "parents" throughout this book with the intent to include mothers, fathers, stepparents, adoptive parents, foster parents, and other forms of caregivers present in children's and adolescents' lives.

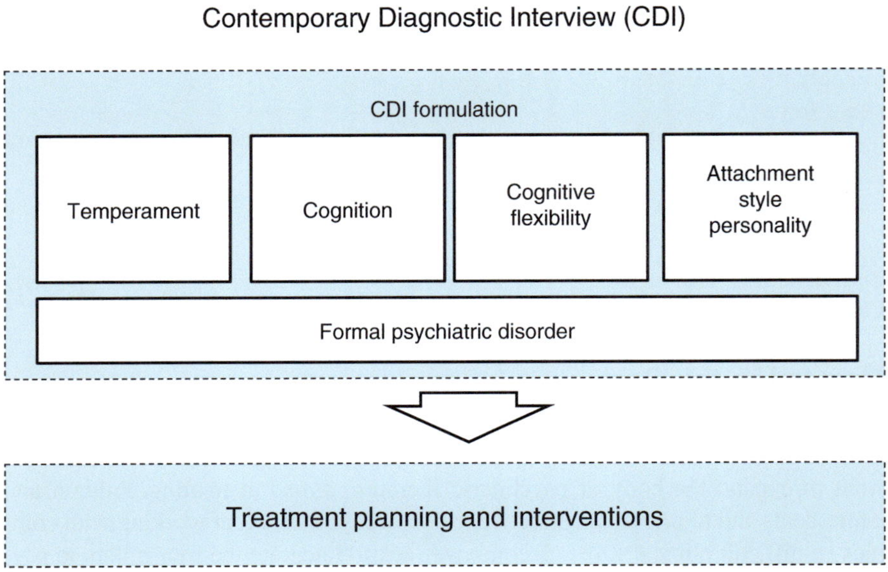

Fig. 1.2 Multidimensional friendly diagnostic tool. (From Delgado SV, Strawn JR, Pedapati EV. (2015) Contemporary Psychodynamic Psychotherapy for Children and Adolescents: Integrating Intersubjectivity and Neuroscience. Springer)

In Chap. 2, *The Four Pillars Through a Contemporary Diagnostic Interview,* we have structured the chapter with the goal of helping the experienced or the newly minted clinician or child and adolescent psychiatrist learn the importance of the four pillars in the child's ability to successfully scaffold the developmental skills needed to succeed. We also provide the reader a how-to on the Contemporary Diagnostic Interview (CDI) model, which provides an integrated developmental approach to allow clinicians to develop realistic and practical treatment recommendations. In Chap. 3, *Temperament: The Building Block of Personality*, we make the case that temperament provides the emotional and behavioral building block on which personalities are constructed. Temperament refers to the stable moods and behavior profiles observed in infancy and early childhood. The individual's capacity to interact with others in an acceptable manner is greatly determined by the how his environment influences matters of reciprocity according to his own unique temperament styles. Additionally, as temperament is shaped by interactions with others, "its regulation is culturally dependent" [22]. Temperament traits in childhood highly correlate with those present after the transition to adulthood [24]. A child's temperament and her adult personality share remarkably similar features, not only in how a person navigates day-to-day interactions with others but also how she manages affect-laden emotional interactions. While temperament and personality are interrelated, they are not one and the same. The former refers to the genetically and biologically based innate behavioral style, while the latter describes how emotions manifest in an individual with a particular temperament.

In Chap. 4, *Intelligence: "Why Don't You Behave?,"* we share an approach that is geared toward understanding the patient from the inside out. We describe a process of evaluating cognition followed by rich case examples in order to illuminate how to apply these concepts to complex children and adolescents. We consider intelligence to be the second pillar within the formulation of our personality. Broadly, it includes all cognitive processes that acquire, process, and act on information or stimuli. In the context of relationships, intelligence includes the capacity and know-how to engage in relationships based on mutual understanding of each other's ideas and intent. Weaknesses in intelligence lead to maladaptive behaviors and emotional dysregulation with increased likelihood of problems with self-esteem, interpersonal conflict, and academic functioning.

Importantly, we will not address the controversies surrounding cultural biases, the choice or quality of psychological tests, or the difficulties using this information to help with educational aspects including advocacy for special education plans. We refer the reader to contemporary sources that present these issues in a balanced manner with practical interventions for parents to use to work with school staff [14].

In Chap. 5, *Cognitive Flexibility: Theory of Mind): "Being in your shoes"*, guides the reader how to assess cognitive flexibility when evaluating children and adolescents. We provide the clinician tools to perform in-the-moment assessments of preschool and school-age youth, as well as adolescents. We also review the many tests available to formally assess cognitive flexibility (CF) and theory of mind (ToM) in youth. Tests used to assess CF and ToM can overlap with the projective tests used in assessing personality. We review tests that we are familiar with, though we note that other available tests offered by collaborating psychologists may be useful as well.

Next, in Chap. 6, *Personality Styles: "My Friends Are Just Like Me"*, we turn our attention to the unique neurobiological underpinnings of personality disorders. Although there is consensus that the precursors of personality disorders occur in childhood and that the clinical presentation during adolescence is similar to that in adults, there continues to be a great deal of reluctance in diagnosing a personality disorder in adolescence. This may be because symptoms are seen as normative in developing adolescents and labeling an adolescent with a personality disorder seems pejorative and stigmatizing. However, when a personality disorder is correctly diagnosed during adolescence, clinicians can encourage early, practical nonpharmacological approaches that can help promote new and more adaptive behaviors. This chapter also presents poignant vignettes that illustrate the in vivo application of these techniques.

Additionally, in Chap. 7, *Putting It All Together: Adapting to Youths' Cognitive Strengths and Weaknesses*, we provide practical interventions for clinicians to share with parents with the goal of promoting emotional, social, and academic success. The interventions are tailored to the specific weaknesses identified by the Contemporary Diagnostic Interview and psychological assessments. The strategies described in this chapter are not intended to replace well-formulated therapeutic interventions, especially for disease-based model mental health disorders. Rather, the strategies presented in this chapter facilitate emotional and social functioning, independent of whether a disorder is present. Youth with weaknesses in their four pillars will have maladaptive patterns of behavior and emotional processing. It would be beyond the scope of this book to review the many educational interventions available for youth with cognitive weaknesses or formal learning disabilities (reading, writing disorders, dyslexia, etc.). We suggest the reader communicate with psychologists or educational specialists for further information regarding these interventions. Finally, in Chap. 8, *Parenting Principles to Help Youths: Debunking Common Parenting Myths,* the first section is a review of fundamental parenting principals helpful for parents with children and adolescents with reasonably good four pillars. The second section provides a brief review of the "myths" that have been passed down through generations and are often viewed as bedrock in parenting, which we believe need to be revised as they do not capture the developmental complexities in youth and at times are even detrimental for children and adolescents emotional and behavioral success.

We recognize that, as with any approach, there will be skeptics about our thinking and way of working. The notion of assessing four pillars—temperament, cognition, cognitive flexibility, and personality style—may not be well received by some mental health clinicians, including those who may be anchored in traditional *DSM–5* disease-based model diagnostic approach. However, we would argue that the traditional *DSM–5* disease-based model must accept the relevance of accrued knowledge from temperament theories, developmental research, as well as cognitive and social psychology. This allows for a more comprehensive understanding of the complexity of the youth's human mind and how it works. Ultimately, this book will have day-to-day clinical relevance to the practicing child and adolescent psychiatrist, advance nurse practitioner, psychologist, social worker, and psychotherapist. Thus, we would argue that this approach, while somewhat more time-intensive, is more cost-effective.

Finally, we apologize to the readers who may feel that we should have written more to further clarify the four pillar clinical concepts or may have wished for more clinical cases with lengthier and more detailed explanations and suggested "in the moment" interventions. To them we say, our work is incomplete; we all have much to learn, and we could have easily taken more time and energy without being able to capture all the nuances of four pillar psychology. Therefore, we kindly encourage the reader to make use of this book as a springboard to further read the many eloquent books and papers referenced throughout the book.

References

1. American Psychiatric Association. Diagnostic and statistical manual of mental disorders. 5th ed. Washington, D.C.: American Psychiatric Association; 2013.
2. Appelbaum PS, Benston S. Anticipating the ethical challenges of psychiatric genetic testing. Curr Psychiatry Rep. 2017;19(7):39. https://doi.org/10.1007/s11920-017-0790-x.
3. Baltes PB, Lindenberger U, Staudinger U. Life span theory in developmental psychology. In: Lerner RM, Damon W, editors. Handbook of child psychology: theoretical models of human development. Wiley; 2006. p. 569–664.

4. Bowlby J. Attachment, 2nd edition, attachment and loss (vol. 1). Basic books Inc., New York. 1999.
5. Bridge JA, Iyengar S, Salary CB, et al. Clinical response and risk for reported suicidal ideation and suicide attempts in pediatric antidepressant treatment: a meta-analysis of randomized controlled trials. JAMA. 2007;297:1683Y1696.
6. Copeland W, Shanahan L, Costello E, et al. Childhood and adolescent psychiatric disorders as predictors of young adult disorders. Arch Gen Psychiatry. 2009;66(7):764–72. https://doi.org/10.1001/archgenpsychiatry.2009.85.
7. Day JJ, Sweatt JD. Epigenetic mechanisms in cognition Jeremy. Neuron. 2011;70:813–29.
8. Delgado SV. Non-adherence to treatment: different rules for different patients. Scientific Pages Fam Med. 2016;1:3.
9. Delgado SV, Strawn JR, Pedapati EV. Contemporary psychodynamic psychotherapy for children and adolescents: integrating Intersubjectivity and neuroscience. Springer, Verlag Berlin Heidelberg. 2015.
10. Delgado SV, Wassenaar E, Strawn JR. Does your patient have a psychiatric illness or nonverbal learning disorder? Curr Psychiatr Ther. 2011;10(5):17–35.
11. Dick DM. Gene-environment interaction in psychological traits and disorders. Annu Rev Clin Psychol. 2011;7:383–409. https://doi.org/10.1146/annurev-clinpsy-032210-104518.
12. Doyle FL, Mendoza Diaz A, Eapen V, et al. Mapping the specific pathways to early-onset mental health disorders: the "watch me grow for REAL" study protocol. Front Psych. 2020;11:553. https://doi.org/10.3389/fpsyt.2020.00553.
13. Dozier M, Bernard K. Attachment and biobehavioral catch-up: addressing the needs of infants and toddlers exposed to inadequate or problematic caregiving. Curr Opin Psychol. 2017;15:111–7. https://doi.org/10.1016/j.copsyc.2017.03.003.
14. Franz C, Ascherman L, Shafiel J. A clinician's guide to learning disabilities. Oxford: Oxford University Press; 2018.
15. Ganna A, Verweij KJH, Nivard MG, et al. Large-scale GWAS reveals insights into the genetic architecture of same-sex sexual behavior. Science. 2019;365(6456):eaat7693. https://doi.org/10.1126/science.aat7693.
16. Goldsmith HH, Davidson RJ. Disambiguating the components of emotion regulation. Child Dev. 2004;75:361–5.
17. Hirsch J. Uniqueness, diversity, similarity, repeatability, and heritability. In: Garcia Coll C, Bearer E, Lerner RM, editors. Nature and nurture: the complex interplay of genetic and environmental influences on human behavior and development. Mahwah: Erlbaum; 2004. p. 127–38.
18. Keenan K, Hipwell A, Chung T, et al. The Pittsburgh girls study: overview and initial findings. J Clin Child Adolesc Psychol. 2010;39(4):506–21. https://doi.org/10.1080/15374416.2010.486320.
19. LeDoux JE. Emotion: clues from the brain. Annu Rev Psychol. 1995;46:209–35. https://doi.org/10.1146/annurev.ps.46.020195.001233.
20. Loughnan RJ, Palmer CE, Thompson WK, et al. Polygenic score of intelligence is more predictive of crystallized than fluid performance among children. bioRxiv. 2019:637512. https://doi.org/10.1101/637512.
21. Morris AS, Silk JS, Steinberg L, et al. The role of the family context in the development of emotion regulation. Soc Dev. 2007;16(2):361–88. https://doi.org/10.1111/j.1467-9507.2007.00389.x.
22. Paulussen-Hoogeboom MC, Stams GJ, Hermanns JM, Peetsma TT. Child negative emotionality and parenting from infancy to preschool: a meta-analytic review. Dev Psychol. 2007;43(2):438–53. https://doi.org/10.1037/0012-1649.43.2.438.
23. Schizophrenia Working Group of the Psychiatric Genomics Consortium. Biological insights from 108 schizophrenia-associated genetic loci. Nature. 2014;511:421–7.
24. Thomas A, Chess S. Goodness of fit: clinical applications from infancy through adult life. Routledge, New York. p. 39–52. 1999
25. Thomas A, Chess S, Birch HG. The origin of personality. Sci Am. 1970;223(2):102–9.

Chapter 2
The Four Pillars through a Contemporary Diagnostic Interview

Tell me and I forget. Teach me and I remember. Involve me and I learn.
— Benjamin Franklin (1706–1790)

The Four Pillars

The four pillars arise from innate and environmental processes and are a scaffold for the child's development and maintenance of self-regulation and implicit relational patterns that guide her successful interaction with others. The first three pillars—temperament, cognition, and cognitive flexibility—form the foundation of the fourth pillar, personality, the interpersonal expression of the internal working model of attachment (IWMA). By understanding the contribution of each pillar, clinicians will have a biopsychosocial understanding of the patient, the patient's needs, and the patient's parents. In this chapter, we introduce these concepts and the way in which they diverge from traditional approaches in understanding psychopathology and how they relate to the Contemporary Diagnostic Interview. The subsequent chapters describe the differences in temperamental styles (Chap. 3), cognition (Chap. 4), cognitive flexibility (Chap. 5), personality styles (Chap. 6), and how understanding and assessing these elements helps us to not only understand the patient and her family but to tailor interventions (Chap. 7, 8).

In thinking about the way in which temperament, cognition, and cognitive flexibility and internal working models of attachment (IWMA) can influence differing presentations, consider three 11-year-old girls: Michelle, Sadie, and Rachel.

Michelle, Sadie, and Rachel each have supportive and nurturing parents in a stable home environment. During the COVID-19 pandemic, each girl experiences the same national trauma, a sudden and difficult life event.

S. V. Delgado et al., *Promoting the Emotional and Behavioral Success of Youths*,
https://doi.org/10.1007/978-3-030-88075-0_2

Michelle understands the risks of the virus and feels happy that her family is healthy and happy. They all follow safety protocols. When her teacher reaches out to ask if she would like to send letters to local nursing home residents who cannot receive visitors, Michelle is pleased and writes supportive letters. She assures her parents that if she goes out, she will wear a mask, socially distance, and wash her hands often. She looks forward to virtual classes.

Sadie is concerned about the virus and repeatedly asks her parents if anyone in the family will get sick or die. She pleads with her parents to avoid going out and demands that they always wear masks when they are not at home. She struggles with sleep and now sleeps on the floor of her parents' bedroom. Sadie's parents make an appointment with a mental health clinician for therapy and consideration of medication.

Rachel ignores precautions related to the virus. She argues with her parents because she does not want to wear a mask or maintain physical distancing when playing at the park. She is unconcerned about her parents' or grandparents' risk of exposure. She looks forward to being reunited with her friends at in-person classes.

When the COVID-19 pandemic began, Michelle, Sadie, and Rachel were the same age; all were provided by their parents with a secure attachment and a stable environment. However, they had different four-pillar profiles that played a significant role in the emotional and behavioral reactions to the pandemic. It is increasingly acknowledged that temperament, cognition, cognitive flexibility, and personality can affect the presentation of childhood well-being or psychopathology [26, 27].

Understanding Michelle, Sadie, and Rachel Psychologically

Michelle understands the risks of the virus and is pleased that her family is healthy and happy. She demonstrates a strong sense of community, caring for others in need and does not need treatment.

Sadie is concerned about the virus and repeatedly asked her parents if anyone in the family will get sick or die and sleeps on the floor of her parents' bedroom. Clinicians may consider that cognitive distortions and anxiety are the primary contributors to the maladaptive behaviors and may suggest cognitive behavioral psychotherapy. While other clinicians will explore whether Sadie demonstrated regressive behaviors due to her temperament and dependent personality traits and may suggest family therapy.

Rachel ignores precautions related to the virus and is defiant when asked to wear a mask. She superficially understands the risk of exposure and is not anxious. Clinicians may believe that although she has supportive parents, Rachel may have had early conflicted childhood experiences that interfered with the development of her emotional regulatory abilities and was a difficult child and her parents struggled to set limits. Thus, the maladaptive behaviors might be best helped with patient-centered psychotherapy for Rachel and family therapy to help her parents set consistent expectations with clear consequences for Rachel.

Understanding Sadie and Rachel from a Disease-Based Model Approach

A clinician using a disease-based model approach might believe that since Sadie and Rachel did not improve with psychological interventions, it means that the maladaptive behaviors might also represent symptoms of a disease-based *Diagnostic and Statistical Manual of Mental Disorders* (5th edition (DSM-5); American Psychiatric Association, 2013) [2] disorder. The clinician might move to develop a diagnostic formulation, recommending pharmacotherapy in addition to the therapeutic process.

Understanding Sadie and Rachel Developmentally

If there is continued lack of improvement with medication, Sadie and Rachel might be described as complex and "difficult patients" that require integrated approaches that combine the careful assessment of the patient and parents. We describe this multidimensional developmental perspective in our previous book, *Contemporary Psychodynamic Psychotherapy: Integrating Intersubjectivity and Neuroscience* [10]. Importantly, the Contemporary Diagnostic Interview allows us to elucidate the "four pillars" and psychological data that contribute to psychological symptoms; we can then improve diagnostic formulations and better tailor treatments.

A child or adolescent's temperament, cognition, cognitive flexibility, and personality style may be the foundation for her maladaptive behaviors, yet these considerations are not always included in the diagnostic formulations. Many clinicians associate cognitive weaknesses with learning disorders in children and adolescents and fail to recognize that cognitive weaknesses can contribute to serious emotional and behavioral problems. Furthermore, when patients or parents provide unreliable information due to their own cognitive weaknesses and unknowingly report maladaptive behaviors inaccurately, this reduces accuracy of diagnosis and can lead to ineffective treatment recommendations. Additionally, in our experience, it is rare that a referral for a psychological assessment is made to help clarify the diagnosis, unless the child or adolescent is struggling academically.

For many mental health clinicians, training related to understanding temperamental and cognitive processes in children and adolescents has been superficial. Yet, these processes are the precursors to adaptive or maladaptive behaviors that cause psychological distress. These aspects of a patient do not fit nicely into a disease-based model diagnostic approach and may lead to ineffective treatments. This is not to say that some youth suffering from clear disease-based model severe mental illnesses (e.g., schizophrenia, bipolar disorder, major depressive disorder) will not have positive and life-changing outcomes with standard pharmacotherapy and psychosocial interventions. Instead, we take issue with lengthy lists of varied psychiatric diagnoses in children and adolescents EHRs (electronic health records) that reflect diagnostic formulations by the clinician's intuitive "best fit" approach—in which the clinician uses whichever signs or symptoms catch his attention. This approach misses the opportunity to assess a youth wholly using the four pillars and then use the arrived findings to understand the patient's emotional and behavioral regulation abilities as these abilities pertain to symptom presentations. This book will address the limited attention given to children and adolescents' varied cognitive abilities as the precursors of their maladaptive behaviors, problems with self-esteem and suicidal ideation.

Take, for example, our hypothetical patient Michelle is securely attached, with a healthy personality structure. She will seek others that model growth-promoting behaviors. Sadie, in spite of a very supportive family that helps her cope with her anxiety, will need medication if her anxiety does not improve with therapeutic interventions. Her family will help her be adherent to treatment recommendations, with a good outcome expected.

Rachel, however, who also has a supportive family, has weaknesses in her four pillars that explain why she often seeks people with similar maladaptive behaviors that may mimic those of a psychiatric disorder [24] in spite of her parents' attempts to set limits.

Rachel ignores precautions related to the virus and is defiant when asked to wear a mask, which may be due to a difficult/feisty temperament. This defiance was likely present before the pandemic and will benefit from behavioral interventions. Furthermore, if she is of average-to-above-average intelligence but has weaknesses in verbal comprehension, working memory, or cognitive flexibility, in addition to a difficult/feisty temperament, these weaknesses are the primary contributors to the maladaptive behaviors and might suggest developmentally informed psychotherapy and family therapy to help her parents modify their expectations and learn how to provide reasonable consequences she can understand, considering Rachel's weaknesses in her four pillars.

Understanding Weaknesses in the Four Pillars of Hospitalized Youth

Weaknesses in the four pillars are evident in youths that have multiple inpatient psychiatric hospitalizations. Many of these patients are frowned upon by inpatient child and adolescent psychiatrists, as well as nursing staff, who may describe these patients as "frequent fliers" or believe there is some secondary gain, they like visiting the hospital. This is unfortunate, as many of these youths have significant cognitive and language problems that impede their functioning in emotionally difficult situations at home, school, or with friends. In a sample of an urban academic inpatient psychiatric facility, more than 80% of youth admissions were due to weaknesses in cognition and cognitive flexibility—two of the four pillars—and half had receptive or expressive language impairments. We assert that the "frequent flier" child or adolescent patient is no different than youths that return to the general inpatient units due to difficulties managing their diabetes, asthma, etc. Both are readmitted due to maladaptive patterns in properly managing their care and not due to the worsening, per se, of their condition. In fact, youths with diabetes and weaknesses in cognitive abilities often struggle managing dosing of insulin; they are seen by their treatment teams as being irresponsible, difficult, or trying to self-sabotage their care when this may not be the case [9]. This short-sided view does not account for the psychological and environmental difficulties youths and their parents experience as a result of weaknesses in the four pillars; these weaknesses interfere with their ability to effectively follow through with treatment recommendations. Furthermore, in some discharge meetings, parents may not understand the information provided. It would be advantageous for inpatient teams to have active collaboration with outpatient clinicians to coordinate care to improve outcomes.

We need to make a concentrated effort to learn what to realistically expect from youths and their parents—and what may not be possible to change. Solutions should be focused on improving health care for youth and their families: connecting families to support groups like National Alliance of Mental Illness (NAMI), International Dyslexia Association (IDA), and having child and adolescent psychiatrists, psychologists, and advanced practice nurses volunteer and give presentations to help destigmatize mental health issues, while also highlighting that a one-size-fits-all approach is not helpful (Table 2.1).

From Psychiatric *DSM–5* to Contemporary Diagnostic Interview

Contemporary clinicians, including child and adolescent psychiatrists, are well trained, familiar, and comfortable with the use of the *Diagnostic and Statistical Manual of Mental Disorders, 5th Edition, disease*-based model (*DSM–5*, [2]) interview style. Clinicians traditionally ask the child and her parents to share the history of the child's current illness, with a timeline that establishes when they first noticed the symptoms, the frequency of symptoms, and variations in the intensity of symptoms over time, along with precipitating and perpetuating factors. Over the course of a traditional psychiatric evaluation, the mental health clinician may quickly focus on elucidating risk factors, identifying predictors of treatment response, and determining which "symptoms" meet threshold criteria for a disorder. Thus, with the standard use of the *DSM–5 [2]*, the diagnosis is based on a collection of signs and symptoms that have been well defined. The clinician or psychiatrist is charged with incorporating the information obtained from the patient, his or her family, and also other multiple sources (e.g., prior medical or psychiatric treatment records) into the formulation of effective recommendations, whether psychotherapeutic or psychopharmacological. The goal of any diagnostic interview is to help the clinician or

Table 2.1 Comparison of disease-based and four pillar approaches

	Disease-based approach	Four pillars approach
Patient's cognitive abilities	May overestimate the cognitive ability of the child to accurately report the onset and severity of the signs and symptoms	Begins by assessing child's ability to accurately describe the sequence of the onset and severity of signs and symptoms
External contribution to the patient's struggles or symptoms	Underestimates the influence of parental, family, societal, and cultural factors that contribute to symptoms	Attends to the parental and family contribution as a potential main factor in the child's struggles or symptoms (e.g., insecure attachments or dysfunctional family)
Early experiences	May limit assessment to developmental delays, early trauma and early signs of disorder (e.g., anxiety, depression, attentional problems)	Assesses for temperament problems, cognitive weaknesses, and the capacity to understand others as innate contributors to signs and symptoms
Pharmacotherapy	Treatment may become focused on individual symptoms	Pharmacological treatment is sequenced in regard to how the four pillars contribute to individual symptoms
Psychotherapy	May match disease state or diagnosis to type of therapy	Matches four-pillar strengths and weaknesses to type of therapy
Parental guidance	May assume that parents are able and willing to accept treatment recommendations or may provide unrealistic advice	Assesses parents' temperament, cognitive abilities and, importantly, their capacity to understand their contribution to the child's maladaptive behaviors

psychiatrist tailor the treatment approaches that best suit the patient and ideally should take a biological, psychological, and social integrated approach [25].

In some contexts, more structured interviews may be desired, and several well-validated tools are available to achieve this, including the Mini-International Neuropsychiatric Interview for Children and Adolescents (MINI Kid) and the Schedule for Affective Disorders and Schizophrenia for School-Age Children: Present and Lifetime Version (K-SADS-PL), which have both been demonstrated to have high levels of interrater and test–retest reliability [19, 30]. Beyond this, today's mental health clinician also has structured clinician-administered inventories including the Young Mania Rating Scale (YMRS, [33]), as well as self and caregiver reporting tools, such as the Screen for Child Anxiety and Related Disorders (SCARED, [5]). Our assertion is not that these methods are invalid or unreliable. Rather, they can limit our understanding of the context of patients' symptoms; these instruments implicitly assume that a child or family's report of symptoms is accurate with regard to time, frequency, and severity. Furthermore, these instruments may fail to capture the context of a patient's symptoms within the family and with regard to her interpersonal life.

It is important to realize, then, that there is considerable heterogeneity in youths' abilities to describe their mental health symptoms. This raises questions about the limitations in using the *DSM–5* [2] disease-based model nosology as it generally does not consider, in its diagnostic formulation, cognitive and psychosocial contributors to mental health stress and situational anxiety in these families.

Existing nosology identifies nondistinct disorders rather than underlying syndromes [16, 21]. The idea that major childhood disorders are discrete categories has long been abandoned, as rates and patterns of co-occurrence, or comorbidity, are far higher than could exist by chance [23].

For example, in several review articles about treatment challenges in pediatric bipolar disorders, a differential diagnosis must include unipolar depression, disruptive mood dysregulation disorder, attention-deficit/hyperactivity disorder, anxiety disorder, oppositional defiant disorder, and post-traumatic stress disorder. We find risks in this approach as it does not consider the many similar symptomatic presentations of children and adolescents with temperamental and cognitive weaknesses that would be best served with behavioral and parental therapeutic interventions. Furthermore, many adolescents meeting symptomatic criteria for depression or a mood disorder may have reading abilities well below a fifth-grade level, which may explain their chronic low self-esteem, labile moods, and state of distress. Accordingly, this makes the information obtained through direct questioning limited at best. Thus, symptoms reported by youths and their families may not be accurate in timing, frequency, or severity of symptoms and/or location where their dysregulated state was triggered.

The emphasis throughout this book will be on helping children and adolescents—and their families—achieve the best psychosocial outcomes possible with respect to their innate abilities. To achieve this, we focus on the four pillars as the foundation of each child's unique personality, emotional regulation style, and cognitive abilities. Universal theories of how people must live and behave are inadequate: they do not differentiate temperamental and cognitive abilities or limitations on how people manage adverse events in their life.

Negative childhood experiences adversely affect physical, emotional, and academic development in children [13]. Although there is limited evidence that screening for these events with standardized questionnaires can help prevent negative childhood experiences, it can alert the clinician for the need to assess the four pillars in child and parents [6]. Knowing the strengths and weaknesses of his patient's four pillars, the clinician can then develop practical strategies to realistically encourage a less conflicted and healthier lifestyle. Treatment interventions for childhood abuse, exposure to violence, and substance use will need to be tailored to each child, adolescent, and parent's strengths, with attention given to their weaknesses.

Trauma-focused interventions are of limited help for youths with verbal comprehension problems. Likewise, behavior modification may worsen actions in youths with difficult/feisty temperament, and substance-use group therapy will not be effective in youths with poor fluid reasoning or low average processing speed. Additionally, treatment failure can have a negative impact in a youth's self-esteem and family support, placing them at risk by seeking others with disruptive behaviors to feel part of a community that understands them; at the most extreme, it can lead to gang involvement. For example, while it may seem logical for clinicians to suggest that parents set clear limits for their child to learn natural consequences, doing so can actually be detrimental in certain scenarios (e.g., giving repeated verbal instructions and reprimands to the child with verbal comprehension weakness or displaying anger toward an adolescent with low average processing speed for not answering questions). This path of action can then lead to increased conflict that could easily be avoided. We will discuss this at greater length in Chaps. 4 and 7.

It is agreed that an integrated biological, psychological, and social interview is valuable when assessing patients to help develop well-thought out-treatment plans [9]. However, as Cardoso Zoppe et al. [7] state, "There is still tension between biological and psychosocial tendencies," and teaching methods are heavily influenced by the setting in which the patient is seen (academic, community mental health center, private practice) and the clinician's school of thought (developmentalist, psychopharmacologist, researcher, or behaviorist), [20].

Case Study: A 12-Year-Old Boy with Possible Pediatric Bipolar Disorder

A 12-year-old boy with frequent emotional outbursts was becoming increasingly agitated at home and at school. His parents seek consultation with a child and adolescent psychiatrist, who diagnoses the child with bipolar disorder and recommends a trial of aripiprazole to address his affective instability. Several months later, his parents share that their son continues to have outbursts and they do not feel that the medication has been helpful. Further, the patient's therapist, who described the child as difficult and having a "poor moral compass," asked the child and adolescent psychiatrist to consider changing medications as the current ones "are not working." The psychiatrist considers if the worsening may be related to rapid-cycling bipolar disorder and suggests a combination of two mood-stabilizing agents, aripiprazole and lithium, which also fails to relieve the patient's symptoms.

In consultation with a colleague, the psychiatrist considers an alternative diagnostic formulation. Using an integrative developmental model, she considers the possibility of cognitive weaknesses as contributing to the patient's impaired affective dysregulation and poor impulse control, especially when he is asked to complete complex tasks like schoolwork, homework, and chores. During the psychiatrist's consultation with her colleague, she shares that her patient's symptoms did not emerge during simple tasks, such as watching television with his parents, playing at the park with peers, and partaking in recreational sport activities. Clearly, there were differences in which context the boy had difficulties. His impaired affective dysregulation and poor impulse control were present only during complex tasks, not during activities he could understand better. Although this was thought to be due to the ebb and flow of a pediatric mood disorder, the differences were suggestive of temperamental and cognitive problems. In short, an integrated developmental approach in the diagnostic formulation of the child had not been taken. A psychological assessment revealed the child to have low average fluid reasoning and working memory abilities, which explained why his behavioral self-regulation problems were present when he was asked to complete complex tasks rather than simple ones.

From a biopsychosocial perspective, we propose that an integrated developmental approach as described above facilitates the complex decision-making needed to outline the sequencing of the interventions to ensure successful outcomes. This approach allows the clinician to grasp of the interplay between the forces of nature and nurture.

In using a traditional *DSM–5* interview, the clinician or psychiatrist's diagnostic formulation is generally based on the assumption that the responses by the patient and parents or caregivers are factual and accurate, unless psychotic processes or developmental disabilities prevents it. However, we highlight in a previous work (2015) the limitations of the *DSM-5*–style interview; namely, that it ignores the patient's temperament, learning abilities or weaknesses; it also fails to consider cognitive flexibilities within the patient's family and social/cultural environment. Herein, the careful assessment of the patient's and parents' innate and relational factors allows the clinician to obtain, in a succinct manner, critical information as to whether the responses provided are actually factual and accurate. He can then use this information to tailor an effective treatment regimen.

Additionally, some feel that the child and adolescent psychiatrist should practice at the "top of their license," in other words evaluating psychiatric *DSM–5* diagnoses, assessing medical comorbidity, pharmacologic treatment, and referral for psychosocial interventions [12]. In our opinion, the integrated approach we advocate in this book provides insight about which signs or symptoms stem from a *DSM–5* disease-based model and best approached with medication, or if the signs and symptoms are due to weaknesses in their four pillars and psychotherapy will be more beneficial and help the patient and family adhere to treatment recommendations.

Case Study: A 12-Year-Old Boy with Poorly Controlled Bipolar Disorder (Continued)

Let's return to the 12-year-old boy with rapid cycling bipolar disorder. His psychiatrist had become concerned that the agitation and behavioral problems were potentially related to temperament and poor cognitive abilities. This new formulation allowed the boy's psychiatrist to understand why her changes in pharmacotherapy failed to improve symptoms. In knowing this, the boy's psychiatrist began to *sequence the interventions*. First, she discontinued medications and requested "wraparound" in-home services to help parents develop visually oriented behavioral strategies (e.g., charts depicting the steps in complex tasks and rewards when completed). Second, she educated the family that that his outbursts were happening because he felt frustrated that he couldn't understand what was expected of him—while implicitly knowing he would likely be reprimanded. The psychiatrist recommended approaching him with one-step requests and then allowing him to repeat them back to confirm his understanding which would reduce his angry outburst for misunderstanding. Further, a psychological assessment was needed in order to identify the nature and severity of his cognitive weaknesses and developed a plan to educate the boy's parents and teachers in terms of psychological and educational needs. Third, his psychiatrist collaborated with his therapist to share the new diagnostic formulation and request that the therapeutic interventions not be insight-oriented, but rather develop practical role-play situations to help the boy learn new skills to use when he felt distressed—for example, he and his parents determined a code word for him to use when he felt angry, so his parents could listen to him and help him be successful. Fourth, the psychiatrist encouraged the boy's parents to share information about his weaknesses with his teachers to help them understand his struggles and form realistic academic expectations.

Although attending to temperament, cognitive abilities or weaknesses, and cognitive flexibilities may initially seem daunting for the mental health clinician, it can promote better outcomes, simplify treatment and avoid ineffective forms of psychotherapy, unnecessary pharmacotherapy or even unnecessary polypharmacy. We don't aim to minimize the lifesaving experiences some children and adolescents have with appropriate therapeutic and medication interventions; rather, we are cautioning about the tension between biological and psychosocial interventions, which can be limiting to a child's future [18].

The Contemporary Diagnostic Interview (CDI)

Although we have identified some of the weaknesses of the traditional *DSM–5*-style structured interview model, our primary goal is to add to and enhance the techniques available to the clinician's or psychiatrist's toolbox to improve the diagnostic reliability needed. However, we don't expect many of the "tools" to initially fit neatly into current clinical practice. The Contemporary Diagnostic Interview is aimed at observing and interacting with patients and their parents or caregivers, and it is designed to capture *a different spectrum* of information that is inaccessible by the standard *DSM–5*-style interview. As with the adoption of any new useful and practical technique, the initial challenge will be overcome through careful study and frequent practice.

The goal of a Contemporary Diagnostic Interview is to facilitate the expression of the patient's and his or her parents' four pillars: temperament, cognition, cognitive flexibility, and the patterns of relating with each other and with others (Table 2.2).

We have found that the Contemporary Diagnostic Interview increases the ability to know when the signs and symptoms endorsed by youths and their parents can be viewed as reliable and accurate, allowing for the development of a comprehensive diagnostic formulation and practical treatment interventions.

The Contemporary Diagnostic Interview is designed to quickly elicit clues about whether the information provided is likely inaccurate or unreliable and to help the practitioner decide when it is best to wait for collateral information or a formal psychological evaluation. Herein, we will outline how to complete a detailed Contemporary Diagnostic Interview for the reader to use in his or her clinical work.

Table 2.2 The four pillars of the Contemporary Diagnostic Interview

Temperament: Stable moods and behavior profiles observed in infancy and early childhood
Cognition: Cognitive processes that acquire, process, and act on information or stimuli
Cognitive flexibility: The capacity to engage in relationships based on mutual understanding of each other's ideas and intent
Personality (internal working models of attachment—IWMA): The style a person uses to attune emotionally to each other within the context of family, social, and cultural norms

Beginning the Interview

We now will review how each of the four pillars can be assessed during a Contemporary Diagnostic Interview. The pillars are outlined in the order in which they emerge in the psychological development of a person. When using a Contemporary Diagnostic Interview, however, the four pillars are simultaneously elucidated. The Contemporary Diagnostic Interview is not based on a standard format to be followed, as is common in a structured interview. Rather, the questions suggested are broad and intended to be of help to child and adolescent psychiatrists and clinicians in discerning, in the here-and-now moments of subjectivity, a youth and her parents' temperament style, cognition, cognitive flexibility, and personality style (models of attachment). Additionally, the clinician will need to consciously delay the use of questions of a *DSM–5* style interview, as this line of questioning may lead the clinician to assume that the patient and parents understand the questions and that their responses reflect the nature and severity of what they endorse.

The interview goes well when the clinician takes a conversational approach to assess the four pillars. There will be plenty of time for a structured interview after the clinician feels he or she has a genuine understanding of the patient and their parents. Initially, the conversational approach may seem nonproductive, but this approach provides the foundation for understanding other people and helps discern whether the clinician's view of the problems is reliable and accurate. The initial 5–10 minutes of the interview should provide the clinician a window into the four pillars.

The reader may wonder which are the most useful comments or questions to use in a Contemporary Diagnostic Interview. While there are many ways to begin a Contemporary Diagnostic Interview, we provide examples to illustrate various approaches. The initial comments and questions that may be used to open the interview can be easily adapted to fit the personal qualities of each clinician.

We emphasize that as part of the initial Contemporary Diagnostic Interview, the first question or comment should not be the reason for coming to the appointment. It is detrimental to begin with open-ended questions about the reasons patients or parents are seeking help, such as: "How can I help you?" "What brings you here?" or "How do you understand your problem?" This style of questioning may make a patient and his parents feel *broken* rather than feeling like people who are seeking help within the context of a larger system. The value in *joining and holding their anxieties* before delving into the stressful aspects of their life is that it facilitates increased reliability, consistency, and accuracy in the description of the signs and symptoms they endorse [10].

Attending to the External Attributes of the Patient and Parents

The initial comment used during a Contemporary Diagnostic Interview is helpful when it attends to the external attributes of the patient and his or her parents—shy, tired, appearing angry, etc.—and the clinician's subjective experience of them. If the patient and family look tired, it is helpful for the clinician to openly acknowledge the experience. On one occasion, a child's mother shared that they had rushed to be on time. She had taken her disabled son to two appointments earlier in the day. "That's why I am late and look so stressed," she said. Without giving attention to nuances of human interaction, their presentation may have easily been misconceived, with the clinician inferring that "this mother is so disorganized"—and that this disorganization contributes to the patient's problems with time management.

It is well received when the clinician gives positive recognition to an outward attribute of the child, such as his age, height, eyeglasses, clothing, backpack, etc. In doing so, the clinician can assess whether the child feels safe interacting with others and his or her capacity to understand the reciprocal nature of typical conversation—something that is not captured in a disease-based model interview.

We remind the reader that the responses not only reflect the patient's in vivo cognitive level of functioning, but they are also influenced by the patient's temperament, cognition, and personality. Herein, the clinician will need to allow the interaction to unfold so as to have the necessary subjective experiences that allow one to use the Contemporary Diagnostic Interview Case Formulation tool.

We cannot emphasize enough that during a Contemporary Diagnostic Interview, the mental health clinician's personal attributes and beliefs will undoubtedly influence what and how the patient chooses to share regarding the problems and symptoms she endorses.

In completing a Contemporary Diagnostic Interview, the clinician may notice feeling frustrated or find that he is asking leading questions, in a rapid-fire manner, hoping the adolescent will eventually "get it right," as if the adolescent is withholding their ability to think clearly. Sadly, this can reinforce the patient's feeling of being limited. In such situations, the clinician should remain focused on understanding the patient's impairments from a multidimensional perspective, as it may be due to weaknesses in the four pillars or from cognitive weaknesses of a disease-based model or, ultimately, both.

Assessing Temperament in the Contemporary Diagnostic Interview

Temperament refers to the "stable moods and behavior profiles observed in infancy and early childhood" [31]. A detailed description of the origin and differences in temperamental styles is provided in Chap. 3, and a description of its use in tailoring interventions is provided in Chap. 7. Briefly, there are three predominant temperamental styles, although presentation can be a mixed form with one style predominant: easy/flexible, difficult/feisty, and slow-to-warm-up.

At times, the maladaptive behaviors for which youth are brought to treatment may be due to temperamental problems which become evident when parents share that they worry about their child or adolescent's "moral compass." If the troublesome behaviors are due to a difficult/feisty temperament with frequent episodes of defiance and irritability, in the initial encounter with the clinician, these youths may say things like, "I hate being here. I am not going to do this; I don't need this." Or they may refuse to speak. In approaching such a patient, the clinician must determine the degree to which the difficult/feisty temperament style is typical, or whether it reflects the child's fear and anxiety related to the evaluation. Some clinicians, when using disease-based model approaches, might notice overlap between a difficult/feisty temperamental style and oppositional defiant disorder, disruptive behavior disorder, and mood disorders. Understanding the core reason for the patient's defiant and oppositional behaviors allows the clinician to provide useful and practical psychosocial interventions for his or her parents.

When the clinician is aware of an adolescent's history of maladaptive behaviors (e.g., hitting others, running away, using drugs, shoplifting), it's helpful to acknowledge this information and wonder aloud, in an empathic manner, if it is correct. This implicit allows the clinician to inquire, in a noncritical manner, about the patient's difficulties within the context of their relational view of the world.

Difficult/feisty temperament, limited cognition, limited cognitive flexibility, and insecure attachment

Julie, 16, arrives for a psychiatric evaluation. She has a prior diagnosis of bipolar disorder. Recently, she learned that her girlfriend had cheated on her. She felt overwhelmed and began having thoughts about taking an overdose of her medication.

Clinician Good morning. I am Dr. Jones. Please come in. *[Tone of voice and body movements demonstrate excitement and vitality of the encounter]*

Clinician *[While walking to the office]* I really like the color of your hair, nice bright green. *[Tone of voice reinforces excitement and vitality of the encounter]*

Patient I don't know why I choose this color. *[Unable to engage in affective reciprocity]*

Clinician What colors have you had before? *[Affectively implying, "I like your hair color"]*

Patient *[Does not respond; appears disinterested in engaging with clinician]*

Clinician I would like to know what you do for fun on weekends.

Patient I am always grounded; my parents don't let me do anything. *[Demonstrates anger]*

Parents: You know why you are grounded. You never do what we ask you to do, and you keep breaking things. *[Voices raised, implying that she is a "bad" adolescent]*

Patient Whatever; you guys are stupid. *[The parents and youth engage with the same implicit relational models used when interacting with others they do not like]*

Clinician Wow, looks like we have some work to do here. *[Subjectively feels that they genuinely do not have the ability for implicit recognition of the clinician's attempt to establish rapport and notes that they rely on established disorganized models of attachment, likely due to difficult/feisty temperaments, limited cognition, and limited cognitive flexibilities]*

Parents She is needy and possessive of the girls she dates and wants them to be with her all the time. She avoids completing her homework. If she doesn't get what she wants, she says she is suicidal to get attention. We are tired of it. *[Continue blaming and using similar interactive patterns the child uses; dismissive of the clinician's opinion]*

Patient I hate school; nobody helps me. I need you guys to get off my back. Between you shouting and Anna cheating on me, I would rather hurt myself than live with you. If you guys would just listen and let me spend more time with my girlfriend, I would not be suicidal.

In this brief interaction, the clinician allowed the patient and parents to demonstrate their implicit interactive style: The parents berate their child in front of the clinician and do not have a spirit of inquiry about why she may be difficult. We see the emergence of a difficult/feisty temperament style in all family members, average cognition and limited cognitive flexibility—lack of understanding that their negative interactions in the presence of the clinician implicitly reveal their inability to view the clinician as helpful (insecure attachment patterns). The clinician now knows that at least some of the information obtained throughout the interview will likely be unreliable, as it is influenced by their temperament and affective states. This makes gathering collateral information even more important.

Mixed temperament (easy/flexible and slow-to-warm-up), good cognition, good cognitive flexibility and secure attachment

Michael, 12, presents for a psychiatric evaluation due to limited response to a trial of several stimulant medications. He has a prior diagnosis of educationally gifted, with attention-deficit/hyperactivity disorder (predominantly inattentive type). He felt overwhelmed at school "because I am too slow and get distracted. I am sad because I disappoint my parents."

Clinician Good morning. I am Dr. Jones. Please come in. *[Tone of voice and body movements demonstrate excitement and vitality of the encounter]*

Clinician *[While walking to the office]* I really like your phone. Is it the new model? *[Tone of voice demonstrates excitement and vitality of the encounter]*

Patient I really like it; I can watch the college basketball games on it. *[Engages with affective reciprocity]*

Clinician What teams do you follow? *[Affectively implying, "I like college basketball as well"]*

Patient I am glad Kansas beat Duke in the last game. They are really good, and the freshmen are amazing. *[Is happy to respond; appears interested in engaging with clinician]*

Later

Clinician Your dad is worried about your problems at school. I wonder what your thoughts are about his worry. *[Assessing for all pillars in this broad question about whether the patient understands his father's concern]*

Patient *[Does not respond. Appears interested in engaging with clinician, but struggles to share. Appears anxious.]*

Parent Michael, tell the doctor why I worry. You know you are a great, smart kid. You just don't speak up. *[Supportive and implying that his son is a "good" adolescent]*

Patient Hmm. *[Appears anxious. Pauses for a few seconds.]* I am not sure what to say.

In this brief interaction, the clinician allowed the patient and father to demonstrate their implicit interactive style: The clinician and father notice the difference in his presentation. When Michael is excited about basketball, he presents with easy/flexible temperament and superior cognitive abilities. When asked about his academic struggles, although his father is supportive, he presents with a slow-to-warm-up temperamental style that may be influenced by slow processing speed that manifests when Michael is challenged by affectively laden situations. Mixed temperament styles present as a combination of the styles, although one style will predominate.

Used clinically, the slow-to-warm-up child can be difficult to engage when thinking about complex situations that require back-and-forth dialogue. Parents and clinician are often puzzled by the discrepancy and may feel frustrated by the lack of a reciprocal dialogue, particularly if there are time constraints. Diagnostically, we think of these patients as those that make the clinician work harder than the patient over the course of the appointment. Such a pattern alerts the clinician of a possible weakness in one or more of the four pillars and that an anxiety disorder is not likely since he is happy most of the time.

Assessing Cognition in the Contemporary Diagnostic Interview

In understanding a patient, clinicians must account for the patient's cognitive ability, particularly with regard to the norms of their age and development (see Appendix A) and should also consider limitations that result from learning disabilities (see Table 2.3).

Table 2.3 Assessing possible learning weakness

Learning disorder/ dyslexia	Suggested questions for youth 8-years-of-age or over and responses that suggest a learning weakness
Written language	*Ask the patient to spell or write in order of complexity: mother, father, school, hospital, bicycle, and giraffe. Can also ask patient to spell or write parents' names and home address.* "I can't spell that good." "Mother, father, sckool, hospital, bysicle, gerafe." "Mother, father, skool, hospital. I can't spell bicycle."
Math	*Ask what coins the patient would use to give the clinician 93 cents.* "Three quarters, two dimes and three pennies." "Two quarters, two dimes, two nickels and three pennies." "Ten dimes and you keep the change."
Reading/ dyslexia	*Ask the patient to read a small paragraph that can be easily used by the clinician to assess reading and comprehension abilities. For example, we use the opening paragraph from* the true story of the three little pigs: *"Everybody knows the story of the pigs. Or, at least they think they do. But, I'll let you in on a little secret. Nobody knows the real story, because nobody has ever heard my story. —By A. wolf."* by third grade, we expect the child to read correctly and possess some ability for abstract comprehension. At this level, the child would understand the story, the role of the author, and how the story is different from the traditional story of the three little pigs. However, with weakness in reading comprehension and abstraction, we might hear responses such as "The pigs don't know who the wolf is." "The three little pigs are not happy."
Nonverbal learning disorder	*Ask the patient about parents' place of employment.* *A patient with a nonverbal learning disorder may respond with a topic vaguely connected to question.* "Not sure where but they like it. I think my dad works in court. I want to be a musician or maybe a lawyer." *[smiling; is embarrassed by her uncertainty. Changes topics, likely without realizing it].* "Why do you have so many toys in your office?" *[changes topics within a few sentences, likely without realizing it.]*

Cognition represents the second pillar in the formation of our personality. Broadly, this pillar includes all cognitive processes used to acquire, process, and discern which information or stimuli to act on when making decisions. Importantly, weaknesses here lead to maladaptive behaviors and emotional dysregulation with an increased risk of developing problems with self-esteem, interpersonal conflict, and academic functioning. However, in thinking about cognition, clinicians will do well to remember that this is multifaceted, dynamic, and influenced by many factors during a child's life. Up to 20% of the U.S. population has some form of cognitive weakness, and up to 40% of those with learning disorders may meet diagnostic criteria for a psychiatric disorder. This will have significant repercussions in how we understand the patient and the treatment recommendations we make [1, 8]. Furthermore, it is estimated that up to 37% of incarcerated youth are eligible for services under the Individuals with Disabilities Education Act (IDEA) [14].

Assessing cognition in more depth is described in Chap. 4. In Chaps. 7 and 8, we describe how being aware of cognitive differences can help the clinician tailor interventions. For years, mental health clinicians have understood that weaknesses in cognitive abilities could lead to problems with self-esteem and behavioral difficulties, although the information provided by intelligence tests was not commonly used for diagnostic purposes or to help develop practical clinical treatment recommendations. Here, we will help the clinician learn how to use the information obtained from a Contemporary Diagnostic Interview with the WISC–V (Wechsler Intelligence Scale for Children, fifth ed.) in mind, to gain a true understanding of their patient from the inside out [32].

The use of a WISC–V full-scale score has been, for decades, the go-to metric to categorize a child's predicted ability for success or impairments. However, the full-scale scores do not capture *the full story* of a child's strengths and weaknesses within the context of interpersonal relationships and emotional regulation. WISC–V is composed of five subtest indices: verbal comprehension (VC), visual-spatial (VS), fluid reasoning (FR), working memory, (WM) and processing speed (PS). Weaknesses in one or more of the indices can often be elucidated through a Contemporary Diagnostic Interview.

Cognitive Weaknesses

Mental health clinicians routinely include qualitative descriptions of cognitive function as they document a mental-status examination (e.g., intelligence, fund of knowledge, insight, and judgment). This style of evaluation/documentation may be disadvantageous, though, as the clinician may remain unaware that core cognitive capacities are the root of the problem.

Identifying Cognitive Weaknesses in the Contemporary Diagnostic Interview

We will briefly outline some interventions we have found helpful in using a Contemporary Diagnostic Interview to tease out matters of cognition and learning in children and adolescents.

The conversational style of interviewing that is leveraged in the Contemporary Diagnostic Interview allows the clinician to assess whether the patient and his parents are able to respond in a developmentally appropriate way or if their responses are poorly formulated due to cognitive weaknesses. When the mental health clinician notices that the patient's and/or the parents' conversations have poor sentence structure (e.g., syntax), malapropisms or paraphasic errors, it should alert the clinician to a few possibilities: lack of education due to socioeconomic or cultural barriers, cognitive limitations, and/or a learning disorder. As such, the clinician will be rewarded by continuing to use a conversational Contemporary Diagnostic Interview approach to tease out these factors in order to become aware of possibility unreliability of reported signs and symptoms, at which point collateral information is essential. Additionally, difficulties in understanding basic humor or typical conversational flow should also alert the clinician to these issues.

There are several ways that a mental health clinician may choose to assess cognitive abilities. As we have said, this is best done using a conversational approach. To illustrate this, we will describe several inquiries that we have found helpful, although other inquiries can easily provide the information needed. We start with the birthday conversation (described in Table 2.4) and follow with the inquiry of the parents' place of employment. This line of inquiry can also be used by asking the patient if they know how their parents choose their name, or what they remember doing as a family to celebrate relevant holidays (e.g., Thanksgiving, Christmas, New Year's). As you read through the examples, note the complex interplay that facilitates an assessment of cognition and provides clues as to the child's temperamental style, cognitive flexibilities, and personality. Using the Contemporary Diagnostic Interview, the clinician also gleans information on possible weakness in visual-spatial abilities.

We should note that in extreme cases of bereavement, depression, or trauma, the patient may present with what may appear as severe cognitive weaknesses. Herein, having a baseline of cognitive functioning is essential.

Birthday Conversation

It is helpful to explore with children over the age of 5 how they celebrated their birthday. These questions are best asked within 2 months of the birthday, which also allows clinicians to assess short-term memory and cognitive flexibility.

Table 2.4 Assessing cognition in the Contemporary Diagnostic Interview

"How did you celebrate your birthday?"	
Cognitive level	Possible responses
Above average	*May reveal a sense of pride and reflect involvement from others.* "I had fun and spent it with my family. Later I went out with my friends." "I had pizza and a birthday cake my mom made."
Average	*Acknowledges event and provides relevant detail [potentially reflecting adequate visual-spatial skills, fluid reasoning, and working memory]* "It was pretty good. I was with my family and friends." "I got some cool stuff.".
Below average	*May reflect frustration, difficulty recalling the temporal aspect of the birthday [possible impairment related to working memory], may be surprised [possible impairment related to fluid reasoning], may lack of interest or depth [possibly reflects verbal comprehension or fluid reasoning].* "Not sure. I know it was okay." "I don't remember what we did.".
Intellectual Disability	*May be not understand the question or concept. The clinician may need to make her question more concrete and in the present tense. The patient's response may relate to senses [what did they see, touch, taste?] rather than the abstract/ conceptual.* "Don't remember." "Don't know." [turns to parents for help].

"What did you get for your birthday?"	
Cognitive level	Possible responses
Above average	*The patient's response to this more specific question reflects strong verbal comprehension [comments on gift], visual-spatial processing [ordering of responses/lists], fluid reasoning [refers to involvement of others], working memory, and processing speed.* "I got gift cards from my family and a new [smartphone, tennis racket, video game, etc.] from my parents." *[Sense of pride]*
Average	*Acknowledges gifts and provides relevant detail [potentially reflecting adequate visual-spatial skills, fluid reasoning, and working memory]* "I think I got money, not sure." "Oh yeah, they got me video games.".
Below average	*Given the more concrete and specific question, the patient's response may suggest weakness in verbal comprehension [lack of specificity or frustration] and/or difficulty with working memory [struggles to recall gifts]. In responding, the patient may be frustrated or appear to lack interest [difficulties with fluid reasoning].* "Not sure. I don't remember." "Probably money or food. I really like pizza."
Intellectual disability	*Is unable to understand the question. The clinician will need to find another form of verbal interaction.*

Parents' place of employment conversation

"Do you know where your mother and father work and what they do at work?"	
Cognitive level	Possible responses
Above average	"My mother teaches fifth grade at St. John's school and my father is a pharmacist at metro hospital." *The patient's response to this more specific question reflects strong verbal comprehension and fluid reasoning [description of type and place of employment].*
Average	*Is aware of parents' occupation and general job description, potentially reflecting adequate visual-spatial skills and verbal comprehension, but may reveal a mild weakness in fluid reasoning [lack specificity in response] and working memory [may not address question completely].* "My mom is a teacher and my dad works at a hospital—In the pharmacy with medicine. I'm not sure exactly what he does." "My dad works in construction and I think he's the boss."
Below average	*May be aware of parents' occupation or title but may not understand work role or place of employment [reflecting impairments in verbal comprehension and visual-spatial processing]. Responses may be concrete or limited to one specific aspect of parents' employment such as travel,* etc. *[reflecting impaired working memory]. May give vague or superficial response that fails to capture abstract aspects of employment [consistent with weakness in fluid reasoning]. The patient may also be frustrated by the question and his or her lack of awareness.* "Mom teaches at a pre-school." [mother reports that she is a teacher's assistant in an elementary school.] "My dad works a lot, but I don't know what he does exactly." "I don't really know.".
Intellectual disability	*Is unable to understand the question. The clinician will need to find another form of verbal interaction.*

Learning Disorders in a Contemporary Diagnostic Interview

It is important to assess the impact cognitive weakness or formal learning disorders can have on how a clinician understands a child or adolescent in a Contemporary Diagnostic Interview. Patients who present with impairment in academic, cognitive, social, and vocational functioning might be struggling with an unrecognized learning disorder. Ten percent of the U.S. population has some form of learning disability, and up to 40% of those with learning disorders may meet diagnostic criteria for a psychiatric disorder [11]. This has significant repercussions in how we understand the patient and the treatment recommendations we make. Moreover, by some reports, 20% of the general population has learning weaknesses, and within this group, many meet diagnostic criteria for learning disorders [1, 8].

Considering these statistics, it is not surprising that children and adolescents with cognitive weaknesses may frequently be described by child and adolescent psychiatrists or clinicians as "difficult to connect with," or as having probable depression or poor motivation. They may frustrate the clinician. Family members who don't recognize the patient's cognitive limitations may also be frustrated with their child. Moreover, at times, the parents' own cognitive weaknesses may prevent them from appreciating their child's struggles.

If time permits, a simple way to assess for possible specific learning weakness can be to ask pertinent questions in each area, taking into consideration age and exposure to school. Although dyslexia or learning disabilities in reading, writing, or math represent a heterogeneous group of conditions, the questions can alert the clinician to possible learning weakness that would benefit from further assessment; he can then give a referral for formal academic testing.

Most children like to attend school, where they develop cognitively, emotionally, and socially. However, many children and adolescents with learning weakness who struggle in school present to mental health clinicians with school refusal, school phobia, and somatic complaints, depending on their age. Children and adolescents with learning weakness typically use their fingers to count and recite the alphabet in song form, in a strategy typical of young children, to recall letters. They typically state that their favorite classes are recess, gym, music, and art. Therefore, it is important that the clinician not conclude that all forms of school refusal are due to disorder-based psychopathology or to psychological or family problems. With a careful assessment of cognition, the approaches developed help the child feel competent and increase his or her motivation to attend school and, once at school, to engage. In difficult situations, the family or clinician may benefit in obtaining psychoeducational testing to provide discrete and quantitative evidence of the child's relative strengths and limitations. With these cognitive/psychoeducational test results in hand (Chap. 4), the clinician can best tailor the treatment interventions and improve the child's self-esteem.

Visual-Spatial Abilities

Visual-spatial ability is having the capacity to understand and remember the position of objects in relation to other objects and to yourself. This skill is required to understand directional verbal descriptions. It's also necessary to know where to find things, such as one's home, to know where things go, and how to get to places. Historically, however, clinicians have undervalued the importance of assessing visual-spatial abilities in children and adolescents (Table 2.5). Unfortunately, weakness in visual-spatial processing may be seen by parents or teachers as stubbornness or moodiness (see Chaps. 4 and 7). This has implications on how these children develop, as they may be criticized or ridiculed, and have chronic low self-esteem. Brief assessments of visual-spatial abilities in youth (Table 2.6).

Table 2.5 Visual-spatial weaknesses

Unable to recall where school assignments are stored
Bumping into familiar furniture repeatedly
Getting easily lost in new school, camping sites, etc.
Limited awareness of important warning signs in parks or swimming pools
Difficulty paying attention to visual tasks or easily distracted by too much visual stimuli (e.g., learning new sport or video game)

Table 2.6 Brief assessments of visual-spatial abilities in youth

Preschool children	Ability to replicate simple block designs or pictures. Stack or spell their name with blocks. Ability to play with LEGOS with ease.
Elementary school age youth	Ability to draw the floor plan/layout of their room. Capacity to enjoy simple magic tricks or illusions with playing cards. Ability to play Jenga, Uno, Connect Four.
Adolescents	Knowledge of directions to their home from the clinician's office. Ability to give details of landmarks near their home.

From Delgado et al. [10]

We frequently ask about landmarks close to an adolescent's home (when the clinician has some familiarity with the area or if parents can confirm for accuracy) to quickly screen for visual-spatial processing difficulties. For example, in the initial encounter, we might ask, "Where do you live?" Then, upon hearing the patient's answer, we might ask which cardinal direction their home sits in relation to the office or clinic, or what routes the adolescent or parents used to come. Alternatively, asking what route the patient takes when going to school can also alert the clinician to problems with attention to direction and detail. The patient's response can reflect their visual-spatial abilities or weaknesses. For example, they may not remember their neighborhood or subdivision name, landmarks near their home or the names of roads. They may remember driving on a highway but display uncertainty about which one. Accordingly, the patient's responses must be viewed within the context of possible verbal comprehension weakness.

A 16-year-old adolescent was asked where she lives.

Lindsay By the schools.
Clinician I am not familiar with your neighborhood. Which school's?
Lindsay Both elementary and high school.
Clinician Thank you. Can you share which neighborhood the schools are in?
Lindsay Both schools are in the neighborhood with lots of streets.
Clinician What grades are getting at school?
Lindsay I am getting As and Bs.
Clinician I would like to call your parents; can you share their phone number?
Lindsay I don't know their number by heart.

This example captures the importance in knowing when cognitive weaknesses may lead adolescents to feel unhappy and overwhelmed with social interactions that may mimic the symptoms of a disease-based model disorder that may not improve with conventional forms of psychotherapy or use of medication. Her grades may be inflated if her teachers do not recognize her weaknesses.

In younger children, we use simple playing-card magic illusions diagnostically, utilizing what we call "wow moments." For example, the child might be shown a simple card trick to assess her attention and visual-spatial abilities in remembering the number and suit of the chosen card (which will later be revealed as the only card in the deck facing up). Alternatively, for younger children, we utilize a coin trick in which a quarter is transferred from the clinician's desk to his right hand. Then, after blowing on his hand, the clinician slowly opens his fingers to reveal that the coin has vanished. Generally, children with above-average and average cognitive abilities and good visual-spatial abilities appreciate the illusions and are genuinely surprised—the "wow moment"—and smile with excitement and request the trick be repeated.

For other children, the same card or coin trick is difficult for them to appreciate due to cognitive or visual-spatial limitations: they may not know what is unusual about what transpired (e.g., the coin has reappeared in another place or the chosen card is the only one in the deck facing up). We encourage mental health clinicians working with children and adolescents to develop their own unique skills that can be useful in a Contemporary Diagnostic Interview for similar diagnostic inquiry.

Another activity that is useful with middle-school and high school-aged adolescents is asking them to draw their bedroom on a blank piece of paper or a small easel board. This permits the clinician to assess both verbal comprehension, fluid reasoning, and visual-spatial abilities. We have known some youths to ask, "Which room? Do you mean this office?" which raises the possibility of verbal comprehension weakness. Additionally, the clinician will look at whether the drawing is simple or if it has many details (e.g., entry door, closet, bed, desk, lamps, TV, computer, etc.). For children or adolescents that are 9 and older, the drawings should have more details [3]). Figures. 2.1 and 2.2.

Cognitive Flexibility (Theory of Mind) in a Contemporary Diagnostic Interview

As part of any evaluation of a patient's cognitive function, the capacity for cognitive flexibility—also referred as social cognition, sense of agency, and theory of mind—should be assessed. Cognitive flexibility encompasses the aspects of cognition that allow the individual to understand another person's state of mind as well as contextually, socially, and culturally appropriate norms [9]. At a minimum, the child and

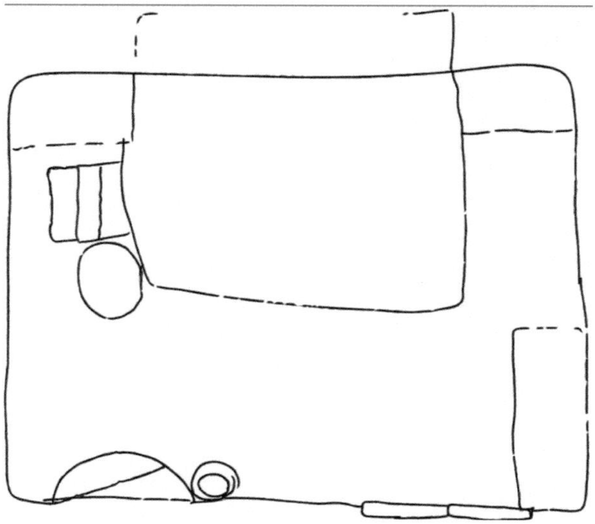

Fig. 2.1 In this drawing by a 13-year-old, the relative size of objects is exaggerated in terms of their importance to him (e.g., large bed). This tendency is typical of the egocentricity seen in younger children (ages 5–7). Regarding details, it is difficult to discern the identify of objects within the room (e.g., desk, lamp, bookshelf). Youth in this age range typically label objects to convey their perspective to the clinician

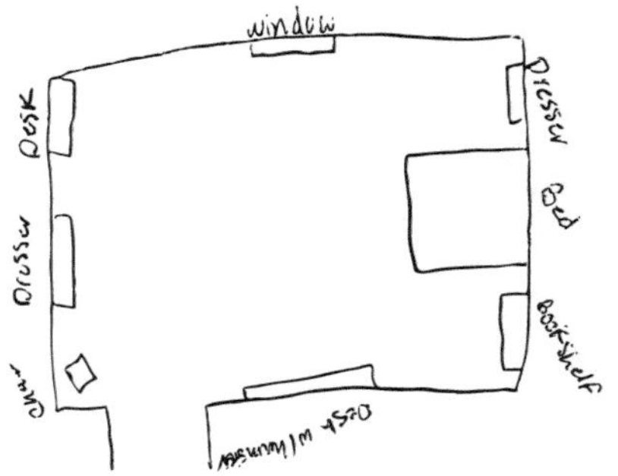

Fig. 2.2 In this drawing, by a 12-year-old boy, objects are lined up around the edge of the room (e.g., grounding). He correctly captures the relative orientation of the furniture and room elements, including walls, doors, window. The limited use of scale should be considered within the context of the assessment, which was brief (1–2 min). Thus, for this typically developing pre-adolescent, time constraints potentially limited his ability to attend to all details and scale

adolescent psychiatrist or clinician should assess whether the patient has the ability to interpret the intent of others. For a detailed description of the assessment of the differences in cognitive flexibility, see Chap. 5. For a description of providing tailored interventions once cognitive flexibilities are discerned, see Chap. 7.

Cognitive flexibility involves several components: executive function, attention, working memory, and emotion regulation [17, 28]. An example of cognitive flexibility would be a child who reacts with glee when he or she infers that it is acceptable to play with the toys in the clinician's office because they are available in an open bin.

Cognitive Flexibility in Adolescents

Assessment in adolescents is less complex than with younger children. Developmentally, adolescents by the age of 13 generally have cognitive capacities similar to those of adults when it comes to understanding themselves and their environment.

A Brief Assessment of Cognitive Flexibility in Adolescents

- History of the adolescent's preferred activities with others, including parents, friends, and those he or she has dated
- History about the adolescent's favorite persons and what attributes they have
- Review achievements and accomplishments they feel proud of
- History of favorite video games and music played; favorite sports events attended
- Review what they are hoping to achieve in the future

Cognitive Flexibility in Preschool and Elementary School-Age Youth

Assessment of preschool and school-age children's cognition and cognitive flexibility for social reciprocity is complex, in that it needs to take into account the norms of their developmental stages (see Appendix A for developmental milestones) and make use of age-appropriate activities (e.g., drawing and coloring books, board or card games, reading). As with any patient, particularly children, there is no one-size-fits-all approach.

In working with children, and at times adolescents with cognitive limitations, the psychiatrist or clinician may wish to utilize a time-tested projective technique: the "three wishes scenario." In this frequently employed technique, children are asked to imagine they find a magic genie's lamp, from which they release a genie who will grant them three wishes. The children are encouraged to request whatever they hope for and why. In using this technique, the clinician can assess the child's cognitive flexibility while helping him avoid the anxiety produced by direct questioning. The patient's responses may be concrete and limited, indicating the impoverished age-related imaginative life of a child with cognitive weakness or formal intellectual disabilities.

A Brief Assessment of Cognitive Flexibility in Preschool and Elementary School-Age Youth

- Elicit the child's recollection of prior birthday parties and favorite gifts received.
- Ask who the child enjoyed having attend the birthday parties.
- Review the child's achievements and accomplishments, as well as other experiences that have made him or her feel proud.
- Obtain a history of the child's favorite toys, games, video games, and movies.
- Use the common projective technique of asking the child, "What would you ask for if a genie granted you three wishes?"
- Ask what the child likes and dislikes about his or her parents.

Another activity that elementary school-age children enjoy is drawing a rudimentary family tree on a small easel board (with the help of the clinician). The clinician asks what the child likes or dislikes about each family member in the drawing. This conveys the child's cognitive flexibility within the context of others in the family, as well as his view of his role in the family.

An alternative way of opening a conversation to assess cognitive flexibility is by making a comment about the child's name and wondering if she knows how her name was chosen, and whether she likes her name. This approach helps in several contexts; it allows the patient to feel recognized as important, it gives context to her experience within her family, and it provides the opportunity to assess whether the patient is able to respond with depth and details or in a cognitively limited manner.

Case Study: A 6-Year-Old Girl with Possible Separation Anxiety Disorder

A 6-year-old girl was seen for possible separation anxiety disorder, as she had been crying on the way to school, although her teachers shared that upon arrival, she stopped crying and adjusted well to school activities and her peers. The clinician approached the child in a jovial manner and stated that he liked her name, Madison, and wondered if she liked it. She cheered up and said that her parents chose her name because her grandmother of the same name, who had passed before her birth, "was a very nice person." She also reported that she liked it because "it is fun to say." The clinician proceeded to wonder if she liked to write her name at school. She replied that she liked writing her name at the top of all her assignments, and that she liked her teacher, who was very funny and polite. During the interaction, her parents nonverbally supported her and encouraged her to feel free to engage in a conversation with the clinician.

In this vignette, the clinician subjectively quickly experiences the child as very likeable, engaging, and easy to affectively attune with. The patient also demonstrates secure attachment, with easy/flexible temperament, above-average cognitive abilities and very good cognitive flexibility. In this quick conversational approach, the clinician has been able to assess many elements of the CDI, and after a few more comments about her personal attributes (e.g., color of hair, height), his subjective experience of her—that she does not have any developmental delays of her cognitive and psychological growth—is reinforced. The clinician recognizes the likelihood of a formal separation anxiety disorder and proceeds with a *DSM–5*-style structured interview to assess the severity and tailor the treatment: cognitive behavioral and/or pharmacological.

Personality: Internal Working Models of Attachment (IWMA) in a Contemporary Diagnostic Interview

At this point, it is important for the reader to appreciate that attachment style—relational patterns that are formed early in life and which drive interpersonal interaction later in life—represents a confluence of three pillars: temperament, cognition, and cognitive flexibility. In this regard, once the clinician becomes familiar using the Contemporary Diagnostic Interview, the differences between a child's responses if securely attached, with good cognitive abilities, compared to a child that struggles with disorganized forms of attachment, poor temperament, and cognitive weaknesses, will be evident. The interaction between the cognition, cognitive flexibility, and temperament between two people highly influences the quality and perception of the attachment itself.

Attachment style and personality disorders are described in more detail in Chap. 6. Information about how knowledge of personality disorders can help the clinician tailor interventions is provided in Chap. 7.

Briefly, there are four attachment styles that have a central role in determining a youth's ability to interact with others.

Secure Attachment Style

A secure form of attachment occurs when the infant experiences caregivers providing coherent attachment patterns, and the child develops a coherent discourse over time. A securely attached child values attachments—whether pleasant or temporarily unpleasant—and can interact with others with a sense of excitement.

Insecure Attachment Styles: Ambivalent/Anxious, Avoidant/Dismissive, and Disorganized

When the primary caregiver does not provide appropriate affective attunement in the early months of life, the infant is at increased risk to develop poor self-regulatory abilities, which become the precursor to a variety of insecure attachment patterns. Insecure attachment is a risk factor for maladaptive interpersonal behavior and formal personality disorders. Insecurely attached adults are more vulnerable to experiencing intense feelings of anger, aggression, and impulsivity, primary characteristics of bipolar disorder [22].

Diagnostic Formulation

After the child and adolescent psychiatrist or clinician has intersubjectively elucidated the patient's and their parents' or caregivers' temperament, cognition, cognitive flexibility, and internal working models of attachment, he or she can embark in formalizing the diagnostic formulation and tailoring the treatment plan sequencing for best outcomes. The integrated CDI has served as the foundation by which the child and adolescent psychiatrist or clinician has identified the reliability of the signs and symptoms endorsed, and the likelihood of the patient and family to adhere with treatment interventions recommended: psychotherapy, pharmacotherapy, or request for formal cognitive testing.

Limitations of the Four Pillars and the Contemporary Diagnostic Interview

Despite the advantages of the approach, we are advocating here, we recognize that, as with any approach, there will be skeptics. Among the arguments that may be levied against our strategy is that diverse approaches cannot be fully integrated. We would argue, however, that these approaches are already implicitly integrated in clinical work, in that the issues related to family systems, personality styles, relational processes, and cognition are part and parcel of everyday clinical work. Our interview style allows to use implicit information in a succinct and systematic way to clinically improve the understanding of our patient's strengths and weaknesses.

To clinicians concerned that this approach would require a prohibitive amount of time, we would note that in difficult cases, the mild increase in time commitment is justified, as cases with high family and patient conflict tend to have more adverse outcomes, longer hospitalizations [29], and a greater likelihood of medical-legal sequelae [4, 15]. Thus, we would argue that our method, while somewhat more time intensive, is more cost effective.

References

1. Altarac M, Saroha E. Lifetime prevalence of learning disability among US children. Pediatrics. 2007;119:S77–83.
2. American Psychiatric Association. Diagnostic and statistical manual of mental disorders. 5th ed. Washington, D.C.: American Psychiatric Association; 2013.
3. Basgul S, Uneri O, Akkaya G, et al. Assessment of drawing age of children in early childhood and its correlates. Psychology. 2011;2:376–81. https://doi.org/10.4236/psych.2011.24059.
4. Beckman HB, Markakis KM, Suchman AL, et al. The doctor-patient relationship and malpractice. Lessons from plaintiff depositions. Arch Int Med. 1994;154(12):1365–70.
5. Birmaher B, Khetarpal S, Brent D, et al. The screen for child anxiety related emotional disorders (SCARED): scale construction and psychometric characteristics. J Am Acad Child Adolesc Psychiatry. 1997;36:545–53.
6. Campbell JA, Walker R, Egede LE. Associations between adverse childhood experiences, high-risk behaviors, and morbidity in adulthood. Am J Prev Med. 2016;50:344–52. https://doi.org/10.1016/jamepre.2015.07.022.
7. Cardoso Zoppe EH, Schoueri P, Castro M, et al. Teaching psychodynamics to psychiatric residents through psychiatric outpatient interviews. Acad Psychiatry. 2009;33(1):51–5.
8. Cooper S, Smiley E, Morrison J, et al. Mental ill-health in adults with intellectual disabilities: prevalence and associated factors. Br J Psychiatry. 2007;190:27–35.
9. Delgado SV, Strawn JR. Difficult psychiatric consultations: an integrated approach. Springer, Verlag Berlin Heidelberg. 2014.
10. Delgado SV, Strawn JR, Pedapati EV. Contemporary psychodynamic psychotherapy for children and adolescents: integrating Intersubjectivity and neuroscience. Springer, Verlag Berlin Heidelberg. 2015.
11. Delgado SV, Wassenaar E, Strawn JR. Does your patient have a psychiatric illness or nonverbal learning disorder? Curr Psychol. 2011;10(5):17–35.
12. Drell MJ. The impending and perhaps inevitable collapse of psychodynamic psychotherapy as performed by psychiatrists. Child Adolesc Psychiatric Clin N Am. 2007;16:207–24.
13. Ford K, Hughes K, Hardcastle K, et al. The evidence base for routine enquiry into adverse childhood experiences: a scoping review. Child Abuse Negl. 2019;91:131–46. https://doi.org/10.1016/j.chiabu.2019.03.007.
14. Gagnon JC, Barber BR, Van Loan CL, et al. Juvenile correctional schools: characteristics and approaches to curriculum. Educ Treat Child. 2009;32:673–96.
15. Halpern J. Empathy in patient-physician conflicts. J Gen Intern Med. 2007;22(5):696–700.
16. Insel T, Cuthbert B, Garvey M, et al. Research Domain Criteria (RDoC): toward a new classification framework for research on mental disorders. Am J Psychiatry. 2010;167(7):748–51. https://doi.org/10.1176/appi.ajp.2010.09091379.
17. Johnson DR. Emotional attention set-shifting and its relationship to anxiety and emotion regulation. Emotion. 2009;9(5):681–90.

18. Kaplan M, Delgado SV. When worlds converge: combining depth psychotherapy and psychotropic medications. Bull Menn Clin. 2006;70:253–63.
19. Kaufman J, Birmaher B, Brent D, et al. Schedule for Affective Disorders and Schizophrenia for School-Age Children-Present and Lifetime Version (K-SADS-PL): initial reliability and validity data. J Am Acad Child Psychiatry. 1997;36(7):980–8.
20. Kontos N, Querques J, Freudenreich O. The problem of the psychopharmacologist. Acad Psychiatry. 2006;30(3):218–26.
21. Kendler KS, Zachar P, Craver C. What kinds of things are psychiatric disorders? Psychol Med. 2011;41(6):1143–50. https://doi.org/10.1017/S0033291710001844l8.
22. Levy KN. The implications of attachment theory and research for under-standing borderline personality disorder. Dev Psychopathol. 2005;17:959–86. https://doi.org/10.1017/S0954579405050455.
23. Lilienfeld SO. Comorbidity between and within childhood externalizing and internalizing disorders: reflections and directions. J Abnormal Child Psychol. 2003;31(3):285–91. https://doi.org/10.1023/A:1023229529866.
24. Matz SC, Harari GM. Personality-place transactions: mapping the relationships between big five personality traits, states, and daily places. J Pers Soc Psychol. 2020; https://doi.org/10.1037/pspp0000297.
25. McConville BJ, Delgado SV. How to plan and tailor treatment: an overview of diagnosis and treatment planning. In: Klykylo WM, Kay J, editors. Clinical child psychiatry. 2nd ed. West Sussex (UK): Wiley; 2006. p. 91–108.
26. Muris P, Ollendick TH. The role of temperament in the etiology of child psychopathology. Clin Child Fam Psychol Rev. 2005;8(4):271–89. https://doi.org/10.1007/s10567-005-8809-y.
27. Shiner R, Caspi A. Personality differences in childhood and adolescence: measurement, development, and consequences. J Child Psychol Psychiatry. 2003;44:2–32.
28. Schmeichel BJ, Volokhov RN, Demaree HA. Working memory capacity and the self-regulation of emotional expression and experience. J Pers Soc Psychol. 2008;95(6):1526–40.
29. Schneiderman LJ. Family demand for futile treatment. Med Ethics (Burlingt Mass). 2001;3:8.
30. Sheehan DV, Sheehan KH, Shytle RD, et al. Reliability and validity of the Mini international neuropsychiatric interview for children and adolescents (MINI-KID). J Clin Psychiatry. 2010;71(3):313–26.
31. Thomas A, Chess S, Birch HG. The origin of personality. Sci Am. 1970;223(2):102–9.
32. Weiss LG, Saklofske DH, Holdnack JA, et al. WISC-V: clinical use and interpretation. 2nd edn: Academic Press, New York. 2016.
33. Young RC, Biggs JT, Ziegler VE, et al. Young mania rating scale. In: Handbook of psychiatric measures. Washington, D.C.: American Psychiatric Association; 2000. p. 540–2.

Chapter 3
Temperament: The Building Block of Personality

Children must be taught how to think, not what to think.
—Margaret Mead (1901–1978)

Temperament

Temperament is defined as the physiological basis for individual differences in reactivity and self-regulation, including motivation, affect, activity, and attention characteristics [21]. Commonly included in the studies of temperament are indicators of frustration or anger, fear (inhibition, withdrawal), approach, pleasure, and positive affect. Self-regulation refers to orienting and executive control of attention and behavior that operates to modulate reactivity, facilitating or inhibiting the physiological, affective, or behavioral response. The dimensions of reactivity, self-regulation and activation of the behavioral inhibition system, reveal individual differences in motivational systems that reflect sensitivity to reward and punishment [12, 13, 21].

Temperament provides the emotional and behavioral building blocks on which individual personalities are constructed. Temperament refers to the stable moods and behavior profiles observed in infancy and early childhood. Though mention of it can be found in ancient Greek texts from two millennia ago, the idea of temperament came to the forefront in developmental psychology and child psychiatry in the 1960s and 1970s [26]. The relevance that temperament styles have in psychiatric work with youths is multifaceted. Although it has been long recognized that temperament has a biological basis, it is also strongly influenced by a person's environment, which triggers which traits become more adaptive than others. As Weiss et al. state, "Clearly, cognition plays a role in every aspect of human functioning and thus can never be fully partialled out of the human factor. Yet, the list of possible noncognitive factors is and encompasses basic temperament" (2016).

S. V. Delgado et al., *Promoting the Emotional and Behavioral Success of Youths*,
https://doi.org/10.1007/978-3-030-88075-0_3

Thomas and Chess confirmed what the British psychoanalyst and father of attachment theory John Bowlby hypothesized: A child's temperament influences how his or her parents experience and interact with the child [2]. This reciprocal relationship exists between the child and parent and diverges from the previously accepted notion that the infant is a passive recipient and product of his or her environment [16]. In essence, attachment theory allowed the child to be seen as a full contributor to the "goodness of fit" between her parents and herself [27]. Children with temperamental vulnerabilities benefit more from positive parenting and are more adversely affected by negative parenting [1]. Thus, children with temperamental vulnerabilities will flounder in the face of negative parenting and flourish in the presence of positive parenting. Parenting and children's temperament characteristics are two important risk factors in the development and maintenance of internalizing problems [12, 13].

While there have been many classificatory schemes, Thomas and Chess [27] are recognized for their landmark scientific contribution to the study of temperament. Their seminal work has achieved general consensus in its finding that temperament expression has been consistent across situations and over time. In their study, Thomas and Chess longitudinally evaluated 141 children over 22 years, from early childhood until early adulthood [25, 26]. Childhood temperament strongly predicted temperament in adulthood, even after taking into account the many interceding factors during such a long follow-up interval. Nonetheless, the authors cautioned that "an ever-present danger … is creating self-fulfilling prophecies" [27]. An individual's capacity to interact with others in an acceptable manner is greatly determined by the how his environment influences matters of reciprocity according to his own unique temperament styles.

Additionally, temperament is shaped by interactions with others, and its regulation depends on cultural factors [20]. Understanding the cultural models' parents use to evaluate the level of success in emotional and social development is crucial, as they can vary in profound ways. For example, research regarding parental perceptions of their young children's temperament suggests that individual variability is culturally structured [23, 32]. Some parents experience youths as difficult if they have low adaptability and negative mood. In contrast, Italian parents may see negative mood as an example of the infant being expressive but become concerned if the infant is slow to warm up in new social situations; they consider this a negative trait [8]. Similarly, in some cultures, academic cognitive abilities are highly valued, while in others, social and creative skills are the most valued. All of this is to say that a youth's cultural environment will have significant impact on the development of her four pillars. A child's age should be considered when evaluating the developmental appropriateness of her response to complex day-to-day situations, but so should her temperament. Most individuals have the capacity to vary in the expression of their temperament traits, although over time one trait will usually dominate the manner in which they approach social situations.

Given that childhood temperament correlates with adult temperament [26], a child's temperament and his adult personality share remarkably similar features not only in how he navigates interactions with others but also in how he manages affect-laden emotional interactions. However, while temperament and personality are interrelated, they are not one and the same. The former refers to the genetically and biologically based innate behavioral style, while the latter describes how emotions manifest in an individual with a particular temperament.

In their work with children with significant psychological problems, Thomas and Chess [25] observed that the family environment and parenting styles were remarkably similar to those experienced by youths who did not have these psychological problems. They noted that "domineering authoritarian handling by the parents might make one youngster anxious and submissive and another defiant and antagonistic." Thus, early on, they recognized that as we try to understand and to work with youths, we must "take into full account the individual and his uniqueness" [24]. Furthermore, both heredity and environmental experiences influence temperament in infancy and early childhood [7]. Around 2 years of age, toddlers begin to develop inhibitory control abilities that are reflective of their temperaments and parental socialization, their moral self [6]. Temperament, neurophysiology, and cognitive development all play important roles that influence emotional regulation capacities in youth. Youth learn about emotional regulation through observation and incorporate the use of specific parenting practices and behaviors related to the socialization. Emotional regulation is affected by the emotional climate of the family, the quality of attachments, styles of parenting, family expressiveness, and the quality of the marital relationship. In essence, the development of emotional regulation is a bidirectional process where children and families mutually influence each other [18]. Consequently, temperament is recognized as pivotal to how we understand the biological, emotional, and social development of youths [15].

Temperament in Twin Girls: Rachel and Elliott

On an early October Saturday morning, twin 6-year-old girls were scheduled to receive their annual influenza vaccines. Both girls began their day happily making a pancake breakfast with their father. Both girls focused on reading the instructions from the pancake mix and proudly announcing the ingredients as they read and discerned the graphical instructions. Rachel checked with her father as she measured the ingredients while Elliott measured ingredients "by herself." When the bowl tipped over, spilling batter onto the counter, both girls said "oops" and helped clean the batter up. Both girls took turns stirring the batter and joked loudly about making the "most gigantic pancake ever made."

When the girls arrived at their pediatrician's office for their scheduled vaccine, Rachel wanted to hand the consent form signed by her father directly to the clinic assistant, whereas Elliott stood very close to and partially behind her father. When it was time to go to the room for the injection, both girls became hesitant, sitting on their father's lap. Rachel asked how much the injection would hurt and told the nurse and her father that she was "a little bit afraid." However, she was proud of herself after having received the "little shot" and wanted to know if the nurse had Barbie stickers. The nurse smiled and retrieved a large basket of stickers from which Rachel could choose. Elliott was also afraid, becoming tearful as she sat on her father's lap. However, she did not easily accept the verbal reassurance from her father or from the nurse. Elliott became agitated as the nurse came closer with the syringe. She turned and buried herself into her father's chest, sobbing and protesting. The nurse, who had just administered the vaccine to Rachel, told Elliott, "If you can't hold still, I'm going to have to get another nurse to hold you down." This enraged Elliott, who hissed at the nurse. Her father also became concerned; he did not want his daughter "held down," knowing that this would likely worsen the situation. With help from Elliott's father, the nurse was able to administer the vaccine, while Elliott cried and protested that it hurt. Elliott did not ask for a sticker. She grabbed her father's hand and pulled him to the door to leave the clinic as quickly as possible.

In reviewing the events, we note that while preparing breakfast with their father, both girls demonstrated easy/flexible temperament traits. They focused on reading the recipe, handled the spilling of the batter in stride, and were able to generally modulate the intensity of their reactions. When the girls arrived at the pediatrician's office to receive their vaccine, Rachel continued to demonstrate an easy/flexible temperament style. She approached the nurse with developmentally appropriate anxiety related to the shot. The nurse engaged with Rachel in a playful way, and Rachel was able to use this playfulness to modulate her anxiety and mood, even in a stressful situation. In contrast, Elliott was fearful and became agitated, clinging to her father. She became intense and loud as she protested in the examination room and struggled to modulate her developmentally appropriate anxiety. When faced with Elliott's temperament and intense reaction, the nurse attempted to help by firmly containing Elliott's reaction instead of flexibly helping her or her father to modulate her fear. Taken together, this suggests a mixed temperament style in Elliott (and in the nurse). Both the nurse and Elliott had predominantly easy/flexible temperament styles, but in the context of an affect-laden situation, they demonstrated difficulties with adaptability, and a difficult/feisty temperament style emerged (Fig. 3.1). This interaction highlights how the expression of temperamental styles can change based on environmental factors and the emotional responses of others [14].

Below we provide a brief review of the nine temperament traits based on a classification scheme developed by the Thomas and Chess research team [28] (Table 3.1).

Fig. 3.1 Temperamental twins

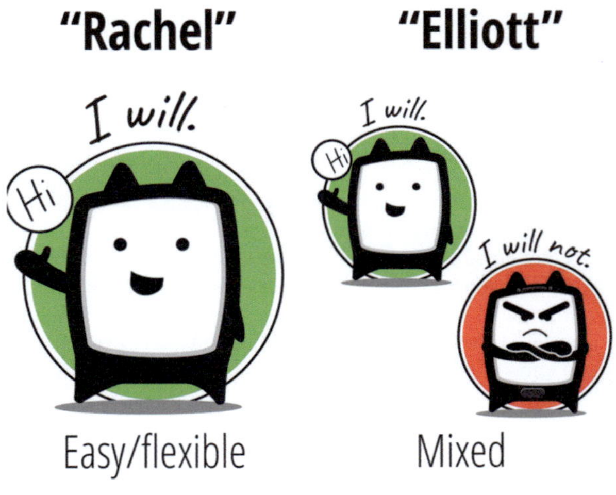

Table 3.1 Temperament traits derived from Thomas et al. [28])

Activity level
Rhythmicity or regularity
Approach or withdrawal responses
Adaptability to change
Sensory threshold
Intensity of reactions
Mood
Distractibility
Persistence when faced with obstacles

Temperament Traits

Activity Level

Activity level is rated as high or low, reflecting whether a person has a tendency to be on-the-go or whether he or she prefers a slower pace, taking a wait-and-see approach. A youth with a high activity level may not have a formal attention disorder, which may explain pharmacological treatment failures. Highly active children may channel their energy into success in sports or theater.

The less-active, calmer youths may become overly thoughtful and unable to decide, within a reasonable amount of time, how to best interact with others; they may be prone to bullying. This can be compounded by slow processing speed, a cognitive weakness discussed in Chap. 4.

Distractibility

This trait, generally rated as "distractible" or "not distractible," refers to the degree of concentration and attention given when embarking on a tedious task or the ability to study or work on team projects without being sidetracked. This trait refers to the ease with which external stimuli interfere with ongoing behavior. This can be compounded by youth with weaknesses in fluid reasoning or processing speed or formal attention-deficit/hyperactivity disorder.

Intensity

This characteristic, described as intense or mild, refers to the strength of a person's emotional response to novel events, whether positive or negative. Intense children are more likely to signal parents about their needs. These children may be gifted in high-intensity sports and artistic activities. Intense children tend to be exhausting to live with.

Rhythmicity

This trait is rated as regular or irregular and refers to the predictability of biological functions like appetite and sleep. Youths with good rhythmicity learn to adapt well to unusual schedules, because they are able to maintain regularity in biological functions such as appetite and sleep. They may do better with lengthy trips.

Sensory Threshold

This aspect of temperament, rated low or high, is related to the sensitivity a person has to physical stimuli. The rating reflects how a child may react (positively or negatively) to sounds when participating in music activities at school or on field trips to an airport or zoo. It is helpful to know if the child has a history of being highly sensitive to noises, lights, and particular types of clothing, as this can alter receptivity to treatment and may be interpreted by the clinician as the patient being difficult. This trait may also be present in youth with sensory sensitivities, neurodevelopmental disorders, and generalized anxiety issues.

Approach/Withdrawal

This aspect of temperament, like the others, is observed early in life and refers to the child's "typical response to unfamiliar people, objects, and situations; the extremes of this dimension define two categories of children called behaviorally inhibited and uninhibited" [22]. Youth with inhibited temperament are more likely to be timid with novel interactions, places, and situations. This is often seen in youth with complex neurodevelopmental disorders. By contrast, uninhibited children may spontaneously approach these stimuli and may approach novel situations with interest and be easily able to engage in healthy and adaptive decision-making.

Adaptability

Adaptability should be thought of as part of a continuum with approach/withdrawal traits; it is rated as "adaptive" or "not adaptive." The patient who is adaptive will likely collaborate actively with family, peers, and teachers to manage transitions between tasks, like switching to a new activity. A child that has difficulties adapting to new people or environments may have complex neurodevelopmental disorders and generalized anxiety issues.

Persistence

Persistence is rated as long or short. This trait refers to the length of time a youth takes when asked to participate in a decision-making process in the face of adversity. A youth who rates "long" in persistence may engage in lengthy discussions and be experienced as stubborn and difficult. There seem to be some common elements of persistence that overlap with the trait of intensity.

Mood

Generally, mood is rated as positive or negative and refers to the emotional response youths have when complex emotional or cognitive information has been delivered to them. When youths demonstrate the capacity to respond positively, this signifies a realistic outlook about their future. When youths respond in a negative mood, it is helpful to clarify if this is typical or if the negativity is new and related to the seriousness of the topics being discussed. Persistent negative moods in youths are difficult for parents to understand as a result of biological factors if they have been successful in raising their other children. They may feel a sense of failure as typical parenting interventions do not provide the relief needed. Youths with negative temperamental moods often bully others.

Many of these dimensions have been related to adolescent externalizing behaviors. In a study by Mrug et al. [19], low flexibility, poor attention regulation, and high activity level were associated with delinquency; negative affect and activity level were related to substance use. Similarly, multiple aspects of temperament distinguished adolescent drug abusers from their peers, including high activity level and negative affect, low attention control and flexibility, and arrythmicity (2012). Negativity is a temperamental characteristic that has showed more externalizing problems when parents provided less guidance and were more hostile or intrusive [3]. Temperamentally "difficult" children, or those high in negativity or irritability, were rated greater on externalizing problems when parents used negative discipline strategies, whereas those whose parents employed more positive discipline techniques were rated with fewer problems [29]. Furthermore, temperamentally difficult children showed larger decreases in externalizing problems over time when their parents were more sensitive [17].

When recognized, certain clusters of temperament traits can be predictive. In a given situation, for example, the combination of negative mood, high intensity, irregularity, and slow adaptability might define a youth as "difficult"—someone who is likely to have and cause problems during his life—whereas the cluster of positive mood, positive approach, and high adaptability usually signifies a successful child. While this may not seem surprising, the knowledge of these temperament styles may guide clinicians in more accurate diagnostic formulations and in creating practical interventions with realistic expectations that are based on an understanding of how genetic and biological factors contribute to the variability of a patient's psychological responses. Recognizing and working with a given person's temperament styles can improve outcomes.

Temperament Styles

Thomas and Chess defined three general temperament styles: 45% of children were classified as "easy or flexible," 15% "slow-to-warm-up," 10% as "difficult or feisty," and 30% as "mixed," a combination of the three (1999). Discerning a youth's temperament style helps identify her ability to develop self-control and self-regulatory capacities, as well as those that will not be able to develop such capacities. Temperament may render children vulnerable for the development of problems regardless of parenting [12, 13].

The Easy/Flexible Temperament Style

This style was found to be present in approximately 45% of the children studied by Thomas and Chess [27]. A person with an easy/flexible temperament style typically has a history of being generally happy and not easily upset by negative news or events. When presented with conflicted situations, youths with this temperament style typically transition from feeling mild, situationally appropriate forms of anxiety to displaying a positive stance and engaging in a cooperative approach with family peers.

The Slow-to-Warm-up Temperament Style

A child with a slow-to-warm-up temperament style (15%) can quickly withdraw when faced with new and difficult situations that involve complex issues with some degree of uncertainty. Youths who present with this temperament style are experienced by the clinician as struggling with anxiety and shyness. These patients may rely on their family members to make decisions for them, which may be frustrating to clinicians. However, we recognize that this temperamental style can be similar in youths with slow processing speed or a formal mental health disorder (e.g. depression, generalized anxiety, etc.)

The Difficult/Feisty Temperament Style

A child with a difficult/feisty style (10%) is often disruptive when interacting with people in new or stressful situations. He or she is often difficult and resistant to reason and creates negative reactions from parents and teaching staff, who hope to be appreciated for the efforts placed to help them.

Infants and toddlers that are temperamentally difficult/feisty are not easy to soothe, placing them at a higher risk for attachment difficulties with their parents. Furthermore, there is evidence that children with difficult/feisty temperamental traits are more vulnerable to adverse effects of negative parenting, which increases the risk of reactive aggression toward the parent by the child [30]. A 2009 study found linkage between difficult/feisty temperament and conduct problems across three generations [11].

Youths with a difficult/feisty temperament style have poor self-control and self-regulation. This temperament subsumes the development of healthy prosocial peer relations and can lead to poor school performance, which contributes to peer rejection, teacher animosity, and conduct problems [4]. Kagan [9, 10] asserts that some parents of youth with difficult/feisty temperaments initially blame themselves for their infant's continued unhappiness and struggle to tolerate feelings of guilt and self-blame. In turn, these exasperated parents may later blame the child for his or her oppositional behavior by assuming a "streak of stubborn anger." Once this takes hold, the hostility between child and his or her parents reverberates and creates a nidus for reactive attachment disorders to develop. These parents might benefit from training in mindfulness strategies for managing their own emotional and behavioral reactions [12, 13]. Additionally, parents benefit from knowing the limitations medication have in youths with this temperamental style.

It is important to note that the maladaptive behaviors in youths with a difficult/feisty temperamental style can present as similar to those caused by cognitive weakness, such as verbal comprehension, fluid reasoning, or working memory as measured by the WISC-V [31] (Chap. 4), poor cognitive flexibility (Chap. 5), and formal mental health disorders (e.g., mood or neurodevelopmental disorders). Additionally, a child with a difficult/feisty temperament style, whose parents have similar temperaments, is likely to be experienced by the parents as "difficult and ungrateful." Such parents provide limited comfort to the child earlier in their life, and in doing so facilitate a pattern of mistrust with frequent use of persistent maladaptive behaviors when interacting with others, the precursors of a borderline personality disorder.

The Mixed Temperament Style

This style of temperament was observed in 35% of children studied by Thomas and Chess [25]. As the name implies, these individuals utilized a mixture of the nine temperament traits. Earlier, we provided an example of mixed temperament styles

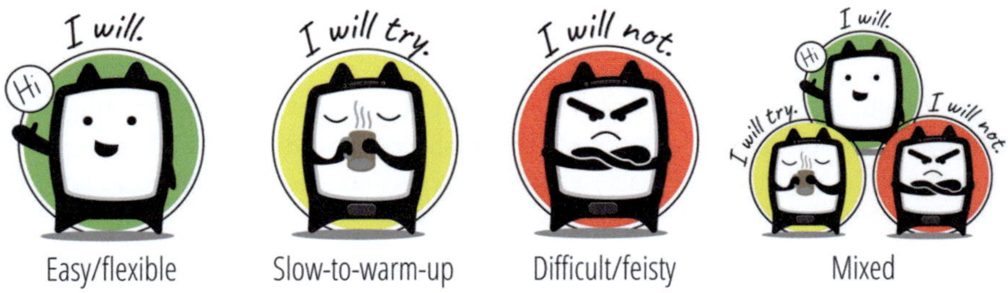

Fig. 3.2 Temperament Styles

in a 6-year-old girl, Elliott, and a pediatrician's nurse. Both have predominantly easy/flexible temperament styles, but in the context of an affect-laden situation, they demonstrated difficulties with adaptability and a difficult/feisty temperament style (Fig. 3.2).

Temperament in Clinical Work

Contemporary temperament researchers assume that vulnerability to psychopathology is characterized by a combination of high levels of emotionality and low levels of effortful control. A stressful life event in youth with high levels of effortful control can regulate these negative emotions by employing more strategic, flexible, and effective coping strategies [5].

For clinicians, understanding their patients' temperament in vivo provides a window into how the patient functions within the family, with friends, and at school. This understanding is a lens through which the clinician can contextualize symptoms as well as the child's strengths and weaknesses across settings. For example, consider a clinician evaluating a child with a difficult/feisty temperament and parents with easy/flexible temperaments that provided secure attachment to their child. The parents may describe their child as "unhappy, even when we bend over backward." The parents may describe their frustration when trying to reassure and calm their child because doing so provides little help. In essence, this dynamic reflects a poor goodness of fit between child and parents—a clashing of temperament styles. In a clinical setting, a clinician may become frustrated with certain young patients due to their temperament; difficulties eliciting information from the patient that has slow-to-warm-up temperament or containing the barrage of criticisms from the patient with a difficult/feisty temperament. We wish to emphasize that a difficult/feisty temperament style and deficits in cognitive flexibility are two main precursors of personality disorders in youths (Chap. 6).

References

1. Belsky J, Pluess M. Beyond diathesis stress: differential susceptibility to environmental influences. Psychol Bull. 2009;135(6):885–908. https://doi.org/10.1037/a0017376.
2. Bowlby J. Attachment. In: Attachment and loss, vol. 1. 2nd ed. New York: Basic Books; 1999.
3. Cipriano-Essel E, Skowron EA, Stifter CA, Teti DM. Heterogeneity in maltreated and non-maltreated preschool children's inhibitory control: the interplay between parenting quality and child temperament. Infant Child Dev. 2013;22(5):501–22. https://doi.org/10.1002/ICD.1801.
4. Delisi M, Vaughn MG. Foundation for a temperament-based theory of antisocial behavior and criminal justice system involvement. J Crim Justice. 2014;42:10–25. https://doi.org/10.1016/j.jcrimjus.2013.11.001.
5. Drabick DA, Ollendick TH, Bubier JL. Co-occurrence of ODD and anxiety: shared risk processes and evidence for a dual-pathway model. Clin Psychol (New York). 2010;17(4):307–18. https://doi.org/10.1111/j.1468-2850.2010.01222.x.
6. Emde RN, Biringen Z, Clyman RB, Oppenheim D. The moral self of infancy: affective core and procedural knowledge. Dev Rev. 1991;11(3):251–70. https://doi.org/10.1016/0273-2297(91)90013-E.
7. Emde RN, Hewitt JK. Infancy to early childhood: genetic and environmental influences on developmental change. Oxford: Oxford University Press; 2001.
8. Harkness S, Super CM, Ríos Bermúdez M, et al. Parental ethnotheories of children's learning. In: Lancy DF, Bock J, Gaskins S, editors. The anthropology of learning in childhood. Lanham: Alta Mira Press; 2010. p. 65–81.
9. Kagan J. The biological contributions to temperaments and emotions. Eur J Dev Sci. 2008;2:38–51.
10. Kagan J. The temperamental thread: how genes, culture, time, and luck make us who we are. New York: Dana Press; 2010.
11. Kerr DCR, Capaldi DM, Pears KC, et al. A prospective three generational study of fathers' constructive parenting: influences from family of origin, adolescent adjustment, and offspring temperament. Dev Psychol. 2009;45:1257–75.
12. Kiff CJ, Lengua LJ, Bush NR. Temperament variation in sensitivity to parenting: predicting changes in depression and anxiety. J Abnorm Child Psychol. 2011a;39(8):1199–212. https://doi.org/10.1007/s10802-011-9539-x.
13. Kiff CJ, Lengua LJ, Zalewski M. Nature and nurturing: parenting in the context of child temperament. Clin Child Fam Psychol Rev. 2011b;14(3):251–301. https://doi.org/10.1007/s10567-011-0093-4.
14. Klein MR, Lengua LJ, Thompson SF, et al. Bidirectional relations between temperament and parenting predicting preschool-age children's adjustment. J Clin child Adolesc Psychol. 2018;47(sup1):S113–26. https://doi.org/10.1080/15374416.2016.1169537.
15. Kochanska G, Kim S. Difficult temperament moderates links between maternal responsiveness and children's compliance and behavior problems in low-income families. J Child Psychol Psychiatry. 2013;54(3):323–32. https://doi.org/10.1111/jcpp.12002.
16. Mahler MS. Symbiosis and individuation – the psychological birth of the human infant. Psychoanal St Child. 1974;29:89–106.
17. Mesman J, Stoel R, Bakermans-Kranenbrug MJ, et al. Predicting growth curves of early childhood externalizing problems: differential susceptibility of children with difficult temperament. J Abnorm Child Psychol. 2009;37:625–36. https://doi.org/10.1007/s10802-009-9298-0.
18. Morris A, Silk J, Steinberg L, et al. The role of the family context in the development of emotion regulation. Soc Develop. 2007;16:361–88. https://doi.org/10.1111/j.1467-9507.2007.00389.x.
19. Mrug S, Madan A, Windle M. Temperament alters susceptibility to negative peer influence in early adolescence. J Abnorm Child Psychol. 2012;40(2):201–9. https://doi.org/10.1007/s10802-011-9550-2.

20. Paulussen-Hoogeboom MC, Stams GJ, Hermanns JM, et al. Child negative emotionality and parenting from infancy to preschool: a meta-analytic review. Dev Psychol. 2007;43(2):438–53.
21. Rothbart MK, Bates JE. Temperament. In: Damon W, Lerner RM, Eisenberg N, editors. Handbook of child psychology: vol. 3. Social, emotional, and personality development. 6th ed. Hoboken: Wiley; 2006. p. 99–166.
22. Schwartz CE, Wright CI, Shin LM, et al. Inhibited and uninhibited infants "grown up": adult amygdala response to novelty. Science. 2003;300:1952–3.
23. Super CM, Axia G, Harkness S, et al. Culture, temperament, and the "difficult child". Eur J Dev Sci. 2008;2:136–57.
24. Thomas A, Chess S. Temperament and development. New York: Brunner/Mazel; 1977.
25. Thomas A, Chess S. The reality of difficult temperament. Merrill-Palmer Q. 1982;28:1–20.
26. Thomas A, Chess S. The New York longitudinal study: from infancy to early adult life. In: Plomin R, Dunn J, editors. The study of temperament: changes, continuities, and challenges. Hillsdale: Lawrence Erlbaum; 1986.
27. Thomas A, Chess S. Goodness of fit: clinical applications from infancy through adult life. New York: Routledge; 1999. p. 39–52.
28. Thomas A, Chess S, Birch HG. The origin of personality. Sci Am. 1970;223(2):102–9.
29. van Zeijl J, Mesman J, Stolk MN, et al. Differential susceptibility to discipline: the moderating effect of child temperament on the association between maternal discipline and early childhood externalizing problems. J Fam Psychol. 2007;22:626–36. https://doi.org/10.1037/0893-3200.21.4.626.
30. Vitaro F, Barker ED, Boivin M, et al. Do early difficult temperament and harsh parenting differentially predict reactive and proactive aggression? J Abnorm Child Psychol. 2006;34(5):681–91.
31. Weiss LC, Holdnack JA, Saklofsk DH, et al. Theoretical and clinical foundations of the WISC-V index scores. In: Weiss LG, Saklofske DH, Holdnack JA, Prifitera A, editors. WISC-V assessment and interpretation: scientist-practitioner perspectives. Elsevier Academic Press; 2016. p. 97–121. https://doi.org/10.1016/B978-0-12-404697-9.00004-2.
32. Zentner M, Bates JE. Child temperament: an integrative review of concepts, research programs, and measures. Eur J Dev Sci. 2008;2(1/2):7–37.

Chapter 4
Intelligence: "Why Don't You Behave?"

As a child in school, things were very hard for me to understand often, and I developed a knack, I think ... I developed a process to simplify things so I would understand them.
—Eric Carle (1929–) illustrator and author of The Very Hungry Caterpillar

Introduction to Intelligence

This chapter will illustrate how weaknesses in intelligence can lead to maladaptive behaviors and emotional dysregulation, with increased likelihood of problems with self-esteem, interpersonal conflict, and academic functioning. We posit that weaknesses in cognitive abilities can lead to problems with self-esteem and behavior difficulties; accordingly, the information provided by intelligence tests is, in fact, clinically useful for developing treatments. Furthermore, this chapter will help the clinician learn to integrate information from psychiatric clinical interviews with intelligence test results to improve the identification of youths who struggle with cognitive weaknesses that are at the foundation of maladaptive behaviors that do not reach the threshold to meet *Diagnostic and Statistical Manual of Mental Disorders* (5th edition (DSM-5); American Psychiatric Association, 2013) [1] criteria for a disease model mental health disorder.

Does Knowing a Youth's Cognitive Abilities Help Parents Have Realistic Emotional and Behavioral Expectations?

It is common for parents to be surprised when their well-adjusted and academically successful youth begins to falter and struggle with social and academic skills. Although struggles appear earlier for some, school difficulties occur most frequently

The original version of this chapter was revised. The correction to this chapter can be found at https://doi.org/10.1007/978-3-030-88075-0_9

S. V. Delgado et al., *Promoting the Emotional and Behavioral Success of Youths*, https://doi.org/10.1007/978-3-030-88075-0_4

when youths enter the fifth grade (depending on the school's curriculum, as well as family and social contexts). Beginning in fifth grade, learning and educational expectations become more complex; they require students to utilize greater abstract reasoning and cognitive flexibility (Chap. 5) to achieve the developmental steps necessary to be happy and successful.

Understanding a youth's cognitive abilities and weaknesses allows clinicians to help the youth's parents have realistic emotional, social, and academic expectations and to develop practical approaches addressing the identified weaknesses. We define and explore intelligence (and, interchangeably, cognition) in an attempt to establish its relevance to the clinician in creating a treatment plan—and to parents in managing their own expectations. Although cognitive weaknesses are mostly permanent, throughout this book, we provide several tools to work around weaknesses and to promote known areas of competency.

The reader may question why we state that cognitive weaknesses are mostly permanent. In general, cognitive capacities can improve developmentally but not beyond innate abilities. However, in certain situations, there are some youths in which there is evidence of some degree of neuroplasticity. The cognitive weaknesses that stem from a traumatic brain injury, treatment of cancer, etc., may return to baseline in some youths. There are a number of situations in which we can see the clear environmental contribution impact on intelligence. For example, a child who lives in poverty or has a medical illness (e.g., Type 1 diabetes) affecting her cognitive ability may see improvements in cognition once social interventions or treatment are provided [10, 14]. Furthermore, in cases of twins raised in families living near or below the poverty level, 60% of their IQ variability is related to the shared environment; in twins living with affluent families, the genetic contribution dominates [28]. Therefore, the clinician assessing cognitive functioning in youths must attend to environmental stressors and consider sequencing psychiatric and cognitive evaluations after the resolution of the stressors for a better representation of the youth's cognitive abilities. Take, for example, an 8-year-old girl who becomes withdrawn when asked to complete her daily chores or homework. During her annual physical exam, her pediatrician notices she has poor eyesight and needs eyeglasses. Once she has eyeglasses, she is happy and is more willing to complete her homework and chores. Had her myopia (nearsightedness) not been identified by her pediatrician, her becoming withdrawn may have been thought to be due to a mental health issue; she also would have struggled with her IQ test.

Intelligence: The Second Pillar

We define *intelligence* (and, interchangeably, cognition) as the second pillar in the formation of personality. Broadly, intelligence includes cognitive processes that we use to understand verbal and nonverbal communication, to learn from experience, and to then use this information to make decisions. Intelligence allows us to adapt to environmental demands and develop successful relationships. Intelligence is also important to academic and professional success. Importantly, intelligence is not simply knowing when to act, but equally, learning to successfully use inhibitory mechanisms to prevent poor decision-making and prevent negative consequences.

As individuals differ physically from one another, they also differ in intelligence. Furthermore, cognitive development is an ongoing and fluid process.

Stable family and social environments, as well as nutrition, sleep, and other factors promote the acquisition of cognitive skills that ultimately scaffold the psychological and social developmental tasks that will ensure success in adulthood. However, the effect of these factors on cognitive development can be positive or negative, as noted by Weiss et al. [30]: "[E]nriching, cognitively stimulating environments enhance intellectual development, whereas impoverishing environments inhibit that growth." Additionally, negative effects from being raised in an impoverished environment can cumulatively and adversely affect cognitive ability [2]. Importantly, weaknesses in intelligence place youths at a disadvantage, as these weaknesses degrade self-esteem, emotional regulation, and academic functioning while increasing the likelihood of interpersonal conflict and maladaptive behaviors. As always, it is important to note that the skills and knowledge needed for success in life vary according to sociocultural context.

The Intelligence Quotient

Currently, the most common measure of intelligence is the "intelligence quotient," known as IQ. IQ measures how a person uses information and logic to answer questions and make predictions. IQ tests measure short- and long-term memory, how well people problem solve, and how well they recall information. IQ measures compare the performance of youths to others of the same age, and the tests are normed for social context and culture. Longitudinal studies suggest that IQ can predict quality of life, including social relationships, educational achievements, and career success [27].

The original IQ instrument, the Wechsler–Bellevue Intelligence Scale, was developed in 1939 by psychologist David Wechsler (1896–1981) the chief psychologist at Bellevue Psychiatric Hospital in New York City from 1932 to 1967. Wechsler defined normal intelligence as the average test score for all members of an age group; the mean could then be represented by 100 on a standard scale. The Wechsler–Bellevue Intelligence Scale—which was standardized for an all-white population—quickly became the most widely used adult intelligence test in the United States until the mid-twentieth century. In 1955, the Wechsler Adult Intelligence Scale (WAIS) was developed; it included 10% minority representation, which he erroneously believed was reflective of the U.S. population at the time. This was revised in 1981, shortly before Wechsler's death.

The Wechsler Intelligence Scale for Children (WISC) was first published in 1949 and, for decades, has been one of the most reliable measures of intelligence in children and adolescents. The last of Wechsler's intelligence tests, the Wechsler Preschool and Primary Scale of Intelligence (WPPSI), was released in 1967, assessing intelligence in children (3 years, 0 months through 7 years, 3 months). The Wechsler intelligence scales continue to be updated and widely used in clinical and educational settings.

The most updated version, the Wechsler Intelligence Scales for Children Fifth Edition (WISC-V) was published in 2014 and is widely used in the United States. WISC-V is composed of five indices: verbal comprehension (VC), visual-spatial (VS), fluid reasoning (FR), working memory (WM), and processing speed (PS). The WISC-V provides information to parents, teachers, and other school personnel about the educational interventions and accommodations needed for the ultimate goal of youths' academic success [30]. For gifted youths, it defines areas needed to promote advanced learning. For learning-disabled youth, it provides specific recommendations for remediation of weaknesses (reading, math, etc.). The WISC-V assesses cognitive functioning, which is closely linked to personality development. Understanding cognitive functioning can help the clinician understand aspects of the patient that relate to his or her suffering even when the patient cannot articulate these weaknesses or is unaware of them [3]. For example, a youth with cognitive weaknesses and a secure form of attachment and personality is more likely to seek help and improve in functioning. In contrast, a youth with cognitive weaknesses and an insecure form of attachment with a dismissive personality will limit his willingness to seek help. The association between personality and cognition has been found to be qualitatively and quantitatively similar in healthy adults between 20 and 90 years of age [25].

While the Wechsler scales of intelligence are the most commonly used, other scales are used in some settings and by some practitioners to assess cognitive abilities, including the Stanford–Binet Intelligence Scales, Cognitive Assessment System, Kaufman Assessment Battery for Children, Woodcock–Johnson Tests of Cognitive Abilities, and the Differential Ability Scales [4].

Throughout this book, we have focused on the WISC-V, as it is one of the most well-established tests, and most frequently used to quantify IQ. We also like that the scores of the indices of the WISC-V can be used to generate a clinical cognitive profile that, when used in tandem with the other three pillars (temperament, cognitive flexibility, and attachment style/personality), can help us understand the basis of emotional regulation difficulties, relational styles, and maladaptive behaviors in youth.

Controversy of IQ Tests

The history of the assessment of intelligence and cognitive processes of youths from different racial, ethnic, cultural, linguistic, and socio-economic backgrounds has been an area of controversy [5, 13]. Psychological assessments have often been criticized for being racially and culturally biased [18]. For decades, it was erroneously assumed that psychological assessments were objective, culture-neutral, and generalizable to racial and ethnic minorities, even though most tests were standardized, validated, and found reliable primarily with White, middle-class, English-language samples [19, 21]. As a result of this thinking, for decades, communities were negatively impacted in their access to educational and employment opportunities. Therefore, it is important to have a reliable way to measure intelligence according to age, social context, and culture. Intelligence tests address these issues as they are adapted in form and content to take into account the differences in adaptive tasks that individuals confront in diverse cultures [26].

Weiss et al. [30] make the case that while racial and ethnic differences exist in the cognitive abilities of individuals, these differences are not due to test bias. They assert that racial and ethnic differences represent a multitude of variables that influence cognitive abilities in psychological assessments, which require future research, for example, disparities in home environment, education, income, and physical and mental health. Undoubtedly, there will continue to be those in favor of and those against psychological assessments. But with increasing immigration of ethnic groups to multicultural countries, the accurate and meaningful assessment of youths' cognitive skills from different backgrounds is imperative.

Finally, it is well established that cognitive growth in youth is greatly enhanced by a secure relational environment that stimulates their social, creative, and intellectual ability. As such, in our four-pillars multidimensional model approach, the information obtained from psychological assessments is helpful only when viewed through a lens that considers the youth's family, social, and cultural context. We have highlighted the importance of context in our book, noting that temperament, cognition, cognitive flexibility, and attachment are shaped by interactions with others and is influenced by cultural factors [20]. Furthermore, parents use cultural norms to evaluate the level of success in emotional and social development. For example, in some cultures academic cognitive abilities are considered most important, while in others, social and creative skills are the most valued. All of this is to say that a youth's cultural environment will have significant impact on the development of her four pillars. While psychological assessments can alert the clinician of a youth's cognitive strengths and weaknesses, the interventions need to be tailored with sensitivity to a youth's family, social, racial, ethnic, and cultural context. The clinical case examples described are drawn from a racially and ethnically diverse group. We do not identify race and ethnicity to highlight the context of the four pillars.

The WISC-V Subtest Indices

The WISC-V usually takes 65–80 minutes to administer, and the scores are typically referenced to a scaled score of 100–the population average. The WISC-V is composed of five indices: verbal comprehension (VC), fluid reasoning (FR), visual-spatial (VS), working memory (WM), and processing speed (PS). For decades, WISC-V subtest indices (Table 4.1) have provided important additional information that can be used to understand a youth's educational strengths and weaknesses and

Table 4.1 WISC-V subtest indices and descriptions

Verbal Comprehension	Fluid Reasoning	Visual-Spatial	Working Memory	Processing Speed
VCI	FRI	VSI	WMI	PSI
The access and application of word knowledge. Ability to categorize and conceptualize information learned verbally. Ability to verbalize meaningful concepts. Long-term retrieval knowledge. Is influenced by education and culture.	Use of reason to solve new problems. Successful manipulation of conceptual rules and relationships. Visual intelligence and abstract thinking. Integration of multiple cognitive abilities.	Evaluation of visual details. Visual-spatial reasoning. Attention to visual detail. Visual-motor integration.	Ability to register, maintain, and manipulate visual and auditory information in conscious awareness. Attention and concentration. Accurate visual and auditory discrimination of information stored in short-term memory.	Speed of sensory and cognitive decision-making. Ability to scan, register, and discriminate information. Short-term memory functions. Ability to rapidly identify, register, and make decisions about verbal and visual information.

to develop interventions for parents and educators to help youths improve their academic efforts. The primary index scores, along with the FSIQ, provide a comprehensive description of the youth's intellectual ability.

Academic Achievement Tests

An essential aspect of a psychological evaluation, in addition to the WISC-V, is the assessment of academic achievement. The instruments used to assess academic skills are designed to identify skills developed in reading, math, written language, and oral language. While these academic tests are beyond the scope of this book, at minimum, the clinician should note if the youth's academic skills are commensurate with his age and at grade level. If the youth's academic skills are below grade level, the clinician can assume that these weaknesses can also contribute his emotional and behavioral difficulties (Table 4.1).

Moving Intelligence out of the Classroom

The psychologist administers and reviews the results of the WISC-V and can determine whether additional psychological tests may provide more insight into the youth's academic performance in regard to her intelligence. Traditionally, mental health clinicians have only cursorily used information about a youth's cognitive abilities or weaknesses and frequently deferred to educators, parents, and tutors on these issues. Although cognitive weaknesses lead to problems with self-esteem and behavioral difficulties, the information provided by intelligence tests was commonly viewed in academic terms rather than as data that could inform diagnostic approaches and clinical interventions. Intelligence testing was thought to mainly identify a youth's educational strengths and weaknesses. It is common for the WISC-V test report to be shared with referring mental health clinicians for their review; however, mental health clinicians are usually more interested in the information provided from the diagnostic rating scales for attention-deficit/hyperactivity disorder, obsessive compulsive disorder, depression, anxiety, etc., giving only superficial attention to the subtest indices of the WISC-V. Consequently, the use of psychological testing results as a psychiatric diagnostic tool has not been used often, aside from when superficially categorizing a youth as intellectually disabled, learning disabled, or having below average, average, or above average intelligence. This approach is problematic, particularly for symptomatic, treatment-seeking youths who struggle with emotional regulation abilities and maladaptive behaviors; in these cases, especially, the information provided by these tests can deepen our understanding of their symptoms as related to a disease-based model disorder or due to cognitive and relational weaknesses.

This added information provides an important insight into a child or adolescent's functioning with regard to her innate abilities, as well as how these abilities contribute to her adaptive and maladaptive functioning within her environment and culture. Psychological assessments are an essential foundation to measure the characteristics of an individual's weaknesses and strengths. Cognitive weaknesses may contribute to poor self-care and capacity to understand treatment interventions.

Finally, many mental health clinicians are hesitant to incorporate the information garnered from psychological tests into their clinical work. There are significant barriers to using psychological testing in our work with patients. Testing can be difficult to obtain, expensive, and not covered by insurance plans. Psychological testing may also be difficult to arrange, frequently requiring in-person appointments. There may also be limited availability of testing in certain geographic areas. For the treating clinician, reviewing the results and discussing the results with the individual who performed the testing may be time-consuming. Also, some clinicians experience the information in testing reports as dense and full of jargon. Consequently, mental health clinicians often focus on the "bottom line" summary of findings as sufficient (full scale IQ; below, average, or above average intelligence; learning disabled or intellectually impaired) and do not review important details of the WISC-V indices that can elucidate the reasons for emotional or behavioral problems in certain contexts.

Variability in Cognitive Assessments

Variation in the results of cognitive assessments is common because their interpretation is influenced by the psychologist or psychometrician's training and expertise [29]. Many psychologists limit the information to that which is related to academic skills or which confirms or excludes a formal learning disorder, while others suggest further assessments to provide a more in-depth guidance for learning problems. Parents and educators assume that if an assessment reports results consistent with expectations given for the youth according to her global estimated cognitive functioning, weaknesses in one or more WISC-V indices (verbal reasoning, working memory, etc.) are not significant contributing factors to emotional, behavioral, and academic struggles. This approach is problematic; for many youths, these weaknesses frequently contribute to their emotional and behavioral struggles beyond the academic setting.

It is important to note that for the last decade, teachers and other school personnel have often reported to parents their youth's level of school functioning, which may be a misrepresentation of the youth's true abilities or limitations. The reason for this discrepancy is complex and relates to multiple factors: more youths in each classroom, limited local support for special education, lowering achievement requirements, grade inflation, and newer teachers having decreased training in cognitive weakness. As such, clinicians should not gloss over information about a child or adolescent's apparent academic performance. Instead, they should consider how information obtained, in vivo, from the CDI (Chap. 2) to assess when a cognitive evaluation is indicated. This enhances a true understanding of a child or adolescent's cognitive abilities to ensure emotional and behavioral success.

Furthermore, some psychologists qualify weaknesses in the WISC-V indices to the referring clinician, stating, "It should be noted that the following results need to be considered in the context of the patient's current psychiatric issues, as such, they may not reflect his optimal functioning, but rather are a snapshot of his current functioning." Suggesting that lower scores may be unreliable because a disease-based model may have interfered with a youth's testing abilities is also problematic. Psychological assessments begin with a clinical interview to help establish rapport, assess the youth's readiness for the tests, and enhance accuracy in the responses given. If a clinician deems a youth unready to give reliable responses, the test should not be administered; this will preserve the integrity of later testing results by preventing the youth from becoming familiar with it.

As we will discuss in this chapter, cognitive weaknesses can be the root of maladaptive behaviors that, when viewed from a disease-based model, can be mistakenly considered "symptoms" of a psychiatric disorder. Herein, we will help mental health clinicians use information from the WISC-V to understand a child or adolescent from the inside out. Armed with this knowledge, the clinician can develop in-depth diagnostic formulations, tailor treatment plans, and provide practical interventions for youths and parents.

Are Full-Scale IQ Scores Clinically Helpful?

For decades, the full-scale IQ score has been the go-to number for clinicians, educators, and administrators who seek to quickly categorize a child or adolescent's ability for success or failure. However, full-scale IQ scores do not capture the full story of a youth's strengths and weaknesses, particularly as they relate to his or her interpersonal relationships and ability to regulate his or her emotions.

Let us consider two 16-year-old boys, Michael and Noah. Both boys have a full-scale IQ of 110 but differ greatly in how they engage with their work at school.

Full-scale IQ scores do not capture the full story

Michael	Noah
Michael has a full-scale IQ of 110 (high average) on the WISC-V. at school, Michael struggles. His teacher is perplexed, noting: "He knows the material; it shouldn't take him that long to complete his assignments." his teacher also wonders if Michael might have anxiety. At home, Michael feels he can't live up to his parents' expectations, and believes his friends think he is "dumb." his parents hope that his pediatrician can prescribe medication for his anxiety: "We know he is smart; he just gets nervous."	Noah has a full-scale IQ of 110 (high average) on the WISC-V. Noah is described by his teachers as a very good student: "He works hard, does well in all his subjects, and turns his assignments in on time." he participates actively in class, gets along well with his parents, and is well-liked by a wide circle of friends. He is active in several sports and takes leadership roles.

While Michael and Noah have the same full-scale IQ, Michael has a processing speed of 83 (low average), which contributes to his struggles completing work at school within the allotted time. This low average processing speed also explains his parents' frustration with his not completing his schoolwork on time, since the teachers report that he understands the material. Knowing that his processing speed is reduced, a clinician could help Michael's parents understand its impact on his day-to-day functioning, conversations, academic work, etc. The clinician could help Michael's parents decrease and avoid conflict by giving Michael extra time to respond to questions or to complete his homework. Importantly, educating Michael's parents about the emotional toll his low processing speed has on relationships will allow them to be vigilant of self-esteem issues and consider psychotherapeutic interventions if needed. Furthermore, Michael would also benefit from accommodations at school (e.g., extra time when asked to participate or to complete his schoolwork). In contrast, Noah has high average scores in all the WISC-V subtests and is

Fig. 4.1 Processing speed

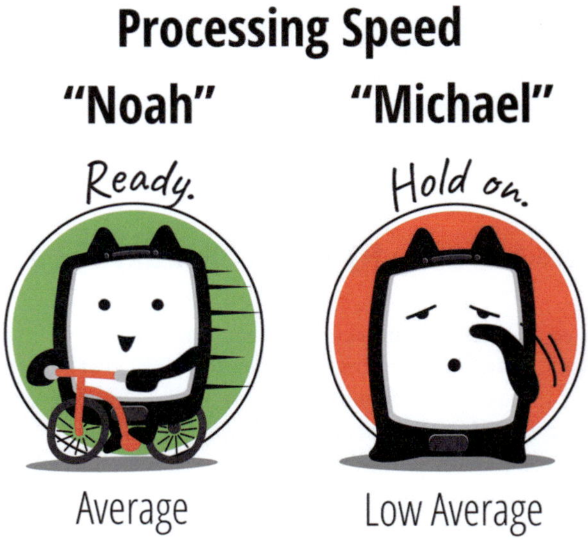

a very good student without any difficulties. Therefore, it is important for clinicians appreciate that full-scale IQ can be misleading and mask significant academic and behavioral difficulties (Fig. 4.1).

Are Full-Scale IQ Scores Clinically Helpful in Inpatient Care?

When we communicated with a lead psychologist of a large urban inpatient psychiatric unit for youths, she estimated that over 80% of the inpatient youths demonstrated cognitive weaknesses that contributed to the emotional and behavioral difficulties that led to their admission. Furthermore, he observed that, in the same unit, nearly 50% of the inpatient youths and 75% of those under 10 years of age failed the speech/language screening. Though research of specific cognitive weakness leading to symptomatic youths remains sparse, surveillance studies of inpatient psychiatric youth cohorts show similar increases in the incidence of cognitive and language difficulties [17]. Being cognizant of patients' cognitive weaknesses can guide treatment teams in developing multidimensional diagnostic formulations and provide tailored interventions to youths and their parents.

Special Evaluations

When working with youths with complex problems and multiple four pillar weaknesses (temperament, cognition [WISC-V], or cognitive flexibility), clinicians should consider requesting speech/language and occupational therapy evaluations. Information from these evaluations can help clinicians determine the impact the weaknesses identified in the four pillars have on the youth's daily activities and relationships. The speech/language therapist will tailor interventions to improve the youth's difficulties with receptive language, expressive language, and/or social-communication skills. The occupational therapist will focus on physical, sensory, or cognitive problems to help the youth gain skills in everyday activities and learn adaptive behaviors and social skills to manage frustration and anger stemming from his or her weaknesses.

The WISC-V Subtest Indices (Continued)

Weiss et al. [30] lightheartedly describe the five subtest indices as "five primary team members of the brain needed to learn facts and relationships among them, remember them when needed, and use them to quickly and efficiently solve problems in life" (Table 4.2). They name the brain team members according to their adaptive function, analogous to what is assessed by the subtest indices (Fig. 4.2).

In keeping with the analogies of Weiss et al. [30], we have added playful descriptions of the brain team members in their adaptive and maladaptive forms in the five

Table 4.2 WISC-V "adaptive" representations

The Librarian	The Detective	The Architect	The Manager	The Clerk
Quickly categorizes and conceptualizes information learned verbally or through reading. Verbalizes meaningful concepts. Uses verbal reasoning; expresses knowledge using words. Has long-term retrieval knowledge Is influenced by education and culture.	Uses reason to solve novel problems. Manipulates conceptual rules and relationships. Has good visual intelligence and abstract thinking. Integrates multiple cognitive processes.	Evaluates visual details Develops visual-spatial reasoning. Attends to visual details. Develops good visual-motor integration abilities.	Registers, maintains, and manipulates visual and auditory information in conscious awareness. Acquires information through attention and concentration to tasks. Has accurate visual and auditory discrimination of information stored in short-term memory.	Displays good skills in sensory and cognitive decision-making. Can scan, register, and discriminate details of information. Has good short-term memory functions Can quickly identify, register, and make decisions about verbal and visual information.

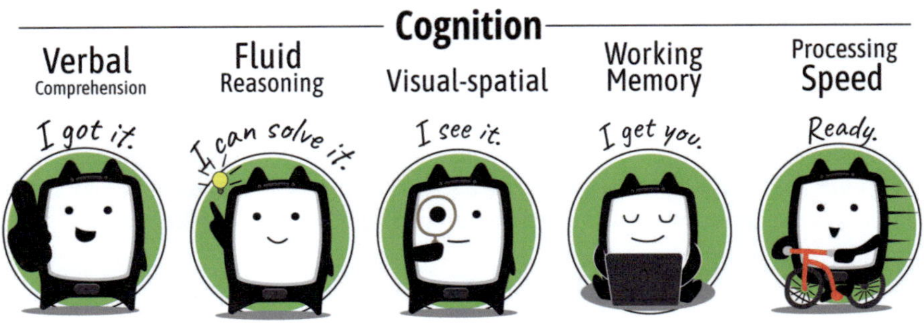

Fig. 4.2 WISC-V "adaptive" representations

Table 4.3 WISC-V "maladaptive" representations

The Impostor	The Demanding Youth	The Worried Builder	The Storm Chaser	The Brave Turtle
Verbal comprehension is in the low average to below average range. Erroneously assumes he knows information received verbally. Gives incorrect or fabricated responses. Finds it difficult to follow instructions and loses track during complicated tasks; may eventually abandon these tasks.	Fluid reasoning index is in the low average to below average range. Has difficulty identifying and applying rules of conceptual relationships, broad visual intelligence, and abstract thinking.	Visual-spatial weaknesses is in the low to below average range. Struggles to evaluate visual-spatial details and reasoning. Has poor visual-motor integration. Avoids playing complex games or sports. Delays learning to drive a car.	Average working memory is in the low to below average range. Struggles to simultaneously process and store information needed to understand the implicit meaning of the ebb and flow of conversations with others. Unknowingly pushes family or friends away due to her inability to understand how they feel and think. Has problems developing a healthy moral compass. Seeks relationships with youths that think and act like her—a precursor for borderline personality disorder.	Processing speed is in the low to below average range. Needs a longer amount of time to reason and integrate social information. Delayed responses are experienced by others as a sign of being defiant or cognitively impaired; a "slow learner." May be bullied or ostracized for slow short-term memory functions.

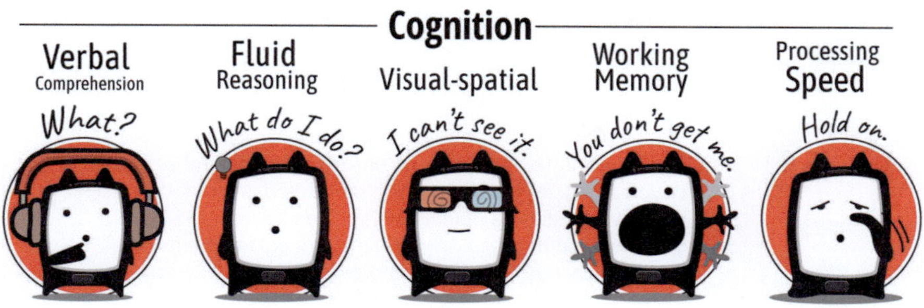

Fig. 4.3 WISC-V "maladaptive" representations

subtest indices. As we have stated, we believe that weaknesses in the low average and very low average range have value in helping us understand the root of a youth's maladaptive emotional and behavioral actions (Table 4.3, Fig. 4.3).

Verbal Comprehension Index (VCI)	
Adaptive 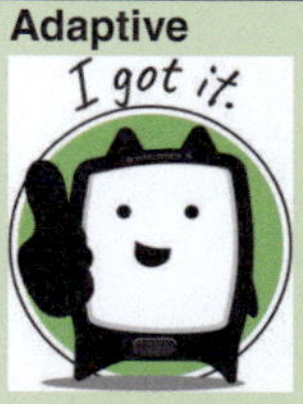	**The Librarian** The verbal comprehension index (VCI) measures verbal reasoning, including the access and application of acquired word knowledge. Much like an actual librarian knows what books the library has and can use that information to help patrons, our librarian has good long-term retrieval functions and the ability to quickly categorize and conceptualize information. She also has the ability to verbalize meaningful concepts. More so than some other indices, the VCI result can be strongly influenced by background, education, and cultural experiences. During this portion of the subtest, youths will be asked to listen to questions, draw from learned experiences, and ultimately express their responses verbally.
Maladaptive 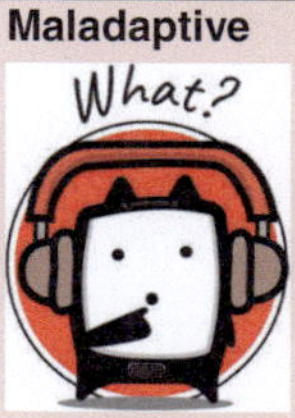	**The Impostor** When a youth's verbal comprehension index is in the low average to below average range, he will struggle with verbal reasoning and have limited abilities to access and apply acquired word knowledge.The impostor erroneously assumes he has mastery over information received verbally; when asked to verbally communicate information about how to solve a problem, he gives incorrect or fabricated responses. He is often in conflict with others, because in conversations he assumes he is correct even when evidence points to the contrary. Impostors have weaknesses in long-term retrieval functions and in the ability to verbalize meaningful concepts, think about verbal information, and express knowledge using words. For example, as youths get older and parents begin to make complex verbal requests (e.g., "How much homework do you have?" or "How long do you think you will be at David's house? You need to pick up your brother at five.") youths will superficially understand the parent requests but will not follow through with them. When parents find themselves frustrated and repeating their requests, youths experience this as their parents' dislike for them. They find it difficult to follow instructions, lose track during complicated tasks, and may eventually abandon these tasks. These youths have trouble with activities that require both remembering and processing information that does not make much sense to them.

Fluid Reasoning Index (FRI)	
Adaptive 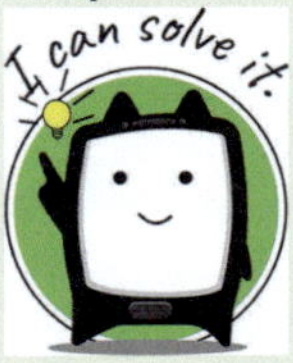 	**The Detective** Fluid reasoning index measures the capacity to think logically and solve novel problems that require the successful integration of multiple cognitive abilities. This ability is independent of acquired knowledge and is an essential component of cognitive development for youths in that it helps them acquire other cognitive abilities. A detective integrates information in a cohesive manner, applying rules of conceptual relationships, broad visual intelligence, and abstract thinking. The detective reviews facts from the librarian (verbal comprehension), the architect (visual-spatial) for orientation of relevant items, and the general manager (working memory) to select or discard facts according to their significance to solving the problem. Fluid reasoning is the cornerstone of human cognition, both during development and in adulthood. Despite this, the neural mechanisms underlying the development of fluid reasoning are largely unknown. Fluid reasoning, in youth, accurately predicts performance in school, university, and cognitively demanding occupations [7].
Maladaptive 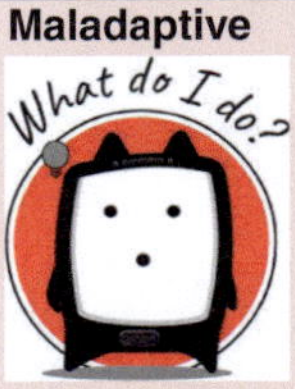 	**The Demanding Youth** Weaknesses in fluid reasoning index in the low average to below average range are seen in youths that are unable to solve novel problems (e.g., learning how to set up their smartphone, adapting to school schedule changes, learning information to pass a driver's licensure test). They demand better treatment when feeling their siblings are not asked to complete similar chores, failing to recognize that their siblings completed the tasks without need for reminders. They have difficulties identifying and applying rules of conceptual relationships, broad visual intelligence, and abstract thinking to day-to-day obstacles. They can become easily frustrated and angry in situations in which they can't identify solutions and demand others tell them how to solve their problem. Attempts to reassure them and suggestions to slow down to consider their options are often experienced as attacks; they then increase the intensity of their demand that others provide solutions. They often state, "I am depressed; this is too much to deal with," without having formal depression.

Visual-spatial Index	
Adaptive 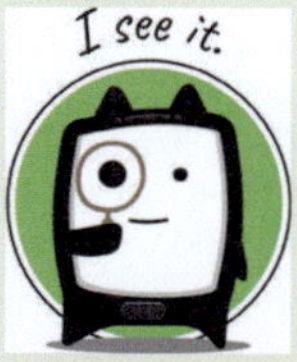	**The Architect** Architects score high in visual-spatial index measures. They have the ability to evaluate visual details as a whole and understand these details within the context of visual-spatial relationships. Architects are able to efficiently use acquired skills in visual-spatial reasoning, attention to visual details, and visual-motor integration (e.g., navigating to their locker or classroom; mastering the ability to parallel park, etc.).
Maladaptive 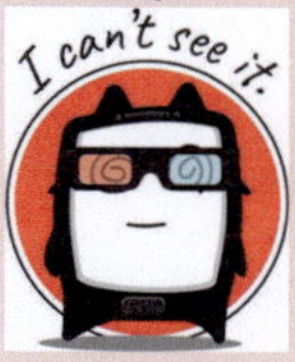	**The Worried Builder** Youths with visual-spatial weaknesses in the low average to below average range struggle to evaluate visual details and consequently struggle in visual-spatial reasoning and visual-motor integration. Young children struggle playing with games like Connect Four or Jenga and worry they will not be liked. In middle school years, they often worry about being late to class due to difficulties finding the classroom, unless they have friends they can follow. Frequently, they delay driving or pursuing team sport activities as they struggle with directions and worry they will be ridiculed. Similarly, youths with nonverbal learning disorders also have weaknesses in visual-spatial skills and require similar emotional, behavioral,and academic interventions.

<table>
<tr><th colspan="2">Working Memory Index (WMI)</th></tr>
<tr><td>Adaptive
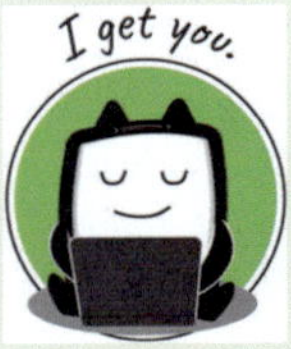
</td><td>The General Manager
Working memory is essential for interactions with others within the context of social norms and culture. This index measures the ability to register, maintain, and manipulate visual and auditory information in conscious awareness. This process requires attention and concentration for accurate visual and auditory discrimination of information stored in short-term memory [15]. Herein, day-to-day conversations are influenced by the ability to translate visual and auditory information, verbal dialogue, and facial expressions within the conversation.
Playing games require working memory: checkers, Monopoly, etc. (Youths with high-level working memory prefer chess, wherein they can hold a plan for several offensive moves while simultaneously holding in their memory how the opponent might respond to each move.) Working memory is predictive of language skills, or the ability to keep track of the ideas presented in long or complex sentences, a skill necessary for actors, musicians, and composers [32]. The reader with good working memory and a good sense of humor will be able to recall what he or she has learned throughout this book.</td></tr>
<tr><td>Maladaptive
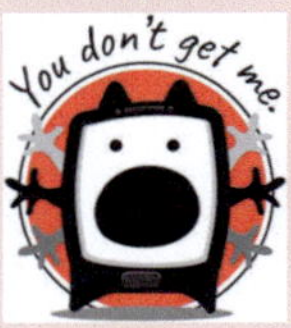
</td><td>The Storm Chaser
Youths with working memory weaknesses in the low average to below average range have significant difficulties interacting with others because they struggle with simultaneously processing and storing information needed to understand the implicit meaning in the ebb and flow of conversations. Consequently, this leads them to unknowingly push family or friends away due to their inability to stay on topic in day-to-day conversations, which ultimately end in conflict. Their inability to appreciate the importance of social norms for successful interactions make them feel that the norms are unrealistic or rigid and defy them (they may, for example, bully others, laugh at the mishaps of others, defy adults' expectations, etc.). The notion of a Storm Chaser captures these youths' unknowing efforts in seeking relationships with other youths who think and act like them with a belief that they are correct in their perception of situations. Consequently, they have problems developing the moral compass needed for understanding and respecting others' thoughts and intents as being different than their own. They lack cognitive flexibility, which can be described as the ability to interpret behavior as both meaningful and based on the mental states and psychological makeup of the self and others, including desires, needs, beliefs, reasons, and feelings (see Chap. 5). They experience others requesting that they adapt to social norms and be have accordingly as bullying. Researchers estimate that 10-15% of school age children struggle with low working memory capacity [8, 10]. At this point,the reader may recognize that weaknesses in working memory abilities is one of the precursors to borderline personality disorder in adolescence.</td></tr>
</table>

<table>
<tr><th colspan="2">Processing Speed Index (FRI)</th></tr>
<tr><td>Adaptive
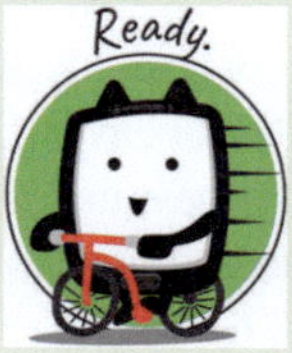
</td><td>The Clerk
The processing speed index measures the ability to rapidly identify, register, and make decisions about verbal and visual information. It requires the ability to visually scan, discriminate, and use short-term visual memory. Processing speed is key to being able to process relevant information between brain regions. As clerks perform a variety of tasks—typing, editing, writing memos, answering phones—our clerk is someone who completes several tasks accurately and efficiently, quickly adapting to different requirements in the tasks. The clerk requires the ability to adjust to a variety of situations, as their duties often change daily.</td></tr>
<tr><td>Maladaptive
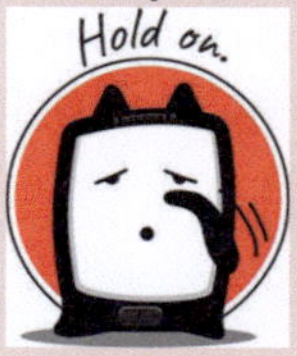
</td><td>The Brave Turtle
Youths with processing speed weaknesses in the low average to below average range require longer amounts of time to reason and integrate social information in daily fast-paced activities with family and peers. As a result, like a brave turtle, a youth with this weakness requires extra time to articulate what he hopes to say to others. Sadly, the delay in response can be experienced by others as a sign of defiance or cognitive impairment.
In clinical settings, parents of youths with processing speed weaknesses often prompt them to answer: "Go ahead, answer the doctor's question; you know the answer." This makes the youth feel inadequate or like a slow learner. These youths are often bullied or ostracized for being slow, with significant consequences to their self-esteem. Importantly, youths with superior or above average intelligence that also have slow processing speed are often thought to have attention deficit hyperactive disorder, predominantly inattentive, although they do not improve with the use of medication.</td></tr>
</table>

Clinical Cases

Having touched on the process and clinical use of intelligence testing, we will now take a brief sojourn to provide the reader with several anonymized clinical cases of youths with emotional problems and maladaptive behaviors that can be best understood by using cognitive test results. These will guide both the clinician and psychopharmacologist's approaches to the patient and her parents (see Chap. 6).

Of note, weaknesses in the subtest indices of the WISC-V have more impact on a youth's emotional and behavioral problems when there is a significant discrepancy in the score results. That is, when a youth has a low or below average score in certain indices, the impact on their cognitive and emotional abilities will be more pronounced if the other indices are in the high to very high average. These youths may expect to perform well in all areas as they may have used their strengths to compensate for their weakness in earlier years and are surprised when they are no longer able to do so.

Verbal Comprehension Weakness: The Impostor

Case 1: Jenna

The Impostor	*Synopsis: Jenna*
Verbal comprehension is in the low average range. Erroneously assumes she knows information received verbally.	Jenna, a 16-year-old adolescent with a history of severe mood swings, was brought by her mother for a psychiatric evaluation after she voiced having suicidal thoughts. Her suicidal thoughts began after discovering that her girlfriend was cheating on her. She became despondent and reported continuously thinking about taking an overdose of her medications. She felt it was a solution to her distress:"I just wanted to hurt [girlfriend]. That's why I thought of taking pills!"
May give incorrect or fabricated responses. Finds it difficult to follow instructions and may eventually abandon tasks.	Jenna's "girlfriend" became worried about what Jenna might do and called Jenna'smother to explain that they were not actually dating. Though she explained to Jenna numerous times that she did not have feelings for her, Jenna continued to hope for a relationship. Jenna's mother was not surprised by this revelation,whichfit with her own experience of Jenna's frequent difficulties with relationships.

DSM–5 Relevant History

Since age 12, Jenna had been in psychotherapy and taking an antidepressant medication for what had been considered depression. Later, she developed behavioral problems, including arguing with parents and teachers, becoming impulsive (getting piercings) and yelling at friends for a perceived lack of loyalty; these behaviors were thought to represent bipolar I disorder. Previous medications and combinations included fluoxetine, sertraline, quetiapine, and aripiprazole. Medications were described by her mother as "ineffective," who noted that the effects were "temporary" because the medications were "not strong enough." Jenna had also participated in cognitive and dialectic behavioral therapies, although she found them difficult "because the therapists talked too much and gave a lot of homework." She had limited insight and judgment regarding her maladaptive actions when she felt distressed. She did not have a history of grandiosity, flight of ideas, increased activity, sleep disturbances, or increased talkativeness. Jenna had no history of any serious medical conditions outside of routine childhood illness.

Jenna had also begun to harm herself, making superficial scratches on her forearms, and her mother was increasingly concerned that she would not be able to care for Jenna at home. Jenna seemed to require increasingly more supervision than her mother was able to provide. Jenna struggled to manage the typical level of increased independence in adolescence (e.g., using a smartphone safely, completing homework and chores, taking her medication, etc.). In addition, her mother knew Jenna did not have any long-standing healthy peer relationships: "She only likes teens who have problems at home and school—like her." Jenna's mother had taken away her smartphone after discovering that Jenna had begun an online relationship and misrepresented her age.

When Jenna began high school, conflicts with her mother frequently spiraled out of control. Because of this, Jenna's clinician referred her to a day-treatment program to help her to learn coping strategies for her emotional dysregulation. Typically, within a day of beginning the day-treatment program, she reported that she felt better and wanted to stop attending the program: "This doesn't help me. I don't like to talk about my problems." However, because she would not make use of the coping skills and safety plans taught, her outpatient therapist and the day-treatment staff felt frustrated by Jenna—a reaction that was similar to that of her mother and teachers.

Contributing Family, Social, and Educational History

Jenna was an only child and lived with her biological mother. Her father divorced her mother when Jenna was 5; he lived in the same city but seldom visited.

Clinicians and teachers who knew Jenna well described her as having poor decision-making abilities, being demanding, and showing emotionally unpredictability. However, Jenna had good moments, too: she could be funny when interacting with younger children and when she engaged in outdoor activities with neighborhood peers.

Educationally, Jenna repeated seventh grade because she failed most of her classes. At the time, this was attributed to the onset of her depression. Currently, she was in tenth grade at a public high school. Despite being a year behind, she struggled with her academic work, including understanding new material and concepts, although she was not identified as an at-risk adolescent and continued in regular education classes. To minimize her struggles, she was assigned to a supervised resource room where she could ask for help as needed. However, Jenna rarely reached out for help instead spending the time drawing. Her teachers observed that she was, at times, calm and pleasant, but her mood could shift suddenly if a teacher corrected her or told her to limit her socializing. In class, she fought with peers who avoided or criticized her and received detention as a result. To help her with her emotional dysregulation, Jenna's teachers allowed her to leave the classroom as needed to go to the school-based social worker's office, but she seldom went.

Contemporary Diagnostic Interview

Jenna was not forthcoming when asked about her difficulties with her girlfriend. She became angry when the clinician attempted to ask about the conflict with her parents. However, when asked to share about her interest in the care of younger children in the neighborhood, she perked up, saying, "I like to teach kids to play. They like me because I don't get too uptight if they get rowdy. I can talk to them and they behave." Her mother confirmed her strengths in caring for younger children. She was also pleasant when speaking about her neighborhood friends: "We get together and ride our scooters in the neighborhood while we talk about who we like."

Regarding her experience with therapists, she did not like them: "They give me too much hard homework (cognitive and dialectical behavior therapies); it doesn't help. They just blame me for my problems with my parents and at school." When asked about her understanding of why she argued and fought with peers at school but did well with them in the neighborhood, she said, "They make fun of me at school because I go to the resource room, and they bully me because sometimes I don't understand the class information or because I'm failing. I get along with friends in the neighborhood because they don't care about grades and because they have problems with their parents, like me."

Formulation

The clinician using the information from a CDI understood Jenna's four pillars as having a mixed temperament (predominantly difficult/feisty when in conflict; easy/flexible when caring for younger children, playing with peers, or when educational demand was low), cognitive weaknesses, varied cognitive flexibility, and secure/dismissive form of attachment. Jenna was referred for a psychological assessment to better understand the nature of her varied psychological functioning.

Session (mixed temperament and varied cognitive flexibility) pearls
Jenna became angry if the clinician attempted to ask about the conflict with her "girlfriend" or her parents [*difficult/feisty temperament*].
On the topic of children, she perked up and cheerfully reported, "I like to teach kids to play; they like me because I don't get uptight if they get rowdy. I can talk to them and they behave" [*easy/flexible temperament, adequate cognitive flexibility*].
Her experience was that her academic limitations were not accurate, and she chose not to care about her education: "I get along with friends that don't care about grades" [*cognitive weakness, limited cognitive flexibility*].

Results of Psychological Testing

FSIQ	VC	FR	VS	WM	PS
100 (50%) Average	89 (23%) Low avg.	109 (73%) Average	122 (93%) Average	91 (27%) Average	100 (50%) Average

Summary of Psychological Testing: WISC-V

Primary Drivers

Low average verbal comprehension.

Secondary Drivers

Mixed temperament (difficult/feisty and easy/flexible), variable cognitive flexibility, and secure/dismissive attachment style depending on context.

Formulation After Psychological Testing

Jenna has an average full-scale IQ and a weakness in verbal comprehension (low average range). Verbal comprehension is required to access and apply acquired word knowledge. This is significant, considering that developing adaptive behaviors and making mature decisions requires the ability to learn verbally from others for day-to-day social interactions.

As early as 12 years old, Jenna often misinterpreted verbal information and experienced her mother and others as disliking her without understanding that they were making efforts to help her develop adaptive behaviors. This is common in youths with weaknesses in long-term retrieval functions who have deficits in their ability to learn and verbalize meaningful concepts, think about verbal information, and express the knowledge by using words.

Under our formulation, Jenna can best be understood as an impostor when engaged in emotionally laden situations. As an impostor, she implicitly assumes that she has accurately learned information provided to her verbally to solve her daily social and academic problems, when she has not. She is rarely aware of her deficiencies and seldom asks for clarification or interpretation of complex conversations. When others attempt to help her with growth-promoting verbal communications, she misunderstands the intended meaning and experiences the comments as critical and rejecting, which leads to feelings of loneliness and emotionally dysregulated behaviors.

With this information, we would expect her complex presentation to be applicable to several diagnostic formulations, when her cognitive weakness is integrated with a mixed temperamental style, varied cognitive flexibility, and secure/dismissive attachment style. The clinician may consider Jenna to have an adjustment disorder with mixed disturbance of conduct and emotion. Furthermore, her cognitive weakness with low average verbal comprehension will interfere in the daily presentation of her cognitive flexibility and executive functions needed for adaptive behaviors and maturity: when in distress, she may be considered to have an impulse control disorder. However, the clinician should capitalize on her strengths and encourage interventions in which she can be pleasant and unknowingly make use of her strengths in temperament, cognition, and cognitive flexibility, that is, caring for younger children, recreational activities with peers or when educational demand is low.

While some clinicians may consider her to have an emerging borderline personality disorder trait, her average fluid reasoning and working memory will help her develop a good moral compass and make matured decisions when others are able to adapt and promote the use of her strengths. Furthermore, her mixed temperament (difficult/feisty and easy/flexible), variable cognitive flexibility, and secure/dismissive attachment style allow for her to have adaptive skills in some contexts. However, if her home and social environment promote maladaptive behaviors, she may later develop more emotional difficulties with a borderline personality disorder of adolescence.

Clinical Highlight

*The Impostor: Low average verbal comprehension (*Fig. 4.4*).*

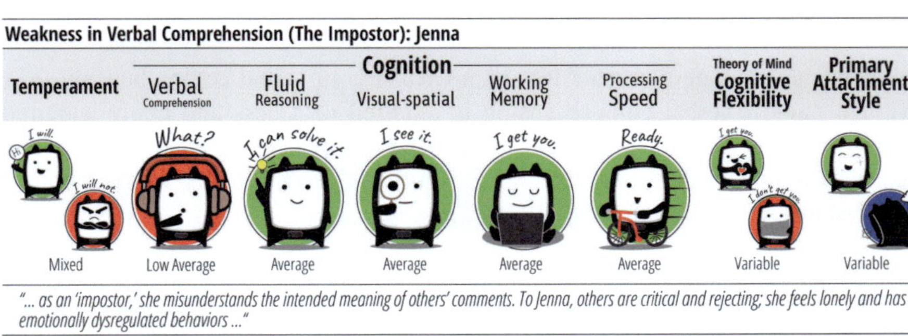

Fig. 4.4 Weakness in Verbal Comprehension (The Impostor): Jenna

Maladaptive Patterns

- Will have difficulties accessing and applying acquired word knowledge; will avoid verbal communication.
- Will often say "What?" or "What do you mean? I don't know what you are saying."
- Reacts with anger when given complex verbal directions.
- Is surprised by how difficult it is to understand conversations with high-school friends, compared to elementary or middle-school years.
- Expects people to be critical and rejecting.
- Experiences individual or group therapy, typical in day-treatment programs, as difficult.

Treatment and Intervention Recommendations

Jenna may benefit from individual art therapy to make use of her strengths (easy/flexible temperament, average intelligence, and elements of good cognitive flexibility) to promote the creative expression of emotions, develop self-awareness, and improve self-esteem. Storytelling with art can foster her social skills. The use of verbal communications will need to be simple and must be used in tandem with visual forms of conceptualization of information.

It is essential to have her mother become engaged in a therapeutic process to be able to learn about the biological underpinnings of Jenna's temperamental and cognitive weaknesses and alleviate any anxiety and self-blame she may experience. Parent therapy can help recalibrate how they interact with each other under distress.

While medications are not specifically indicated, some clinicians might use antidepressants or second-generation antipsychotics to target her anxiety and to reduce emotional upheaval during conflict. However, these medications may not consistently improve her emotional dysregulation or maladaptive behaviors, particularly given that they are related to weaknesses in her four pillars.

Suggested Interventions

- Educate her parents and teachers regarding the nature of her struggles with verbal comprehension.
- When in conversations, stop often to assess her comprehension and intention of the discussion.
- Create emotional word lists to help her verbalize emotions (e.g., upset, unhappy, lonely, not listened to, etc.).
- Provide simple compliments to improve her self-esteem (e.g., thank you for telling me, I will listen now, let's go do something fun, etc.).

- Jenna will be able to accomplish more with written or visual information than with verbal communications, which can improve her ability to develop adaptive behaviors and make mature decisions.
- Encourage the use of nonverbal forms of expression (art, journaling, meditation, texting, etc.)
- Share with Jenna's therapists that she will often misinterpret the intention of verbal communication; they should remember not to assume that her average full-scale IQ reflects good verbal skills.

Relevant Cross-References

- Difficult/feisty temperament: Chap. 3.
- Varied cognitive flexibility: Chap. 5.
- Dismissive attachment style: Chap. 6.
- Interventions for verbal comprehension weaknesses: Chap. 7.

Verbal Comprehension Weakness: The Impostor

Case 2: Daniel

The Impostor	*Synopsis: Daniel*
Verbal comprehension is in the low average range. Erroneously assumes he knows information received verbally. May give incorrect or fabricated responses. Finds it difficult to follow instructions and may eventually abandon tasks.	Daniel is a 16-year-old male whose parents confiscated his smartphone after he destroyed the main home television after not being allowed to connect his video game console. After the smartphone was taken away, he made an impulsive "suicide attempt" in which he jumped out of the window of his second-floor bedroom. Fortunately, he had minimal injuries and was hospitalized in an inpatient psychiatric unit.

DSM–5 Relevant History

Daniel had difficulties at home and school with aggression and irritability. He frequently argued and shouted over minor concerns since he was 13 years old. He received psychiatric treatment (psychotherapy and medication). He had poor response to the use of antipsychotics to curb his aggression and irritability, and they often caused him to feel tired. In addition, his adherence to medication was poor. He had been enrolled in a behavioral after-school program for his impulsive and risk-taking behaviors. During after-school programs, he had difficulty with expressive group work and frequently argued with staff and was unable to articulate the safety plan needed for his discharge.

Daniel's symptom presentation varied depending on context and demand, although symptoms were more pronounced when he had to interact with others verbally. As reflected by his history of varied affective and impulse control problems, it was difficult to capture his difficulties with a single *DSM–5* diagnosis. He had previous diagnoses of oppositional defiant disorder, bipolar I disorder, disruptive mood dysregulation disorder, and impulse control disorder.

Contributing Family, Social, and Educational History

Daniel lived with his biological father and stepmother. Daniel was estranged from his biological mother. His poor grades began in fifth grade, and he required classroom accommodations for his disruptive behaviors. He was thought to be of average intelligence and that his poor grades reflected his mental health issues.

Behaviorally, at home, his parents used a token system that worked well when he was in elementary school. As he got older, he resisted authority and told his parents to "stop lecturing" him. He had few friends in the neighborhood because he was known for his risky behavior. He avoided participating in organized sports because he saw them as "boring," calling them "a waste of time."

Contemporary Diagnostic Interview

Several interactions during his most recent behavioral after-school program exemplified his struggles. Daniel had difficulty understanding how to earn privileges to meet discharge criteria, which made him angry:

> I want to get out of this place; talking doesn't help me. My parents need to be here, not me!

Pointing out that his continued anger with his parents was conflicting with his wishes to be discharged only perplexed Daniel:

> What do you mean? I am doing better than the other patients here.

Formulation

During his evaluation at the program, the clinician, using the information from a CDI, understood Daniel's four pillars as including a difficult/feisty temperament, cognitive weaknesses, rigid cognitive flexibility, and disorganized form of attachment. He was referred for psychological assessment to better understand the nature of his psychological functioning.

Session (difficult/feisty temperament and cognitive weakness) pearls
Daniel would become angry if the clinician attempted to ask about the conflict with others: "I want to get out of this place; talking doesn't help me" [*difficult/feisty temperament*].
Had difficulty with the expressive and speech milieu groups, frequently argued with staff, and was unable to learn what he needed to do to advance his privileges [*rigid cognitive flexibility*].
Pointing out that his continued anger with his parents was conflicting with his wishes to be discharged perplexed Daniel: "What do you mean? *[cognitive weakness]*.

Results of Psychological Testing

FSIQ	VC	FR	VS	WM	PS
89 (23%) Low avg.	89 (23%) Low avg.	94 (34%) Average	107 (55%) Average	91 (27%) Average	92 (30%) Average

Summary of Psychological Testing

Primary Drivers

Low average full-scale IQ and low average verbal comprehension.

Secondary Drivers

Difficult/feisty temperament, rigid cognitive flexibility, and disorganized form of attachment style.

Formulation After Psychological Testing

Daniel's chronic struggles are best explained by his low average cognitive functioning and verbal comprehension weaknesses, which limit his ability to understand his world and to solve problems that require language (including family and peer conflicts). Daniel's verbal comprehension weakness, when combined with his moderate-to-severe form of difficult/feisty temperament, is likely to cause Daniel to demonstrate low frustration tolerance, irritability, and defiance; he is also likely present with disorganized forms of attachment in spite of his parents providing a secure environment. Thus, in our descriptors, he would be understood as an impostor with precursors of narcissistic personality traits.

But why do these youths often get labeled with different disruptive or impulse control disorders? Like Daniel, these youths often struggle to process verbal information and to express concepts using words. They struggle accurately categorizing verbal information received for future use. In the long term, these weaknesses lead to a shortfall of organized information to solve problems. When combined with temperamental difficulties, we see a range of disruptive or impulsive behaviors when the youth is presented with challenging situations. This, however, is a descriptive diagnosis and does not inform about the root of these behaviors: low average full-scale IQ and low average verbal comprehension, difficult/feisty temperament, rigid cognitive flexibly, and disorganized form of attachment style.

The severity of these symptoms can also vary, and in Daniel's case resulted in an impulsive suicide attempt with significant injury.

Clinical Highlight

The Impostor: Low average full-scale IQ and low average verbal comprehension. (Fig. 4.5).

Maladaptive Patterns

- When consequences for his maladaptive behaviors are not understood, in the context of Daniel's difficult/feisty temperament and cognitive impairment, his rapid escalation of disruptive and impulsive behaviors can be expected.
- Authoritarian approaches will elicit resistance and anger.
- Will have difficulties accessing and applying acquired word knowledge.
- Will often say "What?" or "What do you mean? I don't know what you are saying."

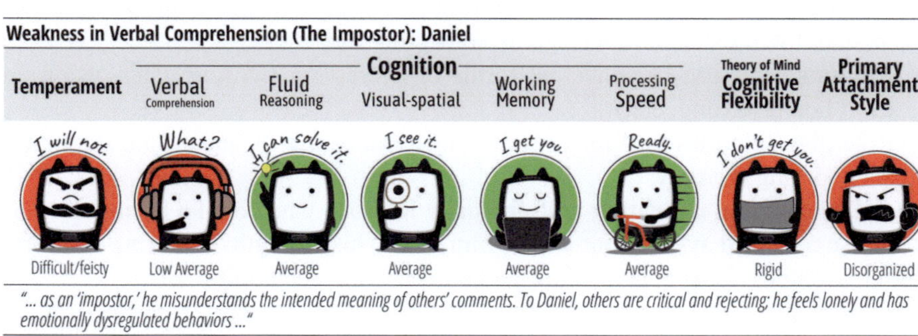

Fig. 4.5 Weakness in verbal comprehension (The Impostor): Daniel

- Reacts with anger when given complex verbal directions.
- Is surprised by how difficult it is to understand conversations with high-school friends, when compared to elementary or middle-school years.
- Expects that people will be critical and rejecting.

Treatment and Intervention Recommendations

While Daniel could benefit from individual visual art therapy, his temperamental difficulties and limited cognitive flexibility will make it a challenging endeavor if he agrees to go. The therapist should remember that establishing a therapeutic alliance will be essential for him to trust that his best interests are served. The use of a verbal communications will need to be simple and must be used in tandem with visual cues.

It is essential that his parents become engaged in a therapeutic process to learn about the biological underpinnings of his temperamental and cognitive weaknesses and alleviate any anxiety and self-blame they may experience. Parent and family therapy can help recalibrate how they interact with each other under distress.

While medications are not specifically indicated, some clinicians might use α_2 agonists or SGAs to address impulse control. However, these medications may not improve emotional regulation or maladaptive behaviors.**Suggested Interventions**

- Educate his parents and teachers regarding the nature of his struggles with low average intelligence and low average verbal comprehension.
- In conversations, pause frequently to assess his comprehension and his understanding of the intent of the discussion: "Let's wait to order the pizza until your mother, brother, and sister arrive so the pizza is warm when it gets here. Does that make sense?" Followed by "When should we call to order the pizza?" If the youth says "now" and did not understand the reason for waiting for family to arrive, rephrase, reducing complexity. "When your mother gets here is when we will order the pizza."
- Provide simple compliments to improve his self-esteem (e.g., thank you for telling me, I will listen now, let's go do something fun, etc.).
- Encourage the use of nonverbal forms of expression (writing notes, using an easel board, texting, etc.)
- Role-play solutions to difficult situations to make use of intact fluid reasoning and working memory.

Daniel's emotional regulation will gradually improve when adults in his environment use a reward system that allows him to use his strengths (working memory, fluid reasoning, visual-spatial skills, and processing speed abilities).

Relevant Cross-References

- Difficult/feisty temperament: Chap. 3.
- Poor cognitive flexibility: Chap. 5.
- Disorganized attachment style: Chap. 6.
- Interventions for verbal comprehension weaknesses: Chap. 7.

Fluid Reasoning Weakness: The Demanding Youth

Case 3: Robert

The Demanding Youth	*Synopsis: Robert*
Fluid reasoning index is in the low average range. Has difficulties identifying and applying rules of conceptual relationships, broad visual intelligence, and abstract thinking.	Robert, a 12-year-old boy, was brought for a psychiatric evaluation because of anxiety. His parents were concerned that he lacked confidence and would give up easily when confronted with difficult tasks at home or school. They were "blindsided" when he failed his quarterly exams and gave him strict consequences, limiting his use of video games or social media to 30 minutes a day, and only allowing him to have his friends over one day a week until his grades improved. A week after he failed his quarterly exams, he confided in a teacher that he was having thoughts of taking his own life because he felt that he had failed in school and his parents were upset. He considered taking ten tablets of ibuprofen, hoping "it would stop my stress," believing that his parents would be happier if he were dead because he was "dumb."

DSM–5 Relevant History

Robert was taken to see a child psychiatrist when he was 7 years old, and his parents noted that he began to isolate and cry because he had failing grades at school. The evaluation concluded that he had a depressive disorder, and Robert began weekly psychotherapy. An antidepressant was started and given for 3 months with increases to reach therapeutic dosing, although there was limited improvement. His parents requested that child psychiatrist "try a different medication to boost his confidence."

In second grade, Robert's academic functioning worsened. His teachers and parents described him being "forgetful" and unserious about his work, and often confronted him on these points. He needed frequent reassurance and was increasingly embarrassed when confronted with failure in his classes, although he was able to maintain grades in the B range. After his teachers and parents completed the Vanderbilt ADHD Diagnostic Rating Scales (VADRS; [31]), Robert's pediatrician diagnosed him with attention-deficit/hyperactivity disorder, predominantly inattentive. Trials of various formulations of methylphenidate and mixed amphetamine salts were ineffective and decreased his appetite and caused insomnia. His parents joined a parent training program for youths with ADHD but found several of the skills taught "difficult to use with Robert. He doesn't remember what we tell him."

When working on a hobby or school project, Robert frequently felt anxious, turning to his parents or friends to ask if he was following the directions correctly. Furthermore, he had problems interacting with his friends because he had difficulties understanding their humor and drawing inferences from information being discussed. He would demand his parents and friends tell him how to do things or explain jokes without understanding the consequences of his "demanding" stance. At times, Robert forgot the rules when playing with his friends in neighborhood sports and became embarrassed, isolating in his room and crying. He was very resistant to participating in any organized sports or school activities.

Contributing Family, Social, and Educational History

Robert lived with his parents, who were both college-educated, and two siblings that were doing well in all psychosocial and academic areas.

Robert attended seventh grade at a local parochial school. He attended regular classes. His teachers found him bright, but his anxiety and fear of failure made it difficult for him to complete his work. He also tended to demand that teachers tell him how to solve problems without putting in much effort.

Contemporary Diagnostic Interview

Robert was visibly upset about being asked to interview. He promptly told the clinician that his teachers "never explain things" and they didn't help with his schoolwork, which was why he was failing some of his classes. His parents interjected that they had gotten him a tutor, although he refused to go. Robert replied, "I don't like the tutor. He doesn't explain things."

The clinician proceeded to ask Robert to share where he lived and the landmarks nearby. His anxiety visibly increased. He asked "Why?" In response, the clinician shared that he liked knowing where his patients lived. Robert said, "It is by the train tracks and the Arby's." After joining comments about eating Arby's sandwiches, the clinician asked Robert about why school was so difficult and why he thought his parents would be better off without him. Robert responded: "I'm not sure. I try hard at school, and I want to have friends. My parents and therapist tell me what to do to feel better, but I forget and then I get mad."

Later in the Interview

The clinician asked what Robert felt he was good at. "I am good at playing video games and sports on my PlayStation 5. I just can't play with my friends. They keep changing the rules," Robert replied.

The clinician, using the information from a CDI, understood Robert as having a slow-to-warm-up temperament, cognitive weaknesses, limited cognitive flexibility, and anxious form of attachment. He was referred for a psychological assessment to better understand the nature of his psychological functioning.

Session (fluid reasoning and visual-spatial) pearls
When asked where he lived and landmarks nearby, his anxiety rose instantly, and although he made an effort, his response was vague: "It's by the train tracks and the Arby's" [*cognitive weakness*].
Fluid reasoning difficulties were noted when Robert reported, "I try hard at school, and I want to have friends. My parents and therapist tell me what to do to feel better, but I forget and then I get mad."
Robert recognized difficulties playing with friends, although he blamed them: "I am good playing video games and sports on my PlayStation 5. I just can't play with my friends. They keep changing the rules" [*limited cognitive flexibility*].

Results of Psychological Testing

FSIQ	VC	FR	VS	WM	PS
93 (32%) Average	100 (50%) Average	82 (12%) Low avg.	89 (23%) Low avg.	91 (27%) Average	114 (82%) High avg.

Summary of Psychological Testing: WISC-V

Primary Drivers

Low average fluid reasoning and low average visual-spatial abilities.

Secondary Drivers

Slow-to-warm-up temperament, limited cognitive flexibility, and anxious form of attachment within the context of a secure home environment.

Formulation After Psychological Testing

Robert can best be understood as having problems adjusting to his cognitive weaknesses and as he reached adolescence—where there is a need for higher cognitive processes—he felt noticeably anxious and overwhelmed when the family, social, and academic demands were difficult for him cope with. As such, a diagnosis of adjustment disorder with mixed disturbance of conduct and emotion (anxiety) secondary to mild cognitive weaknesses in fluid reasoning and visual-spatial abilities is reasonable. This is further complicated by his slow-to-warm-up temperament. Although he has relatively strong cognitive flexibility that helps him know that other people can help him, he becomes overwhelmed if they do not respond to his initial request and quickly demands that others rescue him from his feelings of despair.

Clinical Highlight

The Demanding Youth: Low average fluid reasoning (Fig. 4.6).

Maladaptive Patterns

- Displays an inability to retrieve from memory information necessary to complete complex tasks.
- Becomes easily frustrated and angry when unable to use reason to solve complex problems; demand others tell him how to solve his problems.
- Has difficulties identifying and applying rules of conceptual relationships and abstract thinking to day-to-day obstacles.
- Has difficulties generalizing past to new experiences.
- Has difficulties understanding and evaluating the opinions and views of others.
- Refuses to try new approaches, perhaps because of anxiety.

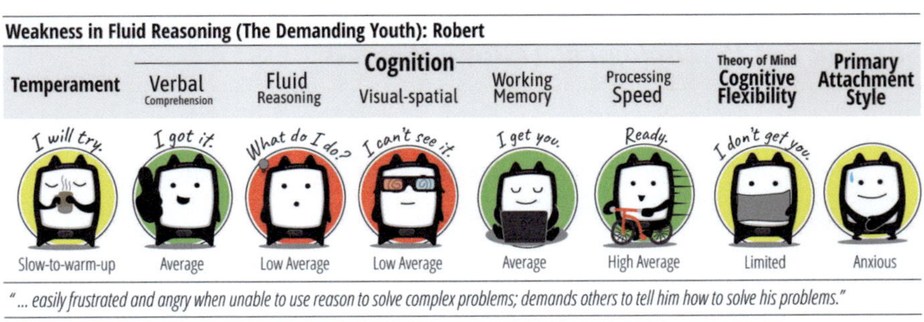

Fig. 4.6 Weakness in fluid reasoning (The Demanding Youth): Robert

- Experience's suggestion to slow down and consider options as an attack on his intelligence.
- Develops generalized anxiety when nervous about learning something new that may be intimidating.

Treatment and Intervention Recommendations

Although there are many forms of psychotherapy that can be considered for Robert, his weaknesses in fluid reasoning and visual spatial abilities may best be served by using supportive individual psychotherapy with attention in promoting interpersonal skills.

Robert will benefit from helping his parents and teachers understand the nature of his struggles with low average fluid reasoning and difficulties knowing how to solve unexpected complex problems (e.g., understanding his homework or new strategies in organized sports practice, etc.). His emotional dysregulation symptoms will improve when his parents modify their approach and model how to manage his interpersonal and academic struggles.

Most importantly, his parents will need help understanding that his difficult/feisty temperament can easily be experienced as defiance and using an authoritarian style will likely worsen his mood.

Suggested Interventions

- Teach Robert how to ask for verbal explanations of new concepts rather than visual instructions to help him internalize the process.
- Educate parents and tutors about how to help him identify useful information when presented with a problem.
- To avoid experiencing others as demanding, Robert will need reassurance before he is asked to slow down and consider alternative options to problems.
- Provide practical behavioral interventions in visual reward form (visual timers, visual diagram of tasks and rewards, etc.)
- Teach his parents how to help Robert de-escalate (e.g., "Let us know what made you angry and then we can figure out together what to do.")

Relevant Cross-References

- Slow-to-warm-up temperament: Chap. 3.
- Limited cognitive flexibility: Chap. 5.
- Anxious form of attachment: Chap. 6.
- Interventions for fluid reasoning and visual-spatial weaknesses: Chap. 7.

Visual-Spatial Weakness: The Worried Builder

Case 4: Kate

The Worried Builder	*Synopsis: Kate*
Visual-spatial weaknesses in low average range. Struggles to evaluate visual-spatial details and reasoning. Poor visual-motor integration. Avoids playing complex games or sports.	Kate is a 13-year-old female with past psychiatric diagnoses of generalized anxiety disorder and dysthymic disorder. Her parents had taken Kate to numerous clinicians and, despite medications and psychotherapy, they noted little improvement and felt clinicians were "missing something." Kate continued to report anxious feelings and low self-esteem, and had begun to engage in mild self-harm behaviors. Her mother requested the psychiatric evaluation, seeking better understanding about the chronicity of her problems, adding, "She is a good kid most of the time."

DSM–5 Relevant History

In fourth grade, Kate began struggling academically and feeling anxious most days. She would comment, poignantly, "I am not good at anything." At school, her peers teased her for being clumsy. She began weekly psychotherapy and was diagnosed with generalized anxiety disorder. Although she attended her sessions regularly and found the therapist likeable, she was unable to use the coping skills learned in therapy to address her anxiety, school challenges, and social difficulties. She was referred to a psychiatrist for a medication evaluation. The psychiatrist believed Kate met *DSM–5* criteria for persistent depressive disorder and prescribed escitalopram, an SSRI, that was titrated over the course of a month to 15 mg daily, an evidence-based, target dose. Kate showed limited improvement in her depressive symptoms.

Contributing Family, Social, and Educational History

Kate lives with her parents, who are caring and attentive to her struggles. She has an older brother who is doing well in all psychosocial areas. There is no family history of psychiatric disorders. Outside of routine childhood illness, Kate had no unusual medical concerns.

Her parents suspected that her clumsy behaviors were due to poor eyesight, but her vision exam was normal.

Kate is successful within her social circles. She is involved in the Junior Optimist Club and sings in the youth choir at her church.

Kate is in the eighth grade at a local charter school. Despite a small classroom size and frequent individual attention from her teachers, she struggles academically. Kate's parents recognize that she pressures herself to achieve at school and worries about grades. Her teachers note that she has difficulty with letter, number, and symbol discrimination. In the past, she was often asked to sit in the front of the classroom as she was easily distracted by visual stimuli. Kate had difficulty paying attention to visual tasks and was easily distracted by too much visual stimuli, which made it difficult to follow the flow of her soccer games and school plays.

Concerned about her inattention and distractibility, her pediatrician requested Vanderbilt ADHD Diagnostic Rating Scales (VADRS, [31]) from her teachers. With this information, her pediatrician noted that she met *DSM–5* criteria for attention-deficit/hyperactivity disorder and began to use of a stimulant with limited results.

Contemporary Diagnostic Interview

Kate engaged easily and was playful during her evaluation. She was pleasant and eagerly gave details about her school struggles, adding, "I know I am slower than my friends at school, but I am a nice person." She was insightful about her weaknesses. The psychiatrist perused her alleged difficulties in visual-spatial abilities by asking her to draw her bedroom (Fig. 4.7). Her anxiety was palpable as she tried to

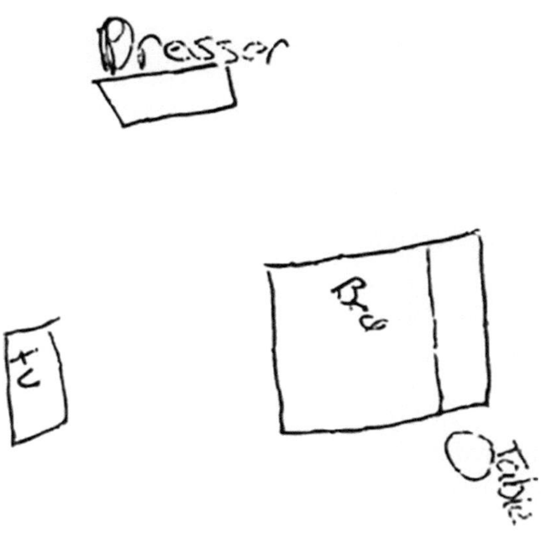

Fig. 4.7 Kate's bedroom drawing

draw, and she repeated more than once that she was not very good at drawing. As she drew her bedroom, she laughed with her mother: "This is hard." At school, it had been difficult for her to make use of visual images in learning. When asked about school difficulties, it took her some time to gather a response. She shared that her anxiety and depressive feelings were intermittent and situational: "When I know I won't do things right, I feel like, why try?"

Formulation

The CDI revealed that Kate had an easy/flexible temperament, possible visual-spatial weaknesses, good cognitive flexibility, and an anxious attachment style within the context of a secure environment. She was increasingly aware that she was not as adept as other adolescents her age and was not proactive in making new relationships. Psychological assessment was requested to clarify cognitive functioning.

Session (visual-spatial processing speed) pearls
As she drew her bedroom Kate laughed with her mother at how difficult it had been for her to draw [*cognitive weakness*].
When asked about school difficulties it took her more time than expected to respond [*cognitive weakness*].
Kate recognized that she was slow: "I know I'm slower than my friends but I am a nice person" [*cognitive weakness and good cognitive flexibility*].

Results of Psychological Testing

FSIQ	VC	FR	VS	WM	PS
98 (45%) Average	108 (70%) Average	100 (50%) Average	86 (18%) Low avg.	103 (58%) Average	86 (18%) Low avg.

Summary of Psychological Testing: WISC-V

Primary Drivers

Low average visual-spatial and low average processing speed abilities.

Secondary Drivers

Anxious attachment style.

Protective Drivers

Easy/flexible temperament, good cognitive flexibility, secure environment.

Formulation After Psychological Testing

Kate has a complex set of weaknesses within the context of a supportive family. Kate's psychological testing identified average intelligence but relative weaknesses in visual-spatial abilities and processing speed. Weaknesses in processing speed, when combined with her anxious attachment style, are consistent with her difficulties socially, which elicit anxiety. Her most recent anxiety, feelings of inadequacy, and her self-harming behavior developed from an increasing awareness of the competency gap (further exacerbated by her visual-spatial deficiencies) between her and her peers. Her low self-esteem is a result of being overwhelmed, anxious, and worried about not meeting the expectations of parents, peers, and teachers.

Diagnostically, it seems reasonable to consider Kate as having an adjustment disorder with anxiety and cognitive weakness.

Clinical Highlight

The Worried Builder: Low average visual-spatial abilities (Fig. 4.8).

Maladaptive Patterns

- Expects people will be critical of her for being slow or clumsy and may resort to isolation.
- Struggles playing visually complex games or sports.
- Has difficulties finding schoolbooks or assignments and easily misplaces objects at home.
- Becomes frustrated when friends ask her to follow complex directions in recreational activities.

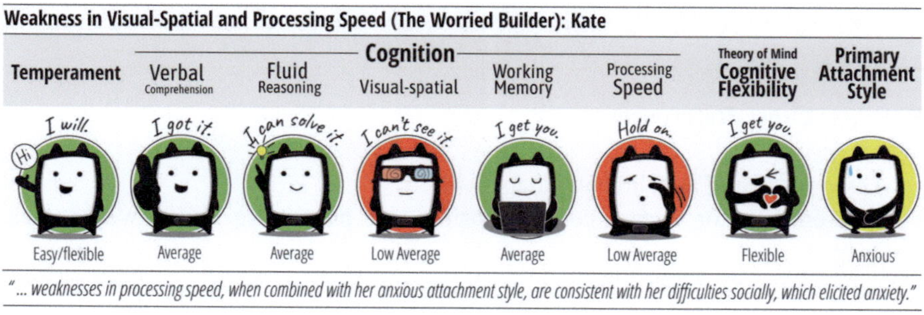

Fig. 4.8 Weakness in visual-spatial and processing speed (The Worried Builder): Kate

- Chooses to withdraw or be unusually quiet in conversations.
- Has difficulties with left and right spatial awareness and visual organization of assignments.
- Avoids learning how to drive.

Treatment and Intervention Recommendations

Psychotherapy, the primary treatment for adjustment disorder with anxiety, will help Kate learn about her limitations and promote skills to manage her anxiety.

Importantly, adults working with Kate may perceive relative strengths in some contexts and attribute her failure in other areas as a lack of motivation or preparation. Supportive parents often pick up on these patterns intuitively, as in Kate's case, and seek help, feeling "something is wrong."

Kate will benefit from helping her parents and teachers understand the nature of her struggles with low average visual-spatial and low average processing speed abilities. Her anxious symptoms will improve when her parents modify their approach and model how to manage her interpersonal and academic struggles.

Most importantly, her parents will need help understanding that her easy/flexible temperament and good cognitive flexibility are protective factors that can help her accept help provided in verbal or written form.

Suggested Interventions

- Educate parents about the nature of her multiple struggles with low average visual-spatial and processing speed abilities.
- Educate parents and teachers about the fact that her cognitive weaknesses will contribute to her situational anxiety and unhappy feelings.
- Role-play opportunities to practice conversations.
- Develop transitional phrases when interacting with others. These can help give context of her thinking process to others, e.g., "I need to think about that;" "That's a lot to think about—give me some time."
- In school, allow written responses to reading passages rather than on-the-spot requests for answers to questions in the classroom.

Relevant Cross-References

- Anxious form of attachment: Chap. 6.
- Interventions for verbal comprehension and processing speed weaknesses: Chap. 7.

Working Memory Weakness: The Storm Chaser

Case 5: Marissa

The Storm Chaser	*Synopsis: Marissa*
Low average working memory. Struggles to store and process information needed to understand the implicit meaning and ebb and flow of conversations with others. Unknowingly pushes family or friends away. Has trouble developing a healthy moral compass and seeks youths that think and act like her, a precursor for borderline personality disorder.	Marissa is a 16-year-old female with history of dysphoria, poor emotional regulation, and disruptive behaviors. Her parents reported the start of her behavioral problems began when she entered high school. She became increasingly irritable and would prefer to be with peers who also had behavioral and academic problems. Her parents felt she was not meeting her emotional, social, and academic potential and were hopeless and frustrated because "she is a master manipulator and hangs around with the wrong crowd." They added that the only people she interacted with were other people "that are depressed and unhappy with their home life."

DSM–5 Relevant History

Marissa began participating in outpatient psychotherapy when she started middle school due to increasing conflict with her parents when they enforced time for homework, set limits on her social media times, and established a curfew. Her defiance and disruptive behaviors escalated at home and school, with Marissa displaying poor reasoning abilities (yelling at others, threatening self-harm, etc.). The psychotherapist referred her to a two-week day-treatment program.

Her parents were frustrated with her behavior and expressed concern because she failed to improve with psychotherapy and day-treatment programs. When they became frustrated with her, they increased restrictions on her social media and peer activity, which resulted in serious conflicts that involved yelling and derogatory comments between Marissa and her parents.

Her parents and psychotherapist did not believe her behavioral problems were due to cognitive issues, as she had been thought to be a bright and high-achieving student until she began high school. In high school, her grades began to drop, and she began to "hang around the wrong crowd." This was initially considered to be "typical adolescent behavior," but when the maladaptive behaviors became persistent, Marissa's parents sought higher level treatment for her.

The psychotherapist diagnosed Marissa with oppositional defiant disorder and later understood her maladaptive behaviors as a manifestation of an underlying depressive disorder and requested a medication evaluation. Later, her behavioral difficulties and irritability escalated, and she disclosed that she had superficially cut her forearm, saying, "It makes me feel better." Her psychotherapist wondered if she had symptoms of a bipolar disorder. Marissa's outpatient psychiatrist, who also cared for her in the day-treatment program, concluded she did in fact have a diagnosis of bipolar disorder in adolescence and used a combination of an SSRI antidepressant and a mood stabilizer. There was some improvement in her labile mood states, but no improvement was noted in her poor decision-making abilities, and she continued to have significant conflict with parents and teachers.

Contributing Family, Social, and Educational History

Marissa lives in a two-parent home with two older brothers who perform well in all areas of functioning.

At the time of her treatment, Marissa was in tenth grade. Her teachers reported that she rarely seemed "present" in the classroom, and that they were concerned about her peer group. The parents were caught off-guard by her recent academic troubles, as throughout elementary and middle school she was a bright and high-achieving student.

Contemporary Diagnostic Interview

Marissa and her parents were asked to come in together for an interview with their new psychiatrist. Her parents reported, "She doesn't follow rules and doesn't want to listen to us." Marissa was initially resistant to the interview, expressing anger toward her parents for enrolling her in a summer school program. She wanted to spend the summer with her friends: "I am only happy when I'm with my friends; they understand me." Her parents' efforts to vociferously interject into the conversation made her more upset, and she stated, "I only get suicidal when I'm at home with my uncaring family." Her parents argued that they could not trust her: "We don't know what she is going to do." Marissa loudly exclaimed, "I would try to kill myself this summer if I had to stay home with you guys. I would drink bleach, slit my wrists, or take pills, and I would not call the police!" Her parents were clearly exasperated. "We feel like hostages," they said. "She doesn't care about the consequences of her bad behavior."

The clinician asked Marissa's parents to briefly leave the room to avoid further escalation between them. Despite her earlier outbursts, Marissa calmed herself. She reported a high degree of distress: "I get depressed all the time unless I'm with my friends. They understand me. My parents don't understand that I need my friends." Though she could superficially explain her needs and what made her upset, she lacked insight about the risks of her dysfunctional social relationships. The psychiatrist used the "joining" technique, acknowledging Marissa's feelings and dilemmas. When the clinician shared that her parents were worried about her because she had sent sexually inappropriate text messages to boys in her class, Marissa calmly replied that her parents were overreacting. She trusted the boys and was surprised when she learned they had shared the pictures with others at school. When asked why her friends would turn on her, she was not able to articulate her perspective. Marissa shifted emotionally, reporting that her friends had turned on her, though she didn't know why. She felt that her friends had begun to bully her; accordingly, she felt angry at them and began to self-harm with superficial cuts on her arm, saying it helped her feel better. The psychiatrist suggested that she needed help developing skills to cope with her emotions and to be understood without being criticized. She responded positively, smiling and asking the psychiatrist to tell her parents she needed help. "They think I'm evil," she said.

Her parents were brought back into the interview. Marissa felt the psychiatrist understood her and hoped he would convince her parents to be more understanding and less critical. She did not realize that his supportive comments helped him assess her limited insight about her own problems. She reported, "This guy [psychiatrist] understands me. He knows my friends turned on me and that it's not always my fault when I get mad. I feel like everybody is mad at me all the time." In addition, it became increasingly clear that Marissa lacked the ability to use caution when involved in unhealthy relationships.

Formulation

During the psychiatric evaluation, the clinician used a CDI-style interview and found Marissa difficult to engage when her parents were present due to her difficult/feisty temperament and poor emotional regulation. When alone, she was much easier to engage, although she was immature in her reasoning abilities. This immaturity likely represents weaknesses in cognition and limited cognitive flexibility, with a dismissive form of attachment suggestive of borderline personality traits. Her parents provide an insecure environment due to their own four-pillar limitations. Marissa was referred for a psychological assessment to better understand the nature of her functioning.

Marissa's parents were clearly contributing to her problems with emotional regulation because of their own difficult/feisty temperaments, poor cognitive flexibility (see Chaps. 3 and 5), and insecure attachment with Marissa. Her brothers were reported as doing very well, suggesting that they had good four pillars and were able to disentangle from the family's dysfunctional style.

Session (working memory and splitting) pearls
"I am only happy when I'm with my friends; they understand me" *[poor cognitive flexibility].*
About her friends, Marissa noted: "They turn on me and I don't know why" *[poor cognitive flexibility].*
"I would try to kill myself this summer if I had to stay home with you guys. I would drink bleach, slit my wrists, or take pills, and I would not call the police!" *[difficult/feisty temperament, poor cognitive flexibility, and insecure attachment].*

Results of Psychological Testing

FSIQ	VC	FR	VS	WM	PS
94 (34%) Average	103 (58%) Average	100 (50%) Average	92 (30%) Average	82 (12%) Low avg.	105 (63%) Average

Summary of Psychological Testing: WISC-V

Primary Driver

Low average working memory

Secondary Drivers

Difficult/feisty temperament, rigid cognitive flexibility with a dismissive form of attachment

Additional Drivers

Parents with difficult/feisty temperaments, limited cognitive flexibility, and a disorganized form of attachment

Formulation After Psychological Testing

Marissa had an average full-scale IQ in WISC-V with low average working memory. We suggest that weaknesses in working memory can be representative of the profile of a "Storm Chaser." We define a Storm Chaser as a person with difficult/feisty temperament, low average working memory, and poor cognitive flexibility (moral compass; see Chap. 6) with a dismissive attachment style. This four pillars profile represents early manifestations of an emerging borderline personality disorder. The Storm Chaser profile aptly captures Marissa in her unknowing tendency to seek relationships with youths that think and act like her, and in her constant conflict with people of authority, as she believes she is correct in her perception of situations. Her weaknesses will lead her to have difficulties with mood regulation and following social norms and will lead her to make use of maladaptive behaviors (aggressive outbursts, poor peer interactions, poor academic performance, self-harm, etc.) without fully understanding the consequences of her actions.

Diagnostically, it seems reasonable to consider Marissa to have borderline personality disorder and cognitive weaknesses.

Clinical Highlight

The Storm Chaser: difficult/feisty temperament, low average working memory, rigid cognitive flexibility (Fig. 4.9).

Formulation of Marissa's Parents

During a meeting scheduled to explain the significance of Marissa's difficult/feisty temperament, working memory weaknesses, and borderline personality disorder, her parents did not agree with how Marissa's cognitive weaknesses contributed to her maladaptive behaviors, but minimized the findings. Instead, they said that until the correct medication was used to help her, they would "clamp down" and restrict all of her social media and peer activities. Consequently, Marissa became extremely agitated and began to shout suicidal threats. The clinician intervened to highlight that the either/or positions each party took was not helpful and suggested working to find common ground, for example, engage in an activity as a family, allow her brothers to help her with homework, allow Marissa to have her smartphone for brief periods of time, etc. Nevertheless, due to the impasse and the rising emotions in all

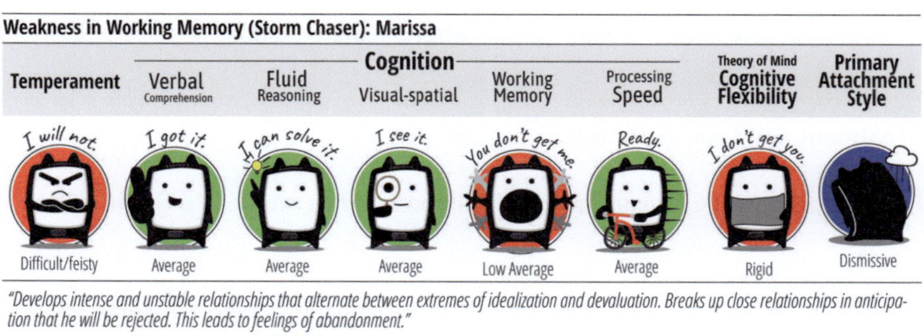

Fig. 4.9 Weakness in working memory (Storm Chaser): Marissa

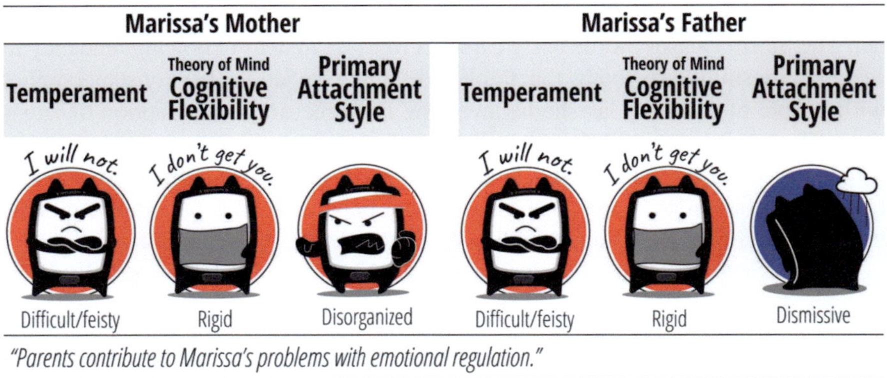

Fig. 4.10 Marissa's mother, Marissa's father

parties, combined with the knowledge of Marissa's tendency to act impulsively, the clinician decided that an inpatient admission was indicated (Fig. 4.10).

When the clinician saw the youth in the inpatient setting the following day, she shared, "This is really helpful. I already made good friends with the other girls." Her comments captured her difficulties making use of her hospitalization to understand the complex relational aspects of what a "friend" is.

Maladaptive Patterns of a Storm Chaser

- Develops intense and unstable relationships that alternate between extremes of idealization and devaluation.
- Breaks up close relationships in anticipation of being rejected and feeling abandoned.
- Feels empty, with fluctuations in self-image that are dependent on specific negative relationships to maintain a sense of identity.
- Experiences intense instability, irritability, or anxiety that may last for several days.
- Projects blame onto others for her problems.
- Recurrent self-injurious and suicidal behaviors are common.

Treatment and Intervention Recommendations

Psychotherapy is the primary treatment for those with a profile of a Storm Chaser.

Specifically, cognitive and dialectic behavior therapies, interpersonal, and group therapy to reduce conflict, improve dialogue, and promote cognitive flexibility are recommended.

While medications are not specifically indicated, some clinicians might use SSRI antidepressants to address anxiety and second-generation antipsychotics (SGAs) or mood stabilizers to target overlapping symptoms of affective dysregulation. However, these medications may improve emotional regulation but are not likely to improve maladaptive behaviors due to temperament, working memory weaknesses, and borderline personality disorder.

Attempts should be made to engage Marissa's parents in a therapeutic process that can help address their own limitations with difficult/feisty temperament, limited cognitive flexibility, and with a dysfunctional environment.

Suggested Interventions

- Help Marissa's parents understand that her cognitive weaknesses contribute to her maladaptive manifestations and emerging borderline personality disorder.
- Engage in case management, when available, to provide her a person to coordinate medical, psychological, and educational appointments, and to help her avoid conflict with her parents.
- Reinforce adherence to psychotherapy.
- Develop solution-focused approaches for family, social, and academic struggles.
- When Marissa is older, she will need help finding and employer that can support her strength in verbal comprehension and limit her need to make complex decisions for positive outcomes (e.g., working with pets, at a florist, packing operations, helping disabled children, etc.).
- Keep in mind that authoritarian approaches will elicit resistance and anger.

Relevant Cross-References

- Difficult/feisty temperament: Chap. 3.
- Poor cognitive flexibility: Chap. 5.
- Dismissive attachment style: Chap. 6.
- Interventions for working memory weaknesses and borderline personality disorder: Chap. 7.

Working Memory Weakness: The Storm Chaser

Case 6: Emilio

The Storm Chaser	*Synopsis: Emilio*
Has low average working memory. Struggles to simultaneously process and store information needed to understand the implicit meaning and ebb and flow of conversations with others. Unknowingly pushes family or friends away due to his inability to understand how they feel and think. Has difficulty developing a healthy moral compass and seeks relationships with youths that think and act like him, a precursor for borderline personality disorder.	Emilio is a 15-year-old male who was seen for an urgent medication evaluation. His mother reported that when he was discharged from his psychiatric in patient hospitalization for anger and suicidal threats a week prior, he had agreed to use coping skills from his dialectic behavior therapy and there was a safety plan in place. He had gone to school for several days and had done well. Nevertheless, while on a walk with his father,the police arrived at his home because Emilio had sent a text to a friend saying he was suicidal. When Emilio saw the police, he laughed and was unapologetic. "My friend overreacts all the time," he said. His father reassured police he would monitor his son, reporting that they had an appointment with his psychiatrist the next day.

DSM–5 Relevant History

Emilio had been engaged in psychotherapy since age 12 for minor but frequent oppositional behaviors. He made some improvement in his behavior and relationship with his parents, but continued to have outbursts of defiance when his parents set limits or asked him to do his chores.

At age 14, Emilio entered high school. His emotional and behavioral difficulties escalated and were initially attributed to disruptive mood dysregulation disorder. His psychotherapy appointments were increased to twice a week and medication was started. He was placed on aripiprazole, with minimal improvement, which was then changed to olanzapine, which provided some decrease in his labile moods, but the response was inconsistent, and the medication was stopped due to weight gain and lethargy. His maladaptive behaviors became more frequent and intense, and he was diagnosed with a bipolar disorder. At home, his father articulated the primary problem as the following: "He gets stuck on certain things and becomes angry when he can't get what he wants; then he claims to be suicidal."

A trial of valproic acid was started during Emilio's first psychiatric hospitalization after he made serious suicidal threats. He had several brief psychiatric hospitalizations after making suicidal statements when he was angry at his father. His father became frustrated: "I am tired of taking him to the hospital every time he has a suicidal thought. He doesn't get better." The psychiatric staff noted that Emilio enjoyed his time while on the unit. After discharge, Emilio continued to attend dialectic behavior therapy groups.

Contributing Family, Social, and Educational History

Emilio is an only child and lives with his parents.

Academically, Emilio initially did well in high school, receiving mostly As. By the second quarter, he began to get Bs and Cs as a result of not completing his assignments at school or at home. This surprised his teachers and angered his parents. "He is a bright kid," they said, "but with those grades he won't get a scholarship. We can't afford his college education."

Socially, Emilio had a wide circle of friends that his parents did not approve of because they were "a bad influence on Emilio. They all argue with their parents and are doing poorly in school." His father attempted to restrict Emilio from his friends because of his poor grades, but Emilio became more moody and verbally aggressive.

Contemporary Diagnostic Interview

Emilio and his father arrived together for the interview with the psychiatrist. His father began by saying, "He is a bright kid, but something must have happened in high school. He doesn't want to follow rules and gets suicidal whenever he's angry at me." Emilio, visibly angry, replied, "Your rules don't help me. You don't care how I feel. I'm happy with my friends; they understand me." His father then shared that he cared very much and that he was at a loss as to how to help him. This made Emilio upset. He said, "Maybe you can figure out that I'm suicidal at home with you and your rules." His father turned to the psychiatrist. "I love him, but I don't know what to do. I can't quit my job to be with him. He doesn't even want me close to him."

To avoid further escalation of emotions between them, the clinician asked Emilio's father to leave the interview for a brief time. Emilio's disdain for his father and other adults in his life was noticeable. Although he was articulate, his comments to the clinician were disrespectful: "You probably want to change me instead of changing my father. He's the problem." The psychiatrist attempted to use "joining" comments, but Emilio proceeded to argue: "You so-called adults make me get depressed. My friends, they understand me. How long will this last?" Though he could explain what made him upset, he did not have the insight needed to know the risks of his dysfunctional social relationships.

When Emilio's father was brought back to the interview, Emilio promptly told him, "You need to stop overreacting." He proceeded to smile, saying sarcastically, "Maybe the psychiatrist can help you understand what I need."

Formulation

Emilio was observed to be irritable and uncooperative with the interview. He displayed a difficult/feisty temperament, poor cognitive flexibility, and a dismissive form of attachment style. However, cognitive weaknesses were suspected, and full psychological assessment was obtained.

Session (working memory and splitting) pearls
"Maybe you can figure out that I'm suicidal at home with you [father] and your rules" [*difficult/feisty temperament, poor cognitive flexibility, splitting*].
"You [father] need to stop overreacting." sarcastically: "Maybe the psychiatrist can help you [father] understand what I need."
Dismissive of psychiatrist: "You so-called adults make me get depressed. My friends, they understand me. How long will this last?"

Results of Psychological Testing

FSIQ	VC	FR	VS	WM	PS
117 (87 %) High avg.	124 (95 %) Very high	109 (73%) Average	114 (82%) High avg.	82 (12%) Low avg.	90 (23%) Average

Summary of Psychological Testing: WISC-V

Primary Drivers

Low average working memory

Secondary Drivers

Difficult/feisty temperament, rigid cognitive flexibility, dismissive attachment style

Protective Drivers

High average full-scale IQ and visual-spatial abilities
Very high verbal comprehension
Secure and supportive home environment

Clinical Highlight

The Storm Chaser: difficult/feisty temperament, low average working memory abilities, rigid cognitive flexibility (Fig. 4.11).

Formulation After Psychological Testing

Emilio's symptoms are context-dependent and poorly fit *DSM–5* criteria for a mood, anxiety, or impulse control disorder. Rather, his "symptoms" are based on context and do not present across several environments. They are consistent with a borderline personality disorder in adolescence, with emerging narcissistic personality disorder traits driven by temperament, weaknesses in working memory, and rigid cognitive flexibility.

The notion of a Storm Chaser captures Emilio. He unknowingly pushes family or friends away due to his inability to understand how they feel and think, with a belief that he is correct in his perception of situations. His moral compass is limited, and he seeks relationships with other youths that think and act like him.

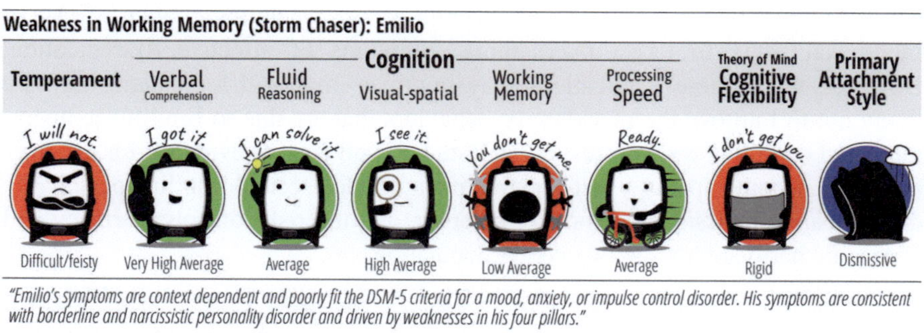

Fig. 4.11 Weakness in working memory (Storm Chaser): Emilio

Maladaptive Patterns of a Storm Chaser

- Develops intense and unstable relationships that alternate between extremes of idealization and devaluation.
- Breaks up close relationships in anticipation of being rejected. This leads to feeling being abandoned.
- Feel empty, with fluctuations in self-image, and is dependent on specific negative relationships to maintain a sense of identity.
- Experiences intense instability, irritability, or anxiety that may last for several days.
- Projects blame onto others for his problems.
- Makes recurrent suicidal comments.
- Displays emerging narcissistic personality disorder traits, flaunting his high average intelligence and feelings of superiority.

Treatment and Intervention Recommendations

Individual psychotherapy is the treatment of choice for those with a profile of a Storm Chaser, specifically cognitive and dialectic behavior therapies—both interpersonal and group formats—to reduce conflict, improve dialogue, and promote cognitive flexibility. However, Emilio has a unique cognitive profile that includes aspects of a narcissistic personality disorder, which will limit the changes that can be achieved with therapy.

Although Emilio may benefit from individual psychotherapy, a key component of early intervention for narcissistic personality disorder, it is essential to engage his parents in the therapeutic process, so that they can understand the biological underpinnings of Emilio's personality disorder and alleviate any anxiety and self-blame they may otherwise experience. Parent therapy can help recalibrate how family members interact with each other under distress.

While medications are not specifically indicated, some clinicians might use SSRI antidepressants to address anxiety and second-generation antipsychotics (SGAs) or mood stabilizers to target overlapping symptoms of affective dysregulation. However, while these medications may improve emotional regulation, they are likely not to improve the maladaptive behaviors that are due to Emilio's temperament and cognitive weaknesses. Overall, there is no current evidence for any specific pharmacotherapy as a first-line treatment of adolescent borderline personality disorder and narcissistic personality disorder, and the risks of polypharmacy and iatrogenic harm are high in this young population.

Suggested Interventions

- Educate Emilio's parents about cognitive weaknesses and how they contribute to his maladaptive manifestations and emerging borderline personality disorder.

- Engage in case management, when available, to provide a person to help Emilio's parents coordinate medical, psychological, and educational appointments, and avoid conflict.
- Remember that authoritarian approaches will elicit resistance and anger.
- Reinforce adherence to psychotherapy.
- Develop solution-focused approaches for family, social, and academic struggles.
- Help Emilio find employment that can support his strengths in high average intelligence and visual-spatial abilities, as well as his very high verbal comprehension abilities to limit interpersonal conflict and to promote positive outcomes (e.g., work as a sports referee, at a theater, as a debate coach, at a sporting goods store, etc.).

Relevant Cross-References

- Difficult/feisty temperament: Chap. 3.
- Poor cognitive flexibility: Chap. 5.
- Dismissive attachment style: Chap. 6.
- Interventions for working memory weaknesses and borderline personality disorder: Chap. 7.

Working Memory Weakness: Not a Storm Chaser

Case 7: Lauren

Very low working memory	*Synopsis: Lauren*
Struggles to process and store information needed to understand the implicit meaning and ebb and flow of conversations with others. Her easy/flexible temperament and good cognitive flexibility help her develop a healthy moral compass.	Lauren is a 12-year-old female whose parents anxiously requested a psychiatric evaluation regarding her chronic feelings of anxiety and depression. Her presenting problems were feeling overwhelmed with homework, loss of interest in social activities, and fleeting suicidal thoughts.

DSM–5 Relevant History

Lauren was evaluated by a child psychiatrist and diagnosed with major depressive disorder with anxious distress; an SSRI was started. However, despite good medication adherence, there was little improvement. She worked weekly in psychotherapy, which she found helpful, but Lauren continued to feel she that she was not a good student. She dreaded Mondays "because my teachers and friends know I am dumb," and only felt competent in art and poetry. Her clinician assumed that her depression interfered with her academic abilities, as she was a high achiever in elementary school.

Contributing Family, Social, and Educational History

Lauren lived with her parents, both physicians, and had two brothers, ages 17 and 9, who excelled socially and academically. Lauren attended seventh grade at a private school. Her teachers commented on her talent and creativity in art and poetry but noted her anxiety and struggle to keep up academically with her peers. Her teachers reported she was inattentive and unmotivated. They were unsure how to help her with her core classes.

Her parents were perplexed by her struggles, especially since the school had been such a good fit for both of her brothers. Given her love of writing and poetry, they were surprised by her struggles in language arts, especially with reading comprehension and classroom discussions. They emphasized that Lauren "does whatever we ask but easily gets lost on how to complete her work; poor kid."

Contemporary Diagnostic Interview

Early observations from the interview suggested that Lauren was of easy/flexible temperament with good cognitive flexibility. She promptly stated that she and her parents were happy the psychiatrist would be able to help her with her anxiety so she could do better in school. She struggled with giving detailed responses to the clinician's questions. She expressed feeling overwhelmed that she could not meet her own and her parents' expectations. She was sad and upset that she did not have as much time to listen to music and spend time with her friends because she was devoting more time to homework "to understand better."

In session, after rapport with the clinician was established, Lauren's good cognitive flexibility and passive style became evident: "Thanks for seeing me," she said. "I'm glad you want to help me." She was open about feeling anxiety on Sunday nights: "I feel so stressed about going to school on Mondays. I take notes and read a lot, but I just don't understand the material. If I ask for help, my teachers will know I'm a bad student." Lauren shared her artwork, and the clinician easily noted her talent (Fig. 4.12).

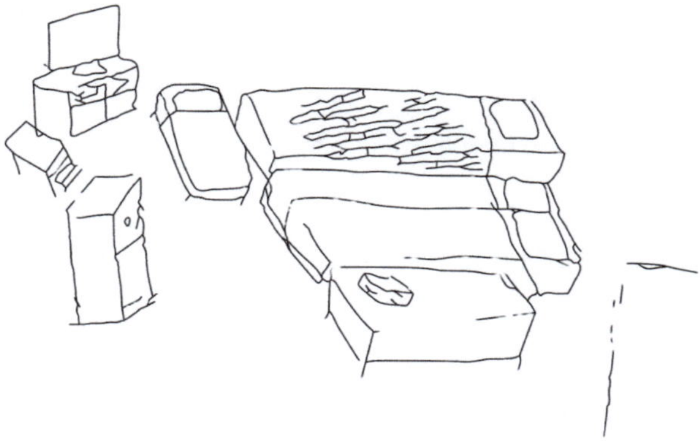

Fig. 4.12 Lauren's artwork

Formulation

Lauren's four pillars were of an adolescent with easy/flexible temperament, good cognitive flexibility, and an anxious attachment style within the context of a secure environment. Her cognitive functioning was difficult to ascertain during the interview but suggested cognitive weaknesses and difficulty processing social information. She did not endorse symptoms of a disease-based model for depression per se; rather, she was overwhelmed with the expectations placed by herself and her parents regarding her school performance. A psychological assessment was ordered for clarification of cognitive strengths and weaknesses.

Session (working memory) pearls
Struggled with giving detailed responses to the clinician's questions [*processing social information*].
Parents state, "She does whatever we ask but easily gets lost on how to complete her work; poor kid" [*cognitive weakness*].
Anxious "because my teachers and friends know I'm dumb." [*cognitive flexibility weakness*].

Results of Psychological Testing

FSIQ	VC	FR	VS	WM	PS
105 (63%) Average	98 (45%) Average	115 (84%) High average	117 (87%) High average	79 (8%) Very low avg.	114 (82%) High average

Summary of Psychological Testing: WISC-V

Primary Driver
Very low working memory

Secondary Driver
Anxious attachment style

Protective Drivers
Easy/flexible temperament, good cognitive flexibility, secure environment
High average visual-spatial, fluid reasoning, and processing speed

Formulation After Psychological Testing

When Lauren's psychological test results were used clinically in tandem with the information of her four pillars, she was best understood as having an adjustment disorder with anxiety due to her working memory weaknesses. Her enrollment in a high-achieving environment allowed several latent weaknesses to surface that were further impacted by her anxious attachment style, which contributed to her passive tendencies (self-imposing the need to meet her perception of people's expectations, despite evidence to the contrary). She had good cognitive flexibility skills and could discern when she had failed meeting others' expectations, which led her to have depressive and anxious feelings, even when others were willing to be helpful.

Lauren had many protective cognitive abilities: high average visual-spatial, fluid reasoning, and processing speed, which allowed her to put effort into her schoolwork. She shared that she created stories in her head, beginning by drawing a story board and then writing the dialogue of the plot, a clear indication that she had intuitively learned to work around her working memory weaknesses. Further academic testing was suggested to tease out the possibility of a reading comprehension learning disability, which would also explain her increased anxious feelings on Sundays before a school week.

Clinical Highlight

The fact that a Storm Chaser profile does not apply to Lauren, despite her very low working memory, highlights the many and complex biological factors that are involved in personality development. Recent research has uncovered some surprising findings regarding the relationship between working memory and creativity. Though this remains an intense area of study, there is substantial evidence that some forms of creative thinking can indeed flourish even in the context of poor working memory [24]. Lauren's good pillar protective factors—easy/flexible temperament,

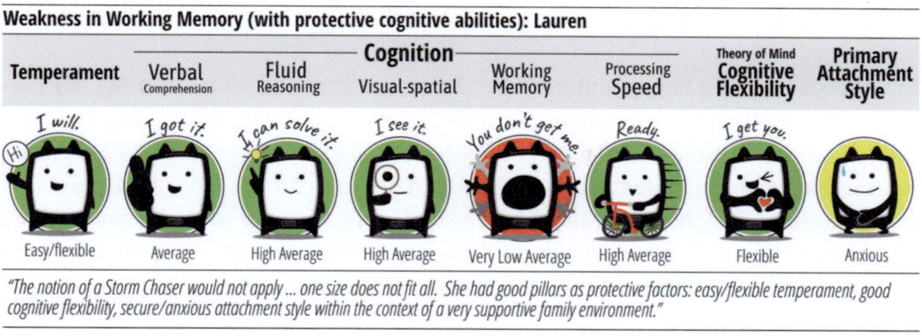

Fig. 4.13 Weakness in working memory (with protective cognitive abilities): Lauren

good cognitive flexibility, secure/anxious attachment style within the context of a very supportive family—helped her to implicitly compensate for her weakness and develop a jovial and creative personality, albeit somewhat anxious at times (Fig. 4.13).

Maladaptive Patterns

- Weakness in working memory will impact her learning abilities, especially in the context of new and challenging material.
- Feels anxious when attending school.
- Avoids expressing feelings that are critical of others due to her anxious attachment style.

Treatment and Intervention Recommendations

Individual psychotherapy will help Lauren recognize the impact her very low average working memory can have on her social and academic activities. Her clinician should help her develop realistic expectations by promoting her high average visual-spatial, fluid reasoning, and processing speed abilities within the context of her good cognitive flexibility skills. Her clinician should also help Lauren develop coping skills to reduce anxious feelings when challenged intellectually.

Suggested Interventions

- Educate parents and teacher of the struggles associated with very low average working memory.
- Provide schooling opportunities that maximize unique cognitive strengths in visual-arts and creativity.
- Encourage Lauren to make use of psychotherapy to improve self-esteem.

Additional Comments

Lauren's story has a happy ending. After learning the results of her testing, her parents understood that it was important to capitalize on her strengths. They enrolled Lauren in a middle school that used a visual approach in teaching (akin to Montessori-based education). Her talents in these areas led her to excel in school, and she found social circles in which she felt more comfortable. Finally, after several months in her new school, she told her therapist that she would like to stop psychotherapy, and politely said, "No offense, but I don't think I need your help anymore."

Relevant Cross-References

- Anxious attachment style: Chap. 5.
- Interventions for working memory weaknesses: Chap. 7.

Processing Speed Weakness: The Brave Turtle

Case 8: Carl

The Brave Turtle	*Synopsis: Carl*
Low average processing speed Needs a longer amount of time to reason and integrate social information Delays in responses may be experienced by others as a sign of him being defiant or a "slow learner." May be bullied or ostracized for slow short term memory functions.	Carl is a 12-year-old male seen in the out patient clinic for concerns of recent social withdrawal and unexpected academic struggles. Socially, Carl has a wide circle of friends and gets along well with them. He is described as the "quiet friend," as he is more of a listener than a talker.His parents began to restrict Carl from his friends as a consequence of his lower grades. In second grade, he was identified as educationally gifted.

DSM–5 Relevant History

In fourth grade, Carl was diagnosed with attention-deficit/hyperactivity disorder, predominantly inattentive type. His parents were unsure if he had benefited from the use of medication (methylphenidate). In seventh grade, he began to struggle completing school assignments that should have been easy for him and which were required to maintain his gifted placement. There was limited improvement with higher dosing of his stimulant medications. His father reported that the medications "stopped working when he entered seventh grade," adding, "I don't understand; he's so bright. Why is he so withdrawn and quiet? Is he depressed?" Carl denied feeling depressed.

Contributing Family, Social, and Educational History

Carl's parents divorced when he was 3 years old. He got along well with his step-parents and stepsister at his mother's house and was also pleased with his parenting schedule.

In second grade, Carl was identified as educationally gifted. In seventh grade at a local junior high school, although his grades were mainly As, he began to get Bs for not completing his assignments in the time allotted, which surprised Carl and his teachers, and also angered his parents, because "he knows the material."

Contemporary Diagnostic Interview

During the interview, Carl was quiet. When asked questions, he looked toward his mother, as if he wanted her to supply the answer. This angered his mother, who said, "You need to talk to the doctor so he can know how to help you." Carl looked back at the psychiatrist and said, in a soft voice, "I have problems at school. I can't finish my work on time." The psychiatrist noted his own initial urge to "speed up" the flow of the conversation; knowing that Carl was gifted, he expected more. However, the psychiatrist recognized that Carl needed more time to answer questions to feel comfortable in the session. After a few minutes, the psychiatrist, who liked college basketball, noted Carl's college basketball cap. He asked Carl about the cap and was surprised by how much Carl knew regarding college basketball. Carl became playful and debated with the psychiatrist which teams would make the NCAA tournament. The psychiatrist later asked Carl to review his understanding of his school difficulties. He again was thoughtful but slow to respond, which angered his mother.

Formulation

In using the information from a CDI, the clinician understood Carl's four pillars as including an easy/flexible temperament. Carl also had signs of slow processing speed when asked about stressful situations; less so when talking about areas in which he excelled due to use of long-term memory functions. He also had good cognitive flexibility and a secure form of attachment. He was referred for a psychological assessment to better understand the nature of his psychological functioning.

Session (speeding up the flow) pearls
The psychiatrist noticed his own urge to "speed up" the flow of the conversation. Knowing that Carl was gifted, he expected more.
Carl knew a great deal about college basketball and became playful and debated with the psychiatrist which teams would make the NCAA tournament [*excelled in use of long-term memory functions and had good cognitive flexibility*].

Results of Psychological Testing

FSIQ	VC	FR	VS	WM	PS
110 (75%) High average	118 (88%) High average	97 (42%) Average	114 (82%) High avg.	125 (95%) Very high avg.	83 (13%) Low average

Summary of Psychological Testing: WISC-V

Carl's psychological assessment revealed that his cognitive skills were in the high average range, and his subtest scores revealed memory, attention, and concentration as relative strengths. However, Carl's processing speed was in the low average range and represented an area of relative weakness.

Primary Driver

Low average processing speed

Secondary Driver

None

Protective Factors

Easy/flexible temperament, high average intelligence (high average verbal comprehension and very high working memory), good cognitive flexibility, and secure attachment.

Formulation After Psychological Testing

Carl's presentation is consistent with the profile of the Brave Turtle. Carl's testing revealed a high degree of cognitive strength that was limited by his low average processing speed. A weakness in the speed of processing routine information may make the task of comprehending information more time-consuming and difficult. Youths with weaknesses in processing speed may have more difficulty with tasks that require reasoning ability, both of which are important to the acquisition and understanding of information. Processing speed weaknesses require more time and increased mental effort for a person to understand new, complex information.

It often goes unnoticed that youths with processing speed weaknesses require additional time to process social information, including conversations, facial expressions, and group activities. For Carl, especially if others in his classroom have above average processing speed, he may appear withdrawn or uninterested. Often, as Carl's mother did during the interview, teachers or peers may ask Carl to promptly answer questions.

Carl's cognitive strengths will allow him to succeed in gifted classes, but he will require extra time to articulate what he hopes to say to others and to complete assignments. Additionally, at home, although his parents will appropriately have high expectations, it will be important for them to give Carl time to respond when asked questions or requests and to not assume he is being defiant. This should be considered when formulating his diagnosis, as this can easily be erroneously thought to be indicative of an attention-deficit/hyperactivity disorder, predominantly inattentive type. In addition, because of his low average processing speed, he will have a proclivity to feel anxious, which can be mistaken with symptoms of a generalized anxiety disorder, for which he does not meet *DSM–5* criteria.

Clinical Highlight

The Brave Turtle: Low average processing speed (Fig. 4.14).

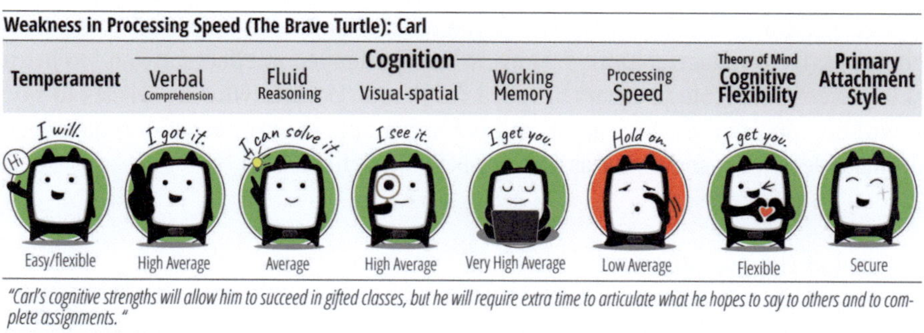

Fig. 4.14 Weakness in processing speed (The Brave Turtle): Carl

Alternative Formulations

Youths with weaknesses in processing speed combined with other indices in the low or below average range will have significantly more problems in understanding new information with their day-to-day reasoning ability. Consequently, they are at risk for emotional and behavioral problems that will not be adequately captured when viewed through the lens of a disease-based model diagnosis. Their maladaptive behaviors will be noted in contexts that require fast-paced, complex reasoning, and parents or teachers may assume they are being defiant. However, when their indices are above average, they may do well in situations that capitalize on their cognitive strengths, so long as the situation provides additional time to process social information (e.g., visual arts with visual-spatial strength, organization with working memory strength, etc.).

Maladaptive Manifestation

- Feels insecure and may appear to be shy.
- Has a slow processing speed, which can be viewed as defiance, increasing anxiety.
- Looks to others to answer questions that cause him anxiety.
- Has problems processing social information, including conversations, facial expressions, and group activities.

Treatment and Intervention Recommendations

Individual psychotherapy will help Carl recognize the impact his low average processing speed can have on his family, social, and academic activities. His psychiatrist should help promote his high average intelligence, good cognitive flexibility, and secure form of attachment. His psychiatrist should also help Carl to develop coping skills to reduce anxious feelings when challenged intellectually and to learn skills to communicate to others his need for time to process what he wishes to say. It will be important for his parents to give him ample time to respond to questions or make decisions, and to not assume he is being defiant.

Suggested Interventions

- Educate parents and teachers about Carl's struggles with low average processing speed. Parents should share with family and friends the reasons for Carl's slow responses. ("Please give him time to explain what he means.")
- Provide Carl additional time to process social information, including conversations, facial expressions, and group activities.

- Teach Carl skills to communicate to others that he needs time to process what he wants to say.
- Provide schooling opportunities that maximize his unique cognitive strengths.
- Teach him how to monitor time (an hourglass or digital timer is helpful).
- Encourage Carl to make use of psychotherapy to improve self-esteem.

Relevant Cross-References

- Interventions for processing speed weaknesses: Chap. 7.

Special Situations

Dyslexia and Nonverbal Learning Disorder (NLD)

Youths that have dyslexia or nonverbal learning disorders are a unique population. They may have average intelligence in the WISC-V, as will be seen in the cases below. Furthermore, they often score at grade level in academic achievement tests; their difficulties with reading comprehension are often not detected because they may have good vocabulary knowledge and the ability to deduce correct answers even if they do not understand what they are reading. The tests needed for these diagnoses require independent, specially trained psychologists who know how to interpret tests needed beyond a WISC-V. Furthermore, these psychological assessments are costly and often not covered under parents' insurance policies, as dyslexia and nonverbal learning disorder are unfortunately considered an educational diagnosis and not a clinical one. In short, the mental health effects that dyslexia and nonverbal learning disorder have on a youth's self-esteem and social interactions have not received the attention deserved. Furthermore, the psychological assessments needed for the diagnosis of dyslexia and nonverbal learning disorder are not part of school-based evaluations. Finally, some students with learning problems do not qualify for special education services if they perform at expected age or grade level.

Clinically, dyslexia and nonverbal learning disorder may be first diagnosed as attention-deficit/hyperactivity disorder, anxiety disorder, disruptive mood dysregulation disorder, bipolar disorder, or autistic spectrum disorder, with limited response to initial treatment [6, 23]. Clinicians must learn to distinguish dyslexia and nonverbal learning disorder from conditions that may exhibit symptomatic or syndromic overlap.

Given the number of youths with these disorders and with significant emotional, social, and behavioral difficulties, we provide the clinician a brief review of dyslexia and nonverbal learning disorder. This is followed by a clinical case of each condition to alert clinicians about the effects these conditions can have on a youth's development of emotional and behavioral skills necessary for success.

Despite increased awareness of dyslexia and nonverbal learning disorder in youths for more than 50 years, there is scant literature about the emotional, social, and behavioral consequences these conditions have on youths. These conditions affect 10–20% of the general population [23]. Herein, familiarity with dyslexia and nonverbal learning disorder has become remarkably important for the practicing clinician. The *DSM–5* [1] classifies dyslexia as an impairment in reading under the specific learning disability (SLD) category. Unfortunately, nonverbal learning disorder does not fit the category of a specific learning disability (SLD) and therefore is not included in the *DSM–5.* Moreover, nonverbal learning disorder is not a disability covered by the Individual with Disabilities Education Act [12], the special education law that ensures students with disabilities are provided free appropriate public education tailored to their needs.

Dyslexia

Dyslexia—the most common learning disability in children—varies in severity from mild to severe. Earlier identification of dyslexia produces the best outcomes. In 1968, the World Federation of Neurologists defined dyslexia as "a disorder in children who, despite conventional classroom experience [32], fail to attain the language skills of reading, writing, and spelling commensurate with their intellectual abilities." Furthermore, the International Dyslexia Association emphasizes that dyslexia has a neurobiological origin and "Typically, difficulties in patients with dyslexia stem from weaknesses in phonological components of language that are unexpected in relation to other cognitive abilities and the provision of effective classroom instruction [15]." As such, youths with dyslexia have difficulties with accurate and/or fluent word recognition and by poor spelling and decoding abilities. They can become frustrated as they learn to read, and as a consequence can develop behavioral problems that can appear to be symptoms of depression or mood dysregulation disorders. These children may lose interest in school-related activities and appear to be unmotivated or lazy. They may act out in order to draw attention away from their learning difficulties.

Case 9: David

David, a 7-year-old second-grader, disliked school. In first grade, he was happy going to school and played well with his peers, although his teacher noted his difficulty reciting the alphabet, although he liked learning about numbers and excelled in visual-spatial tasks, for example, playing Jenga, drawing animals for class, etc. His teacher noted his delay in reading skills and that he would memorize new words, hoping to know how to use them in later reading. When asked what letter a word started with, he would become confused. He preferred to draw his stories rather than write them, as requested by his teachers. By the fourth grade, he avoided schoolwork, which led to conflict with his parents. He began to experience physical symptoms, particularly on school days, and his parents and pediatrician were concerned about the possibility of an anxiety disorder.

DSM–5 Relevant History

David was treated with an SSRI for what was thought to be a generalized anxiety disorder. He initially felt better and was able to complete more of his schoolwork in the subjects he excelled in, although his reading skills did not improve, and his anxiety persisted on weekdays. An increase in his SSRI dosing did not improve his apparent anxiety. He began to have difficulties in social situations as he did not understand the implicit information exchanged during the ebb and flow of conversations.

Formulation

After limited response to medication for his anxiety, family conflicts around academic issues, and David receiving failing grades and showing a continued dislike for school, the psychiatrist referred David for a psychological assessment to better understand the nature of his cognitive weaknesses.

Results of Psychological Testing

FSIQ	VC	FR	VS	WM	PS
100 (50%) Average	89 (23%) Low average	109 (52%) Average	122 (93%) High avg.	91 (27%) Average	100 (50%) Average

Formulation After Psychological Testing

David's WISC-V results revealed a full-scale IQ score in the average range with verbal comprehension in the low average range, which did not explain the severity of his difficulties at school and home. Fortunately, his teachers shared with his parents that they had the impression he was not understanding his reading material. This encouraged his parents to pursue further academic testing, which revealed that his general reading abilities were in the low average range, and contextual fluency was below grade level. The scores of his subtests in conjunction with academic testing revealed that he had dyslexia (Specified Learning Disorder, with impairment in reading).

Diagnostically, it seems reasonable to consider David as having an adjustment disorder with anxiety due to the impact of dyslexia on his self-esteem.

Primary Driver

Impairment in reading: dyslexia

Protective Factors

Easy/flexible temperament, average intelligence, good cognitive flexibility, and a secure form of attachment.

Treatment and Intervention Recommendations

Individual psychotherapy is recommended to help David accept his dyslexia and recognize the impact it has on his family, social, and academic activities. His parents, clinicians, and teachers should help him use his average intelligence, good cognitive flexibility, and secure form of attachment to improve his self-esteem and develop coping skills to reduce his anxious feelings when challenged intellectually. Tutoring is important so he can learn the skills needed to communicate to others his need for extra time to process what he reads. It will be important for his parents to give him ample time to read and review material; they should not assume he is being defiant.

Suggested Interventions

- Educate parents and teacher about David’s struggles with dyslexia to facilitate schooling opportunities that maximize unique cognitive strengths; have him work with a person who is experienced in helping students with disabilities.
- Use visual organization strategies at home to keep track of Daniel’s chores and the family schedule.
- Encourage David to use active listening and note-taking software to keep track of tasks (sports practice or work schedule) or assignments.
- Recorded books are recommended.
- Provide additional time for David to process written information. Help him generate detailed outlines for writing; help him organize ideas and develop a plan for writing assignments.
- Use email to communicate with family and friends about important information; this will allow him to avoid anxiety if he forgets.
- Encourage David to make use of psychotherapy to improve his self-esteem.

David attended a learning center for youths with dyslexia, where they helped him develop practical learning methods, and accommodations were made at school to improve his educational needs. His parents were taught how to discern behavioral and academic difficulties present in youths with dyslexia and were able to modify how they approached David, providing rewards for his efforts to learn. His self-esteem improved, and he was able to have a better relationship with his parents without feeling anxious about not meeting their expectations. He was able to meet other peers his age with learning disabilities and socialized with them after school, which he enjoyed.

Nonverbal Learning Disorder (NLD)

It is generally agreed that verbal learning disorders affect academic and cognitive areas, but lesser recognized are the influences of nonverbal learning disorders (NLD or NVLD) on the social–emotional functioning of youth. Nonverbal learning disorders may be as prevalent as dyslexia, and, like other learning disabilities, cluster in families. Common features of nonverbal learning disorders include deficits in nonlinguistic information processing, speech prosody deficits, deficits in reading facial expressions, and associated impairment in interpersonal functioning. Furthermore, the severity of these deficits will vary among individuals with nonverbal learning disorders [6]. Youths with nonverbal learning disorders often have strengths in rote verbal memory, spoken language mechanics or form, and word reading. Youths may rely on their verbal skills as a principal means for social relating and anxiety relief and may withdraw from social situations as they become aware of their deficits. Youths with nonverbal learning disorder have difficulty playing and making friends and, as such, may often feel socially isolated. Critical skills of social reciprocity or understanding social context may lead to many superficial friendships but a lack of deep relationships.

Table 4.4 Differences between NLD and autistic spectrum disorder without intellectual disability

Clinical features	Nonverbal learning disorder	Autistic spectrum disorder without intellectual disability
Visual-spatial cognition	Difficulties having clear sense of direction	Precise knowledge of where objects or places are located
Math and reading comprehension	Recognize words and have good reading skills, although poor math and reading comprehension	Good age and grade level math and reading comprehension
Interests	Sustained attention to one topic for short periods, frequent changes of topic in conversations	Restrictive interests
Interpersonal actions	Mostly aware of shortcomings, a degree of mind sharing, empathy	Pedantic and blame others for social difficulties
Affect regulation	Easily overwhelmed by peer group social interactions. Often do not recognize when use of humor is offensive	Often have social anxiety and avoid being near nonfamily members

Source: Adapted from Delgado et al. [6] Does your patient have a psychiatric illness or nonverbal learning disorder?" Current Psychiatry

Individuals may commonly experience chronic low self-esteem, anxiety, and mood symptoms due to their limited capacity to express their feelings within the context of social reciprocity.

Importantly, youths with nonverbal learning disorders have social interaction difficulties that appear similar to those with autistic spectrum disorder. Overlapping behaviors, similar cognitive processes, and coexisting conditions may challenge even experienced clinicians ([6]; Table 4.4). However, impairments are more severe in autistic spectrum disorder and will present as early as age 4. Youths with autistic spectrum disorder show difficulty communicating, often engaging in pedantic or one-sided discussions of topics that are unusual for the age group, with poor attention to social cues. By contrast, communication difficulties in youths with nonverbal learning disorder are not apparent until after they start school. Youths with nonverbal learning disorder may be easily overwhelmed by peer group interactions but remain emotionally aware of their shortcomings. Youths with autistic spectrum disorder may have specific skills, such as expertise with directions and spatial reasoning, whereas youths with nonverbal learning disorder may get lost even when traveling to familiar places or may have difficulty relaying directions. Both groups likely will have good reading skills, but youths with nonverbal learning disorder will have trouble comprehending and integrating the material. However, these two disorders may be comorbid, thus complicating the diagnostic process. Early recognition of nonverbal learning disorder may, in some cases, prevent internalized psychopathology and loss of self-esteem [6]. Additionally, the social (pragmatic) communication disorder in *DSM–5* addresses the pragmatic language and communication deficits in these youths although it does not capture their weaknesses in math and visual-spatial abilities.

Case 10: Abby

Abby, a 12-year-old girl, was seen by a child psychiatrist because of her suicidal thoughts. Several months earlier she had felt "really sad, anxious, and depressed" and she texted her girlfriend photos of pills, a knife, and a person hanging, stating: "I need help." At that time, she began weekly psychotherapy, and although her mother noted that "her therapist said she really doesn't talk much in therapy," Abby reported that her depression was "getting better." Her mother noted that Abby improved over the summer and worsened at the beginning of the school year. Abby voiced that she didn't like school saying it was "too hard." Her mother did not think this was due to learning difficulties, as "she is a bright kid; she just needs to be motivated." Abby had a wide circle of friends and was liked for being jovial and having a good sense of humor, although her parents noted that her peers sometimes complained that she did not know when to "stop joking" when matters were of a serious nature.

During the school year, Abby struggled keeping up with classes. She became overwhelmed, and began to doodle on her assignments without completing them. She would say she was depressed because her parents were mad at her: "My grades are bad, and I don't know what to do." Her parents restricted her use of the smartphone and her activity with friends. She began to have increased difficulties in social situations, not understanding the ebb and flow of conversations, and she began to express feelings of anger toward her friends for being "mean to [her]."

DSM–5 Relevant History

When Abby was 11 years old, she was diagnosed with a generalized anxiety disorder. Sertraline was started and increased to 150 mg/day, with unclear results. She struggled making use of psychotherapy because she didn't "know what to talk about." Her therapist had voiced frustration to Abby's parents: "Abby is not being serious about it. She talks a lot, but about topics that are not related to her problems."

Formulation

Abby was very likeable, although the experience of talking with her was like talking with a younger child. She struggled to discuss her problems, and it was difficult for her to articulate her thoughts; she was literal and had trouble recalling the events that contributed to her sadness. She struggled to understand metaphors and was surprised when the clinician, attempting to empathize, shared that he understood how it felt "to have people think you are lazy, when, in fact, you work hard." She turned to her parents with anger: "Did you hear what he said? He thinks I am lazy and don't work hard." This simple example captures how Abby felt misunderstood by the clinician. Because of her difficulties with self-esteem and academic-related family conflicts, her psychiatrist referred Abby for a psychological assessment to better understand the nature of her cognitive and emotional weaknesses.

Results of Psychological Testing

FSIQ	VC	FR	VS	WM	PS
108 (70%) Average	111 (77%) High average	109 (73%) Average	122 (93%) High average	115 (84%) High average	108 (70%) Average

Formulation After Psychological Testing

The results from her psychological assessment revealed that Abby's cognitive skills were in the high average to average range. Despite this, her academic and emotional difficulties alerted her parents to the need to take Abby to an education specialist for further academic testing. This revealed that Abby had a nonverbal learning disorder, with her verbal skills stronger than her nonverbal skills, her verbal memory stronger than her visual memory, and a relative weakness in arithmetic.

Abby will be at an increased risk for depression because of failures in coping, loss of self-esteem, internalized psychopathology, and other social and emotional strains. In addition, individuals with nonverbal learning disorder may experience multiple psychosocial impairments, including difficulty maintaining employment, achieving goals, and maintaining relationships [6, 22].

Primary Driver
Nonverbal learning disorder

Secondary Driver
Limited cognitive flexibility

Protective Factors
Easy/flexible temperament, average intelligence, secure form of attachment.

Treatment and Intervention Recommendations

We recommend individual psychotherapy to help Abby recognize the impact her nonverbal learning disorder can have on her family, social, and academic activities. Her psychotherapist should encourage her to develop coping skills when anxious and to better communicate to others. It will be important for her parents to understand that her nonverbal learning disorder will affect her social and academic skills, which will contribute to anxious feelings and difficulties maintaining friendships. They should also not assume she is being defiant.

Suggested Interventions

- Educate parents and teacher of Abby's struggles with a nonverbal learning disorder.
- Provide Abby additional time to process verbal information.
- Encourage Abby to use individual psychotherapy to improve self-esteem.
- Recognize Abby's inability to accurately interpret nonverbal language, social norms, and interpersonal expectations, which interferes with her academic and social skills.
- Make teachers aware that Abby struggles with tasks that require higher level processing and understanding nuanced verbal information, comprehension of language structures, and abstract verbal directions and instruction.
- Socially, Abby's parents can help by teaching and modeling social skills, with attention to appropriately expressed emotions. This can be facilitated by actively watching movies or attending group activities together.
- Frequent informal assessments will be necessary to determine if Abby has grasped the information given.

- Ask Abby to repeat back instructions or demonstrate understanding to assess her comprehension, particularly as she navigates social situations.
- Use printed texts and materials to complement verbal presentations for subject areas that rely heavily on verbal presentation; this instructional format may be difficult for Abby.
- During group work at school, ensure specific social expectations are clearly stated, not assumed. Make directions and communications clear and concise.
- During conflicts, teachers and parents should be aware that Abby's failure to respond (or inappropriate responses) must be interpreted within the context of her difficulty understanding nonverbal and implicit aspects of communication. Unexpected behavioral responses should be considered a misinterpretation until proved otherwise.
- Use written lists, diagrams, and charts to help Abby learn new information. Abby is more likely to understand the relationship of concepts if they are represented in a visual chart or display rather than embedded in a verbal context.

Abby's parents learned to recognize behavioral and academic difficulties in youths with nonverbal learning disorder and were able to modify how they approached her, providing rewards for her efforts to learn. Abby's self-esteem and her relationship with her parents improved. She also felt less anxious when she did not meet their expectations. At Abby's school, teachers provided more frequent informal assessments to determine if she grasped the information given and asked her to rephrase instructions or demonstrate understanding to assess her comprehension. In history and language arts—classes in which Abby relied heavily on verbal presentations—teachers provided additional written text. They also provided visual charts or displays of information rather than embedding information in a verbal context. Abby's parents helped her to engage in weekly tutoring, which improved her academic skills and ultimately her self-esteem and anxiety. However, her teachers were flexible and were able to make shifts in their instructional approach after recognizing her difficulties understanding the structure and meaning of nonverbal information and social contexts. Unfortunately, it should be noted, not all schools accept nonverbal learning disorder as a valid diagnosis, and often do not provide the accommodations needed to improve an affected student's educational needs.

Closing Remarks

In this chapter, we shared an approach that is geared toward understanding the patient *from the inside out*. We consider intelligence to be the second pillar within the formulation of our personality. Broadly, it includes all cognitive processes that acquire, process, and act on information or stimuli. In the context of relationships, intelligence includes the capacity and know-how to engage in relationships based on mutual understanding of each other's ideas and intent. We describe a process of evaluating cognition followed by rich case examples in order to illuminate how to apply these concepts to complex children and adolescents. Weaknesses in intelligence lead to maladaptive behaviors and emotional dysregulation with increased likelihood of problems with self-esteem, interpersonal conflict, and academic functioning.

Importantly, we did not address the controversies surrounding the choice or quality of psychological tests or the difficulties using this information to help with educational aspects including advocacy for special education plans. We refer the reader to contemporary sources that present these issues in a balanced manner with practical interventions for parents to use to work with school staff [7].

References

1. American Psychiatric Association. Diagnostic and statistical manual of mental disorders. 5th edn DSM–5. American Psychiatric Association: Washington, D.C. 2013.
2. Blair C, Raver CC. Poverty, stress, and brain development: new directions for prevention and intervention. Acad Pediatr. 2016;16(3 Suppl):S30–6. https://doi.org/10.1016/j.acap.2016.01.010.
3. Bram AD, Peebles MJ. Psychological testing that matters: creating a road map for effective treatment. Am Psychological Assoc. 2014; https://doi.org/10.1037/14340-000.
4. Campbell JM, Brown RT, Cavanagh SE, et al. Evidence-based assessment of cognitive functioning in pediatric psychology. J Pediatr Psychol. 2008;33(9):999–1020. https://doi.org/10.1093/jpepsy/jsm138.
5. Council of National Psychological Associations for the Advancement of Ethnic Minority Interests. Testing and assessment with persons & communities of color. Washington, D.C.: American Psychological Association; 2016. Retrieved from https://www.apa.org/pi/oema.
6. Delgado SV, Wassenaar E, Strawn JR. Does your patient have a psychiatric illness or nonverbal learning disorder? Curr Psychol. 2011;10(5):17–35.
7. Franz C, Ascherman L, Shafiel J (2018) A Clinician's Guide to Learning Disabilities. Oxford, University Press.
8. Ferrer E, O'Hare ED, Bunge SA. Fluid reasoning and the developing brain. Front Neurosci. 2009;3(1):46–51. https://doi.org/10.3389/neuro.01.003.2009.
9. Fried R, Chan J, Feinberg L, et al. Clinical correlates of working memory deficits in youth with and without ADHD: a controlled study. J Clin Exp Neuropsychol. 2016;38(5):487–96. https://doi.org/10.1080/13803395.2015.1127896.
10. Hair NL, Hanson JL, Wolfe BL, et al. Association of Child Poverty, brain development, and academic achievement. JAMA Pediatr. 2015;169(9):822–9. https://doi.org/10.1001/jamapediatrics.2015.1475.
11. Holmes J, Gathercole SE, Dunning DL. Adaptive training leads to sustained enhancement of poor working memory in children. Dev Sci. 2009;12(4):F9–15. https://doi.org/10.1111/j.1467-7687.2009.00848.x.
12. Individual with Disabilities Education Act. 1990. Retrieved from https://sites.ed.gov/idea/.
13. Jones N. Analysis of African American and White American cognitive profiles for language and cultural influences. Educational Specialist. 2016;108. https://commons.lib.jmu.edu/edspec201019/108
14. Lin A, Northam EA, Werther GA, et al. Risk factors for decline in IQ in youth with type 1 diabetes over the 12 years from diagnosis/illness onset. Diabetes Care. 2015;38(2):236–42. https://doi.org/10.2337/dc14-1385.
15. Lyon GR, Shaywitz SE, Shaywitz BA. A definition of dyslexia. Ann Dyslexia. 2003;53:1–14. https://doi.org/10.1007/s11881-003-0001-9.

16. Mather N, Wendling BJ. Essentials of psychological assessment series. Essentials of dyslexia assessment and interveention. Hoboken: Wiley; 2012.
17. Merikangas KR, Nakamura EF, Kessler RC. Epidemiology of mental disorders in children and adolescents. Dialogues Clin Neurosci. 2009;11(1):7–20. https://doi.org/10.31887/DCNS.2009.11.1/krmerikangas.
18. Neisser U, Boodoo G, Bouchard TJ, et al. Intelligence: knowns and unknowns. Am Psychol. 1996;51(2):77–101. https://doi.org/10.1037/0003-066X.51.2.77.
19. Olmedo EL. Testing linguistic minorities. Am Psychol. 1981;36:1078–85.
20. Paulussen-Hoogeboom MC, Stams GJ, Hermanns JM, et al. Child negative emotionality and parenting from infancy to preschool: a meta-analytic review. Dev Psychol. 2007;43(2):438–53.
21. Reynolds CR. Methods for detecting construct and predictive bias. In: Berk RA, editor. Handbook of methods for detecting test bias. Baltimore: Johns Hopkins University Press; 1982. p. 192–227.
22. Rourke BP, Young GC, Leenaars AA. A childhood learning disability that predisposes those afflicted to adolescent and adult depression and suicide risk. J Learn Disabil. 1989;22(3):169–75.
23. Siegel LS. Perspectives on dyslexia. Paediatr Child Health. 2006;11(9):581–7. https://doi.org/10.1093/pch/11.9.581.
24. Smeekens BA, Kane MJ. Working memory capacity, mind wandering, and creative cognition: an individual-differences investigation into the benefits of controlled versus spontaneous thought. Psychol Aesthet Creat Arts. 2016;10(4):389–415. https://doi.org/10.1037/aca0000046.
25. Soubelet A, Salthouse TA. Personality-cognition relations across adulthood. Dev Psychol. 2011;47(2):303–10. https://doi.org/10.1037/a0021816.
26. Sternberg RJ, Grigorenko EL. Intelligence and culture: how culture shapes what intelligence means, and the implications for a science of well-being. Philos Trans R Soc Lond Ser B Biol Sci. 2004;359(1449):1427–34. https://doi.org/10.1098/rstb.2004.1514.
27. Squalli J, Wilson K. Intelligence, creativity, and innovation. Intelligence. 2014;46:250–7. https://doi.org/10.1016/j.intell.2014.07.005.
28. Turkheimer E, Haley A, Waldron M, et al. Socioeconomic status modifies heritability of IQ in young children. Psychol Sci. 2003;14(6):623–8.
29. Wahass SH. The role of psychologists in health care delivery. J Family Commun Med. 2005;12(2):63–70.
30. Weiss LG, Saklofske DH, Holdnack JA, et al. WISC-V: clinical use and interpretation. 2nd ed. San Diego: Academic Press; 2016.
31. Wolraich ML, Lambert W, Doffing MA, et al. Psychometric properties of the Vanderbilt ADHD diagnostic parent rating scale in a referred population. J Pediatr Psychol. 2003;28:559–67.
32. World Federation of Neurology. Report of research group on dyslexia and world illiteracy. Dallas: World Federation of Neurology; 1968.
33. Zhou H, Chen B, Rossi S. Effects of working memory capacity and tasks in processing L2 complex sentence: evidence from Chinese-English bilinguals. Front Psychol. 2017;8:595. https://doi.org/10.3389/fpsyg.2017.00595.

Chapter 5
Cognitive Flexibility (Theory of Mind): "Being in your Shoes"

There are three ways to ultimate success: The first way is to be kind. The second way is to be kind. The third way is to be kind.
–Fred Rogers (1928–2003).

Cognitive Flexibility/Theory of Mind

Cognitive flexibility or theory of mind (ToM) encompass aspects of cognition that allow us to psychologically approach new social interactions with openness knowing that our experience will be influenced by the others' state of mind. Cognitive flexibility also allows us to tolerate uncertainty when we interact with others. Interactions with others are influenced by social context and culturally appropriate norms [7].

Cognitive flexibility involves executive function, attention, working memory, and emotion regulation [13, 23]. As Koole [14] eloquently notes, "emotion regulation emerges as one of the most far-ranging and influential processes at the interface of cognition and emotion." Cognitive flexibility precedes the language development and typically emerges between 2 and 5 years of age [4]. Individuals with good cognitive flexibility handle complex situations by seeing them as growth opportunities rather than as personal threats. For example, when a child with good cognitive flexibility sees her mother at the door carrying balloons and a cake with candles, she knows that the balloons, cake, and candles are being brought to celebrate a birthday; she infers that her mother is happy to celebrate her birthday. Importantly, fluid reasoning and working memory (Chap. 4) are essential components of cognitive flexibility; these elements improve cognitive control and allow us to make inferences about difficult situations. Distributed networks subserve adaptability of thought and relational patterns, and functional magnetic resonance imaging (fMRI) studies implicate left hemispheric white matter (e.g., superior longitudinal/arcuate

S. V. Delgado et al., *Promoting the Emotional and Behavioral Success of Youths*,
https://doi.org/10.1007/978-3-030-88075-0_5

fasciculus) which connects frontal, parietal, and temporal cortical regions. Thus, the neurostructural foundation of cognitive flexibility is broad and distributed but is integrated and overlaps with the neural substrates with working memory, fluid reasoning, and processing speed [3].

For school-age children, we observe cognitive flexibility when they engage in meaningful conversations with peers and develop social competencies. This enhances their ability to share affectively detailed narratives with others. Additionally, the capacity to maintain intimacy in relationships, resolve conflicts, and adapt in novel and unfamiliar situations requires cognitive flexibility. Ultimately, cognitive flexibility is needed by child and parent to have reciprocal implicit growth-promoting communications.

> Tamara, a 6-year-old girl finishes a glass of milk and walks away from the kitchen table and leaving her glass on the table. Her father, in a supportive tone says: "Tamara" with the implicit intent of alerting Tamara that the glass should not be left on table and should be placed in the sink. Tamara looks back, implicitly understands and says, "Sorry, I forgot" and takes the glass to the sink.

Tamara implicitly infers mental state her father—a process that involves perceptual (explicit) and cognitive processes (implicit) [19, 22]. The explicit representation of the others' mental states requires understanding language and higher order reasoning [18]. Implicit processes comprise decoding of socially relevant information, e.g., facial expression, voice, and body motion. Ultimately, it is important to develop the ability to understand others mental states to feel happy, trusting, embarrassed, guilty, and shame, which are conducive to adapted behavior in groups [6].

In this chapter, we focus on conditions in youth in which the impact of cognitive flexibility deficits fluctuate based on situations and interactions. The deficits in cognitive flexibility appear to others as rigid behaviors. Youth with limited cognitive flexibility struggle to shift and adapt their perspectives during certain social interactions although not in all. In other words, we will describe cognitive flexibility in day-to-day, emotionally laden interactions in which difficulties understanding how others feel and think limit individuals' ability to predict the social consequences of their behaviors. However, these youth have periods of good cognitive flexibility when not in emotionally charged interactions, as will be described. We refer the reader elsewhere to understand and intervene in cases of *pervasive* cognitive and behavioral rigidity that characterize autism spectrum disorder (ASD), cluster A and C personality disorders, and obsessive-compulsive disorder (OCD) [10, 20].

Executive Functioning

Although executive functioning and cognitive flexibility overlap considerably, there are important differences. The inhibitory aspects of executive functioning are important to manage information input through cognitive flexibility [9]. Executive functioning consists of four domains: inhibition (self-control), interference control (resist distracting stimuli), working memory (planning), and cognitive flexibility (several ways to approach situations). Cognitive flexibility, while a component of executive functioning, is strongly influenced by temperament styles (Chap. 3), working memory, and fluid reasoning (logical thinking to solve problems independent of acquired knowledge) (Chap. 4).

Mentalization

At this point, you may wonder whether there are differences between cognitive flexibility/ToM and mentalization. Mentalization has long-standing roots in the psychoanalytic tradition [24] and gained popularity when Peter Fonagy, a psychoanalyst and developmental researcher, linked mentalization and attachment theory. Mentalization is a well-known concept that describes the ability to interpret behavior as meaningful and is based on the mental state of both "objects" the self and others, taking into account desires, needs, beliefs, reasons, and feelings [2].

Mentalization and cognitive flexibility/ToM fundamentally differ. Mentalization involves a person holding "mind (of the other) in mind (self)" and develops from object relations (i.e., the notion that a person incorporates others [objects] into his psyche and reacts to these objects). By contrast, cognitive flexibility/ToM takes into account the personal experiences people have, as well as the world in which they live and is influenced by temperament, executive function, attention, working memory, and emotion regulation as it relates to social context and to recognize the appropriate affect given various social contexts. In essence, cognitive flexibility/ToM promotes a cohesive and more flexible way of reflective abilities to know what works for healthy social reciprocity with implicit aspects of morality [8].

Cognitive Flexibility/ Theory of Mind Clinical Assessment

Clinicians request assessments of youth's cognitive flexibility or theory of mind competencies for many reasons. These assessments help clinicians know whether a child or adolescent can implicitly understand other's thoughts and behavior. Additionally, if assessments identify deficits in cognitive flexibility, clinicians can help parents to understand how these deficits may lead their child to have emotional and behavioral difficulties and how to approach these difficulties. We provide the reader an in vivo assessment approach for cognitive flexibility/ToM in preschool and school-age children, as well as adolescents in Chap. 2. In this chapter, we provide a brief review of the psychological tests often used to formally assess cognitive flexibility/ToM. The choice of test is influenced by the school of thought of the psychologist. We follow this with rich case examples with deficits in cognitive flexibility/ToM and are complimented by formal cognitive testing (Fig. 5.1).

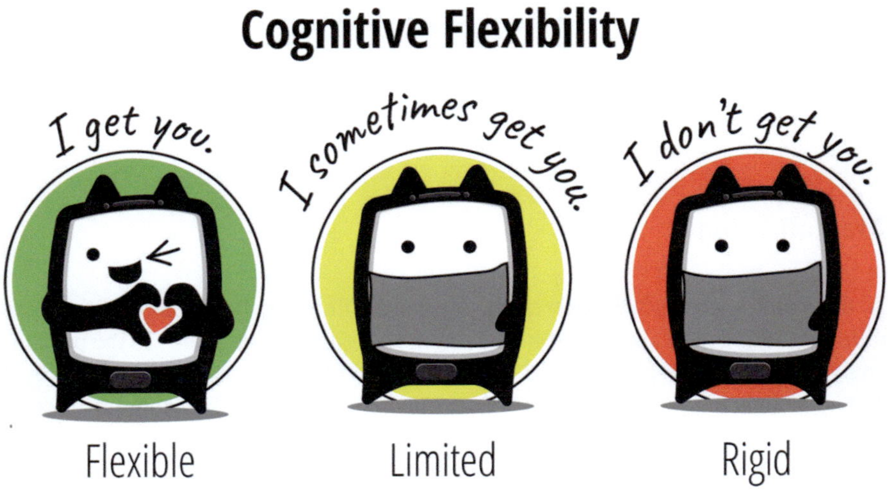

Fig. 5.1 Cognitive Flexibility

Cognitive Flexibility/Theory of Mind Testing

There are many tests available to formally assess cognitive flexibility/ToM in youth. These tests rely on language comprehension and will be undoubtedly difficult for youth with verbal comprehension and language problems. Therefore, it is important to have the cognitive flexibility/ToM psychological assessment sequenced after a WISC-V to confirm verbal comprehension abilities. However, some tests used to assess cognitive flexibility/ToM can overlap with projective tests that are used to assess personality styles or disorders (Chap. 6). In general, the test that is employed is chosen by the expertise psychologist who will administer it.

Rorschach Test | Ages 6+

The Rorschach, a projective test, consists of a series of black and white and color "ink blots" that have been used to assess personality, emotional functioning, unconscious conflict, and psychopathology. It was widely used in the psychoanalytic circles to assess intrapsychic functioning, e.g., ego functioning, quality of object relations, sublimation abilities, superego integration, motivation for treatment, etc. [5]. Some believe that Rorschach can be useful in assessing cognitive flexibility/ToM. The test involves showing the individual being tested five black-and-white inkblots and five color inkblots. The person is asked to describe what he or she sees (project) in each inkblot. The answers are then coded by taking all of the text transcribed during the test administration and turning it into numeric scores to be used later in the structural summary, and ultimately, for interpretation. The Rorschach test is perhaps the most famous and most controversial projective psychological test because Wood et al. [25] observed that when the Rorschach was administered to "healthy" individuals, almost half had Rorschach interpretations that suggested distorted thinking. Thus, false-positives are common with the Rorschach, and it should be used cautiously. In fact, some predict that the Rorschach test is on the brink of extinction in clinical and academic settings due to its decreasing use because of its psychoanalytic roots [21].

Theory of Mind Task Battery | Ages 2–18

The Theory of Mind Task Battery was designed to assess the cognitive flexibility/ToM in children and adolescents (age 2–18) with various cognitive and linguistic profiles and has excellent test–retest reliability [12]. This test can be used with nonverbal individuals; the person being tested can indicate responses either verbally or by pointing. This battery consists of 15 questions embedded within 9 tasks. The tasks are presented in short vignettes that begin to increase in difficulty. The tasks are presented in a story-book format with each page having colored illustrations and accompanying text. The short vignettes portray different scenarios and increase in complexity as it progresses, from the ability to identify facial expressions to the ability to infer false beliefs. The characters in the vignettes come from a range of races and ethnicities.

Behavior Rating Inventory of Executive Function, Second Edition- BRIEF2 | Ages 5–18

The Behavior Rating Inventory of Executive Function Second Ed (BRIEF2, [11]) is a self-report scale for children and adolescents aged 5–18 years and consists of eight scales that measure executive function. Used primarily across clinical, psychoeducational, and research settings, the BRIEF2 evaluates everyday behaviors associated with executive function in home and school. Clinicians may struggle to find convergence across forms and raters. As with many rating scales, the BRIEF2 asks respondents to describe how frequently they experience certain behaviors. Given the limited number of questions and frequency ratings on the measure, some behaviors may not be captured adequately.

NEPSY-II | Ages 3–16

NEPSY (A developmental NEuroPSYchological assessment) consists of a series of tests used to assess neuropsychological development in children ages 3–16 years in six functional domains. The NEPSY is grounded in developmental and neuropsychological theory and practice. The original English version of the NEPSY was published in 1998 and was superseded by the NEPSY-II in 2007 [15–17]. It was designed to assess cognitive functions not typically covered by general ability or achievement assessments. Most subtests are brief and useful in busy clinical settings. The NEPSY briefly evaluates six domains: (1) attention and executive functions; (2) language and communication, (3) sensorimotor functions; (4) visuospatial functions (5) learning and memory; (6) social perception (added in the NEPSY-II). NEPSY allows for selective assessment enabling the selection of certain subtests based on clinical need which helps reduce testing time. The subtests in the NEPSY-II that are relevant to the social perception domain are Affect Recognition and Theory of Mind.

Affect Recognition

Affect recognition is designed to assess youths' (1) ability to read emotional expression in others (happy, sad, anger, fear, disgust, and neutral), which is an important component of reciprocal social interactions; (2) capacity to follow nonverbal instructions or cues; (3) ability to recognize the impact of their behavior on others; and (4) ability to know how to alter their behavior to achieve the goal of the social interaction. Lower scores on this domain suggest poor recognition and identification of emotion in facial expressions.

Theory of Mind

Theory of Mind assesses youths' ability to understand mental functions, such as belief, intention, deception, emotion, imagination, and pretending. It also assesses the youth's ability to understand that others have their own thoughts, ideas, and feelings that may be different from their own. It further assesses how a child or adolescent is able to understand how emotion relates to social context and to recognize the appropriate affect given various social contexts. Low scores suggest difficulty in comprehending others' perspectives, experiences, and beliefs.

The results of the NEPSY-II describe and characterize youths' skills, but they should not be used to determine diagnosis. However, in our experience, the NEPSY-II can be used in conjunction with the CDI and subtest indices from the WISC-V, to provide a broader understanding of a child or adolescent's cognitive strengths and weakness when interacting with family and friends.

Cases

Youth that are representative of deficits in cognitive flexibility/ToM are those with borderline and narcissistic personality disorders. These deficits can exist with or without weaknesses in their intelligence. In essence, this confirms the several neurobiological pathways of personality disorders.

Adolescent with Low Average Working Memory, Below Average Theory of Mind Struggles Engaging in Psychotherapy

Synopsis: Mason is a 16-year-old male with extensive history of outpatient treatment for disruptive behaviors since he was 12 years.

DSM–5 Relevant History

- Previous diagnoses of attention-deficit/hyperactivity disorder, predominantly combined type; disruptive mood dysregulation disorder; oppositional defiant disorder; and a mood disorder, was considered.
- Initially his treatment consisted of individual and family therapy, and when his disruptive behaviors escalated, he was treated symptomatically with medications.
- Stimulants were stopped due to increased agitation and poor sleep; mood stabilizers (quetiapine and risperidone) were stopped due to drowsiness and weight gain; alpha-adrenergic agents (guanfacine ER) provided some improvement of his impulsive behaviors, but he would refuse to take.
- Discharged from psychotherapy due to his refusal to engage and his oppositional behavior during sessions.

Contributing Family, Social, and Educational History

- Mason lived with his biological parents.
- Mason was a social child until he was 6 when he became more isolated and less social although he would tell his parents that he had many friends even though it was clearly not accurate.
- In elementary school, he would text his peers, but they would not respond.
- When around adult family members he would intrude in conversations and would boast how likeable and smart he was.
- His parents had wondered if his being manipulative was to "annoy others and get what he wants" and if his disruptive behaviors were a symptom of depression.

- In adolescence, his defiant behaviors increased and his parents noted, "He doesn't appear to care about us or anyone else" and were hoping someone could "get into his mind and tell us why he is so difficult."

Contemporary Diagnostic Interview

History

- In term of attachment style, he had a long history of difficulty forming trusting relationships with adults or peers.
- He had few friends but tended to demand that others admire his intellect.
- Difficulties considering his parents and others' perspectives about his problems.
- Believed his problems were his parents' fault for not providing what he demanded and because they were "too uptight about my behavior."

Formulation

During his psychiatric evaluation, the clinician using a CDI style interview found Mason difficult to engage with. The clinician understood Mason's pillars as having a difficult/feisty temperament, average cognition, limited cognitive flexibility with a dismissive form of attachment with narcissistic personality traits. Mason was referred for a psychological assessment to better understand the nature of his functioning.

Session (in the moment) pearls
Used his intellect to dismiss the attempts made by the clinician to empathically join in learning his point of view regarding his problems, "you won't be able to understand me. I am sure you don't see bright kids like me."
Later
"Your resident isn't very good. She didn't know what to say when I told her I was smarter than her." [*he noticed the resident had gathered background history including academic abilities, before the psychiatrist entered the room*]. "I do not want to talk to her anymore, she needs to leave!" [*in spite of reassurance to Mason from the psychiatrist and his parents, he did not agree and it was best for the resident to leave the interview*].

Results of Psychological Testing

FSIQ	VCI	FR	VS	WM	PS
94 (34%) Average	103 (58%) Average	100 (50%) Average	92 (30%) Average	82 (12%) Low avg.	105 (63%) Average

Summary of Psychological Testing–WISC-V

Primary Driver
Low average working memory.

Results of Cognitive Flexibility/ToM Testing

NEPSY–II	
Affect Recognition	**Theory of Mind**
At Expected Level	Below Average

Summary of Cognitive Flexibility/Theory of Mind–NEPSY-II

Secondary Driver
Below average theory of mind.

Discussion of NEPSY-II

In the subtest of affect recognition, Mason was able to recognize the impact of his behavior on others and how to alter his behavior accordingly in a way that is consistent with others his age.

In the Theory of Mind subtest, Mason poorly understood others' perspectives, experiences, beliefs, and feelings as being different from his. In this area, he was noted to function poorly in day-to-day, emotionally laden interactions, particularly if these interactions occurred when there were other demands that he needed his attention. His difficulties understanding other's views contributed to social problems related to a limited or delayed ability to understand how others feel and think in different situations. Moreover, he had difficulty predicting the social consequences of his behaviors or understanding the impression other people have of him from his behaviors.

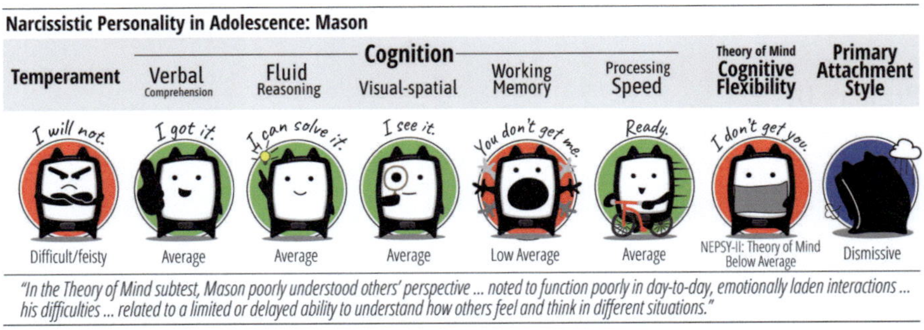

Fig. 5.2 Narcissistic Personality in Adolescence: Mason

Formulation After Psychological Testing

Mason was best understood as having low average working memory (Chap. 4) and below average cognitive flexibility (moral compass), with emerging narcissistic personality disorder traits and a dismissive attachment style (Fig. 5.2).

Maladaptive Manifestation

- Feelings of superiority and excessive need for admiration.
- Sense of entitlement.
- Low frustration tolerance.
- Willingness to take advantage of others to achieve goals.
- Lack of understanding and consideration for other people's thoughts and feelings.
- Projecting blame onto others for his mishaps.

Treatment and Intervention Recommendations

Psychotherapy is the primary treatment for narcissistic personality disorder.

- Individual, e.g., Mentalization-Based Therapy–Adolescent (MBT–A), family and group therapy to promote cognitive flexibility.

Goals

- Relate to others in a positive way.
- Have more realistic expectations of others.
- Listen to others reasoning.

Suggested Interventions

- Educate parents of Mason's struggles with low average working memory.
- Listen to Mason's reasoning without necessarily agreeing and diffuse conflict by asking about something to occur in the future.
- Engage in redirecting conversations to areas of mutual agreement.
- Redirect Mason when making negative comments in front of others, "Mason, let's talk about something else like ..."
- While medications are not specifically indicated, some clinicians might use SSRIs to address anxiety or affective symptoms, as well as $\alpha 2$ agonists to address impulse control and affective dysregulation. Additionally, antipsychotics or "mood stabilizers" to target overlapping symptoms of affective dysregulation. However, these medications may not improve emotional regulation or maladaptive behaviors.

Relevant Cross-References

- Working memory: Chapters 4 and 7.
- Narcissistic personality: Chap. 6.

Adolescent with very low average working memory and processing speed, well below average theory of mind and low average fluid reasoning and visual-spatial abilities

Synopsis: Brooke, an 11-year-8-month-old girl, described feeling depressed and reported loss of interest in school and persistent suicidal ideation with superficial cutting on her arms.

DSM–5 Relevant History

- Since the age of 6, Brooke had been treated as an outpatient for her on-going aggressive and disruptive behaviors at home and school.
- Brooke had been previously diagnosed with reactive attachment disorder, disruptive mood dysregulation disorder, mood disorder, and oppositional defiant disorder.
- Her parents noted an increase in both severity and frequency of her problematic behaviors after she entered middle school.
- Over the years, SSRIs and later an SNRI, in combination with weekly supportive and dialectical behavioral psychotherapy provided limited improvement.

- Brooke's subsequent psychopharmacologic treatment included olanzapine, risperidone, quetiapine aripiprazole, and augmentation with lithium. Medications were frequently changed as a result of minimal benefit and frequent side effects.
- She had two short 3-day inpatient psychiatric admissions for impulsive aggression (hitting and tearing up her sister homework daily, threatening to set fire in her room).

Contributing Family, Social, and Educational History

- As a result of neglect, Brooke was placed in foster care when she was 18 months of age.
- Brooke was adopted by her parents at 20-months-of-age and had a history of in-utero exposure to alcohol, nicotine, and opiates.
- By age 4, she had attempted to start fires and would hide her sibling's medications and laugh when caught.
- Brooke had some protective factors. She had a positive attitude when caring for special needs younger children and elderly family members.
- She had a great singing ability and liked going to the church choir.
- She had dexterity for sports although she struggled complying with the coach's requests.
- Academically she was unmotivated and demonstrated poor attention and poor academic functioning.

Contemporary Diagnostic Interview

History

- She maintained relationships with peers that were similar to her who had conflict with adults and peers although her parents would try to restrict her interactions with them.
- She was aggressive toward siblings whom she experienced as receiving more parental attention.
- Argued with certain peers that she felt were "fake and back-stabbers."
- Dreaded going to school because she struggled educationally and displaced the blame on others, "my teachers and friends are dumb."

Formulation

Brooke presented to the clinician based on the information obtained from a CDI, with a defiant attitude capturing in-vivo her hardwired difficult/feisty temperament. Due to her apparent weaknesses in cognitive and cognitive flexibility functioning, the clinician chose to use brief assessment of cognitive flexibility questions typically used in elementary school-age children (Chap. 2). Brooke experienced the questions as difficult and intrusive. She began to escalate and said she would no longer talk to the clinician and would be drawing, and he should ask her parents questions if he needed more information. Since she enjoyed drawing, the clinician empathically asked if she could draw her bedroom which she complied and stated, “This is fun, just don’t ask me lots of stupid questions like other people.” Her drawing was simple, like a younger age child’s”, suggesting visual-spatial difficulties (Fig. 5.3). Her dismissive attitude toward affect-laden issues suggests impairment in her cognitive flexibility and demonstrated a dismissive style of attachment. Her new consulting child psychiatrist requested a psychological assessment given the years of failure of outpatient management and evidence of dangerousness at home.

Session (in the moment) pearls
Brooke enjoyed drawing, the clinician empathically asked if she could draw her bedroom which she complied and stated, “this is fun, just don’t ask me lots of stupid questions like other people.”
Suggestive weakness in working memory and fluid reasoning when feeling that nonthreatening inquiring questions are “stupid” e.g. “Don’t ask me lots of stupid questions like other people.”
Simple and rudimentary drawings suggest weakness in visual-spatial abilities.

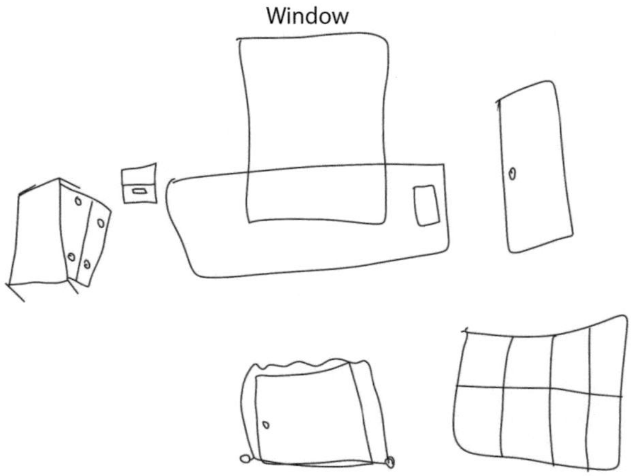

Fig. 5.3 Drawing of bedroom: The relative size of objects is exaggerated in terms of their importance to her (e.g., large bed). This tendency is typical of the egocentricity seen in younger children (ages 5-7)

Results of Psychological Testing

FSIQ	VCI	FR	VS	WM	PS
91 (27%) Average	100 (50%) Average	82 (12%) Low Avg.	84 (14%) Low Avg.	79 (8%) Very Low Avg.	75 (5%) Very Low Avg.

Summary of Psychological Testing–WISC-V

Primary Drivers
Very low working memory and processing speed.

Results of Cognitive Flexibility/Theory of Mind Testing

NEPSY-II	
Affect Recognition	**Theory of Mind**
At Expected Level	Well Below Expected Level

Summary of Cognitive Flexibility/ToM Testing –NEPSY-II

Secondary Drivers
Well below average theory of mind.
Low average fluid reasoning and visual-spatial abilities.

Discussion of NEPSY-II

In the subtest of affect recognition, Brooke demonstrated an ability at expected level to recognize the impact of her behavior on others and how to alter her behavior accordingly.

In the Theory of Mind subtest, Brooke scored at a well below average level which indicated poor comprehension of other's perspectives, experiences, beliefs, and feelings as different from hers. Her skills in this area are likely much poorer in day-to-day emotionally laden interactions if they involve a significant amount of reasoning ability. Her weakness will contribute to social problems and will have difficulty predicting the social consequences of her immature behaviors.

Results of Personality Testing

Due to Brooke's age, 11 years and 8 months, the M-PACI (Million Pre-Adolescent Clinical Inventory) was administered.

Primary Drivers

- Emerging personality structure with affective and interpersonal instability due to an immature, nebulous, and wavering sense of identity.
- She may exhibit extended periods of dejection and apathy interspersed with spells of irritability, anxiety, or resentment.
- When feeling cheated, and unappreciated, her underlying ambivalence makes her struggle between feelings of anger and shame.
- Resentment toward others may be turned against herself in a self-critical, condemnatory manner that can lead to self-harm and suicidal thoughts.
- When others become increasingly frustrated with her behavior, the more her self-deprecatory and self-harm behaviors are likely to arise.
- Her unstable personality organization predisposes her to episodes of emotional, cognitive, or behavioral dysfunction related to mounting internal pressures or overwhelming external demands.
- May attack others capriciously for their lack of support and for what she sees as their unreasonable expectations and demands.

Formulation After Psychological Testing

Brooke's test results are complex. In situations where there is high scatter (significant variation in individual domains), a full-scale IQ is not reported. This was the case for Brooke based on her very low scores in working memory and processing speed relative for verbal comprehension and perceptual reasoning that are within the "normal range." Instead, a General Abilities Index (GAI) is reported in situations where there is such significant variation, as it provides an estimate of intellectual functioning than the full-scale IQ. As we reviewed in Chap. 4, an individual with working memory weaknesses that are accompanied by difficult/feisty temperament may appear exhibit relational patterns, distress, and emotional instability that look clinically like borderline personality disorder in adolescence (Chap. 6).

Brooke's symptoms as well as the severity of her symptoms vary depending on the complexity of the demands within the context of her abilities. As such, capturing her symptoms and presentation as a single (or even multiple) *Diagnostic and*

Statistical Manual of Mental Disorders (5th edition (DSM-5); American Psychiatric Association, 2013) [1] diagnoses would be difficult and it is likely that a clinician using such an approach would diagnose Brooke as having a mood disorder and/or impulse control disorder, although a diagnosis of oppositional defiant disorder might also be rendered given that this would capture many of Brooke's behaviors. However, these diagnoses do not capture the etiology of these symptoms.

Although tempting to consider Brooke having a reactive attachment disorder, as stated in Chap. 6, the genesis is always due to active trauma; specifically, the severe emotional neglect which occurred before she was adopted at 20 months of age and she has lived in a nurturing and stable environment for 11 years, acquiring many protective factors: positive attitude when caring for special needs younger children and elderly family members; a great singing ability and liked going to the church choir and dexterity for sports activities. We can be sure that her history of in-utero exposure to alcohol, nicotine, and opiates had an impact on her four pillar development, but as described not all were affected negatively.

We can best understand Brooke as having significant cognitive difficulties that contribute to her maladaptive and immature behaviors (very low working memory and processing speed, as well as low average fluid reasoning and visual-spatial abilities, Chap. 4). When combined with her difficult/feisty temperament and cognitive rigidity, she is likely to be irritable and difficult to reason with. Furthermore, she has below average cognitive flexibility with a dismissive style of attachment and emerging traits of borderline personality disorder in adolescence.

These youth frequently struggle to know the importance in being able to adapt to social norms and develop a healthy relationship. They struggle to accurately categorize information for future use. In the long-term, these weaknesses will lead to difficulty organizing themselves to solve interpersonal problems. When combined with temperamental concerns and when presented with challenging situations, we would expect a range of affective responses ranging from reactive depression, irritability, and mood lability. The severity of these symptoms can vary, and in Brooke's case resulted in her making superficial cuts on her arms and thighs in times of distress and intense affect (Fig. 5.4).

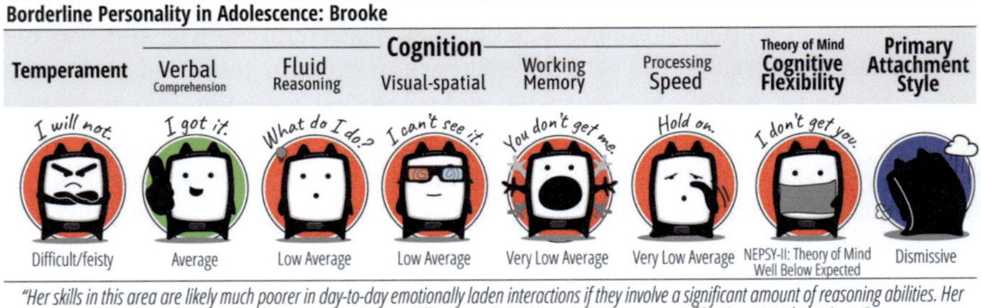

Fig. 5.4 Borderline Personality in Adolescence: Brooke

Why Are Youth like Brooke Labeled as Having Affective Disorders?

In short, the parents of these youth try to help when their child experiences turmoil. However, this approach does not help clinicians to recognize these youths' strengths and adaptive skills. For example, Brooke has a positive attitude when she cares for special needs children, younger children, and elderly family members. She excels in singing and enjoys singing in the church choir and is athletic. For Brooke, the triggers of her mood dysregulation are specific to her cognitive and psychological weaknesses and emerge when she confronts complex situations that overwhelm her ability to manage them. She quickly returns to an adaptive emotional state when she finds her parents, peers, and others as understanding and nonthreatening. By contrast, in an affective disorder, one can expect that episodes of mood dysregulation are chronic, severe, and not predominantly tied to cognitive abilities.

Maladaptive Patterns

- Expects that people cannot be trusted and will not be available to support her. This leads to her feelings abandoned.
- Develops intense and unstable relationships that are alternate between extremes of idealization and devaluation.
- Breaks up close relationships in anticipation that she will be rejected.
- Feels empty and has fluctuations in self-image and feels dependent on specific negative relationships to maintain her sense of identity.
- Intense instability, irritability, or anxiety that may last for several days.
- Projects blame onto others for their mishaps.
- Recurrent self-injurious and suicidal behaviors.

Treatment and Intervention Recommendations

- Psychotherapy is the primary treatment for borderline personality disorder.
- Individual, e.g., Cognitive Behavior Therapy (CBT), Dialectical Behavior Therapy-Adolescent (DBT-A), Interpersonal Therapy-Adolescent (IPT-A), family, and group therapy to promote cognitive flexibility.
- Kinesthetic yoga can also help Brooke to increase body awareness, self-regulation skills using movement and breath.

Goals

- Identify cognitive distortions about relationships and self-image.
- Relate positively to others.

- Have realistic expectations of others.
- Develop coping skills that reduce stress and conflict.

Suggested Interventions

- Educate Brooke's parents so that they understand that her cognitive defects contribute to her maladaptive manifestations and borderline personality disorder.
- Engage in case management, when available, to provide her a person to coordinate medical, psychological, and educational appointments, and avoiding conflict with her parents if they were to enforce them.
- Reinforce adherence to psychotherapy.
- Develop solution-focused approaches for family, social, and academic struggles.
- When Brooke is older, help her to find employment that can support her strength in verbal comprehension and limit interpersonal interactions for positive outcomes (e.g., working with pets, flower shop, packing operations helping disabled children, etc.).
- Authoritarian approaches will elicit resistance and anger.
- While medications are not specifically indicated, some clinicians might use SSRIs to address anxiety or affective symptoms, as well as α_2 agonists to address impulse control and affective dysregulation. Additionally, antipsychotics or "mood stabilizers" target overlapping symptoms of affective dysregulation. However, these medications may not improve emotional regulation or maladaptive behaviors.

Relevant Cross-References

- Working memory, processing speed: Chapters. 4 and 7.
- Borderline personality disorder: Chapters. 6 and 7.

References

1. American Psychiatric Association. Diagnostic and statistical manual of mental disorders. 5th ed. Washington, DC: DSM-5. American Psychiatric Association; 2013.
2. Allen JG, Fonagy P, Bateman A. Mentalizing in clinical practice. Washington, DC: American Psychiatric Publishing Inc; 2008.
3. Barbey AK, Colom R, Grafman J. Architecture of cognitive flexibility revealed by lesion mapping. NeuroImage. 2013;82:547–54.
4. Blackwell KA, Cepeda NJ, Munakata Y. When simple things are meaningful: working memory strength predicts children's cognitive flexibility. J Exp Child Psychol. 2009;103:241–9.
5. Bram AD. The relevance of the Rorschach and patient-examiner relationship in treatment planning and outcome assessment. J Pers Assess. 2010;92(2):91–115. https://doi.org/10.1080/00223890903508112.

6. Cotter J, Granger K, Backx R, et al. (2017) social cognitive dysfunction as a clinical marker: a systematic review of meta-analyses across 30 clinical conditions. Neurosci Biobehav Rev. 2018;84:92–9. https://doi.org/10.1016/j.neubiorev.11.014.
7. Delgado SV, Strawn JR. Difficult psychiatric consultations: an integrated approach. Springer; 2014.
8. Delgado SV, Strawn JR, Pedapati EV. Contemporary psychodynamic psychotherapy for children and adolescents: integrating Intersubjectivity and neuroscience. Springer; 2015.
9. Diamond A. Executive functions. Annu Rev Psychol. 2013;64:135–68.
10. Geurts HM, Corbett B, Solomon M. The paradox of cognitive flexibility in autism. Trends Cogn Sci. 2009;13(2):74–82. https://doi.org/10.1016/j.tics.2008.11.006.
11. Gioia GA, Isquith PK, Guy SC, et al. BRIEF2: behavior rating inventory of executive function. Second Psychological Assessment Resources. 2015;
12. Lutz FL, Hutchins TL, Prelock PA, Bonazinga LA. Psychometric evaluation of the theory of mind inventory (ToMI): a study of typically developing children and children with autism spectrum disorder. J Autism Dev Disord. 2012;42:327–41.
13. Johnson DR. Emotional attention set-shifting and its relationship to anxiety and emotion regulation. Emotion. 2009;9(5):681–90. https://doi.org/10.1037/a0017095.
14. Koole SL. The psychology of emotion regulation: an integrative review. Cognition Emotion. 2009;23(1):4–41.
15. Korkman M, Kirk U, Kemp S (1998). NEPSY: a developmental neuropsychological assessment. Retrieved December 10, 2008, from the mental measurements yearbook database.
16. Korkman M, Kirk U, Kemp S. NEPSY-II: administration manual. San Antonio, TX: Harcourt Assessment; 2007a.
17. Korkman M, Kirk U, Kemp S. NEPSY-II: clinical and interpretive manual. San Antonio, TX: Harcourt Assessment; 2007b.
18. Meinhardt-Injac B, Daum MM, Meinhardt G, et al. The two-systems account of theory of mind: testing the links to social- perceptual and cognitive abilities. Front Hum Neurosci;12:25 Published 2018 Jan 31. 2018; https://doi.org/10.3389/fnhum.2018.00025.
19. Mitchell RL, Phillips LH. The overlapping relationship between emotion perception and theory of mind. Neuropsychologia. 2015;70:1–10. https://doi.org/10.1016/j.neuropsychologia.2015.02.018.
20. Paast KZ, Memari AH, et al. Comparison of cognitive flexibility and planning ability in patients with obsessive compulsive disorder, patients with obsessive compulsive personality disorder, and healthy controls. Shanghai Arch Psychiatry. 2016;28(1):28–34. https://doi.org/10.11919/j.issn.1002-0829.215124.
21. Paul AM. The cult of personality: how personality tests are leading us to miseducate our children, mismanage our companies, and misunderstand ourselves. New York Free Press; 2004.
22. Schaafsma SM, Pfaff DW, Spunt RP, et al. Deconstructing and reconstructing theory of mind. Trends Cogn Sci. 2015;19:65–72. https://doi.org/10.1016/j.tics.2014.11.007.
23. Schmeichel BJ, Volokhov RN, Demaree HA. Working memory capacity and the self-regulation of emotional expression and experience. J Pers Soc Psychol. 2008;95(6):1526–40. https://doi.org/10.1037/a0013345.
24. Target M. Commentary. In: Busch F, editor. Mentalization: theoretical considerations, research findings, and clinical implications. London: Analytic Press; 2008. p. 261–79.
25. Wood JM, Nezworski TM, Lilienfeld SO, et al. What's wrong with the Rorschach?: science confronts the controversial inkblot test. San Francisco, CA: Jossey-Bass; 2003.

Chapter 6
Personality: "My Friends Are Just Like Me"

Personality is like a charioteer with two headstrong horses, each wanting to go in different directions.
—Martin Luther King, Jr. (1929–1968)

Personality

Personality refers to individual differences in patterns of thinking, feeling, and behaving within the family, social, and cultural context. As Meltzoff [50] observed, "We are not born social isolates. We are fundamentally connected to others right from the start, because they are seen as being 'like me.' This allows rapid and special learning from people." He later adds, "Social cognition rests on the fact that 'you' are 'like me,' differentiable from me, but nonetheless enough like me to become my role model and I your interpreter." Herein, as attachment theory posits, a secure environment allows an infant to explore how to interact with others, which represents an important step for the developing brain architecture, self-regulation abilities, and forming attachments with others. Secure, organized attachments develop when an emotionally available caregiver responds consistently to the infant's distress. Over time, the child makes use of growth-promoting and challenging experiences, and gradually becomes able to self-regulate rather than relying on his or her caregivers; the child effectively becomes himself or herself [26].

The first three pillars—temperament, cognition, and cognitive flexibility—contribute to the development of personality. Current evidence suggests the transition from adolescence to young adulthood is characterized by continuity of personality and increasing maturity; adolescents develop more control and social confidence, and less anger and alienation [37, 62, 64].

S. V. Delgado et al., *Promoting the Emotional and Behavioral Success of Youths*, https://doi.org/10.1007/978-3-030-88075-0_6

Attachment Theory

Attachment theory assumes that a secure attachment develops when the infant can successfully regulate his or her emotional state. This secure attachment is initially learned through early nonverbal communication with the parent. This process helps the infant learn how to tolerate positive and negative nonverbal emotions and, over time, the ability to regulate these emotions verbally. It is internalized during this process, leading to the development of the internal working model of attachment (IWMA) to others [24]. However, when the infant is unable to internalize early regulatory experiences because of weaknesses in the first three pillars or because of traumatic experiences, he or she may develop insecure internal working models of attachment and obstruct functional regulation of emotions. Attachment style is critically relevant to the development and persistence of personality disorders in youth. Accordingly, we will briefly review the relevant aspects of attachment theory that help us understand personality disorders.

The "father of attachment theory," British psychiatrist and psychoanalyst John Bowlby (1907–1990) posited that infants need to develop a relationship with at least one primary caregiver, regardless of gender, for healthy psychological development to occur. Through his work with infants, Bowlby described an evolutionary, innate wish infants desire for close, shared experiences with their primary caregivers for survival, growth, and development (1999). According to Bowlby, this biologically rooted urge, developed early in life, creates attachment behavioral systems that allow the infant to assess whether his caregiver is available not only physically, but emotionally. Bowlby further suggested that the quality of the attachment between the infant and the parent or primary caregiver predicts a child's later social and emotional facility [11]. The parent or caregiver strongly influences how the infant develops the capacity for emotional regulation of his or her feelings, creating an "internal working model of social relationships" that serves as a template when relating to others [14]. Attachment theory subsequently provided a longitudinal view on how early dyadic relationships, between infants and their mothers or primary caregivers, shape the quality of emotional relationships the child has with others throughout his or her lifespan. Bowlby believed that working models of attachment were related to many forms of emotional distress and personality disturbance and that attachment difficulties underlie a wide range of adult dysfuntions, including personality disorders [14] (Fig. 6.1).

Attachment Styles

Here, we briefly review the four attachments styles seen in children and adolescents. A youth's attachment style plays a central role in determining his or her ability to interact with others.

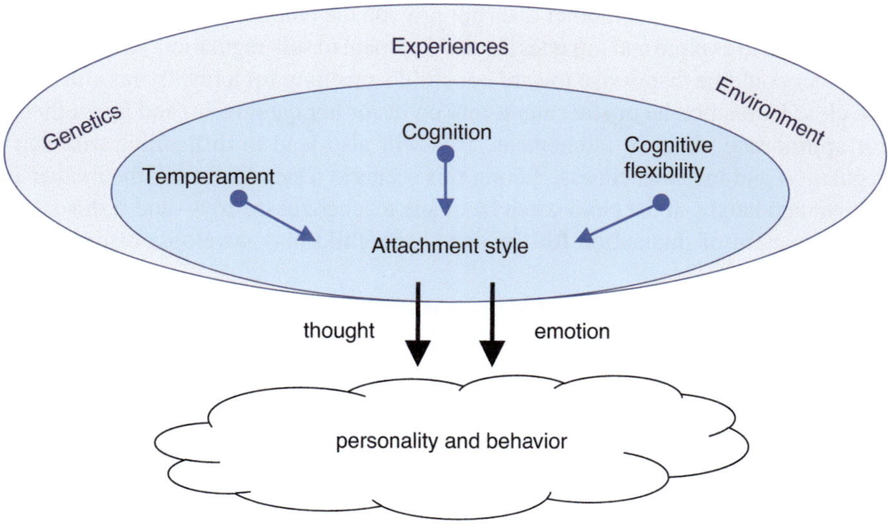

Fig. 6.1 Contributions of intrinsic factors to attachment

Secure Attachment

A secure form of attachment occurs when the infant experiences caregivers as providing coherent attachment patterns and relate with a playful sense of reciprocity. The caregiver also exhibits empathic attunement and helps the infant to handle normal periods of distress with comforting responses (e.g., holding, soothing with touch, rocking rhythmically, or singing). The child develops a coherent discourse over time, values attachments—whether pleasant or temporarily unpleasant—and can provide others a sense of reciprocity.

> A 3-year-old girl is taken to the zoo and becomes anxious and fearful near the elephant exhibit. She tells her father, "I am afraid of the elephants." Her father reassures her and says, "Let's sing 'If You're Happy and You Know It' and stomp like elephants. I bet the elephants will laugh at us." The child begins to laugh and accepts her father's reassurance, implicitly understanding that singing "If You're Happy and You Know It" recalls prior happy moments of a secure attachment

Insecure Attachment

When an infant's primary caregiver does not provide appropriate affective attunement in the early months of life, the infant may fail to develop the ability to self-regulate his or her emotions; this serves as a forerunner to a variety of insecure attachment patterns. Consider an infant whose mother is very anxious and has difficulty tolerating the child's struggle to reach for a toy. His or her mother reaches and gives the toy to the child, thereby preventing signs of distress that might make him or her anxious. This mother does not provide the emotional availability needed for the child to explore and impedes the development of self-regulation. Alternatively, a mother could be dismissive toward her child's reaching for a toy. In this situation, the child learns that he or she cannot rely on his or her caregivers (and later others) for appropriate affective attunement. This will also lead to difficulties with self-regulation and interrelatedness. Taking this scenario a step further, if the mother is critical and laughs at the child when he or she reaches for the toy—and if this is the typical pattern of interaction for the dyad—the child may develop a disorganized attachment style [24].

These examples illustrate implicit patterns of relating that will over time form internal working models of insecure attachment, which is a considerable risk factor for maladaptive interpersonal behavior and formal personality disorders. Insecure forms of attachment are known to be precursors of personality disorders. Adults with insecure attachment are more vulnerable to experiencing intense feelings of anger, aggression, and impulsivity, primary characteristics of borderline personality disorder [43].

Insecure Attachment Styles: Ambivalent/Anxious, Avoidant/Dismissive, and Disorganized

Ambivalent Attachment/Anxious

The ambivalent/anxious type of attachment occurs when an infant feels anxious because his or her caregiver's availability is unpredictable and inconsistent. The infant develops patterns of relationships based on superficiality. He or she grows to wish for closeness with others, but often avoids reaching out for fear of criticism or rejection. For example, a child remains close to her mother and declines to engage in playful activities when visiting cousins. When the child is invited to have a jovial conversation, his or her mother states, "You can talk with them if you want," although subjectively conveys she prefers him or her not to. This form of attachment is a precursor for cluster A and C personality disorders.

Avoidant Attachment/Dismissive

The avoidant/dismissive type of attachment occurs when an infant is in constant fear due to the unpredictability of the quality of the relationship with his or her caregiver and cannot develop a stable internal working model of social relationships [14]. Youths with avoidant/dismissive attachment styles develop patterns of self-sufficiency and frequently have difficulties with day-to-day social interactions. They may withhold verbal communication with others and are accordingly frequently rejected, repeating the original pattern established with their caregivers. Clinicians may become frustrated attempting to gather the information needed to organize their narrative. Most believe this is an early precursor of mild to moderate forms of cluster B (borderline, histrionic, and narcissistic) personality disorders.

Disorganized Attachment

Disorganized attachment occurs when an infant's caregiver provides unpredictable attachment patterns with a poor sense of reciprocity. There is common history of abandonment or trauma in youths, who grow to be frightened of commitment and have significant vulnerabilities that prevent them from sustaining stable relationships, causing a repeating cycle of their incoherent life discourse. They often are bullied by parents and consequently bully others, with limited appreciation of the impact it has on others. As adults they are prone to relational trauma and dissociative experiences. This form of attachment is an early precursor for severe forms of borderline personality disorder, conduct disorders, and antisocial personality disorder (Table 6.1) (Figure 6.2).

Attachment Theory Across Lifespan

Attachment theory helps us understand how early childhood experiences contribute to not only attachment patterns in children and adolescents, but across a person's lifespan [56]. In fact, substantial evidence suggests that early attachment patterns

Table 6.1 Experiences expected from others according to attachment styles

Attachment Style	Experience of others	Typical interaction with others
Secure	I know and feel cared by my family and friends. I know that when I need help, I can ask others to help me.	Interacts well with parents and peers. Is in sync with emotional states of others and follows themes of conversations. Recognizes when to ask for help.
	Insecure	
Anxious	My parents don't like me because I worry all the time. I do not think I am good enough. I can't please anybody.	Avoids initiating interactions. Shares many somatic complaints and uses these to avoid being in school or social activities. Prefers to be near parents.
Dismissive	I am ignored by the adults in my life. They always think I am a failure.	Gives one-word answers. Demonstrates lack of interest in others. activities or discussions.
Disorganized	I will be yelled at. Nobody loves me.	Demanding of age-inappropriate privileges, i.e. activities without supervision, late curfew, smoking with parents, and use of weapons.

From Delgado et al. [24]

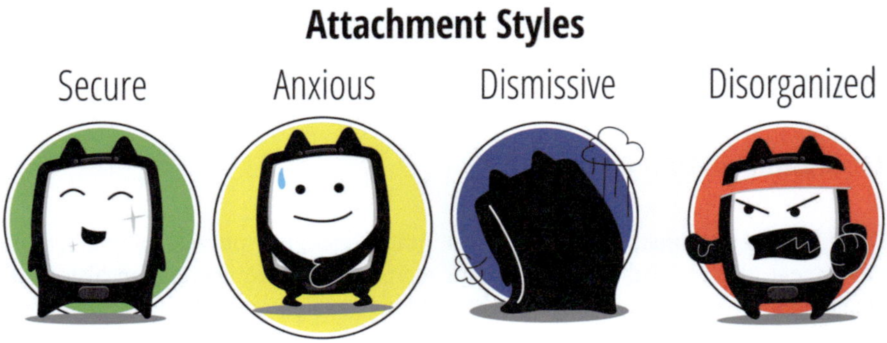

Fig. 6.2 Attachment styles

predict the characteristics of later romantic relationships [65]. Adolescents who describe themselves as having secure, ambivalent, or avoidant styles of attachment in their current relationships had similar patterns as children in their families of origin.

Personality Disorders (Attachment Disturbances)

We will not review reactive attachment disorder. The genesis of reactive attachment disorder is always trauma: specifically, the severe emotional neglect commonly found in institutional settings, such as overcrowded orphanages, foster care, or in homes with mentally or physically ill parents [29]. The absence of adequate nurturing results in poor language acquisition, impaired cognitive development, and contributes to behavioral dysfunction [69]. As such, reactive attachment disorders are developmental disorders in which the assessment of the four pillars is limited, since the pillars will be in flux depending on when a child is removed from a neglectful or traumatic environment.

A personality disorder is "an enduring pattern of inner experience and behavior that deviates markedly from the expectations of the individual's culture, is pervasive and inflexible, has an onset in adolescence or early adulthood, is stable over time, and leads to distress or impairment" (*Diagnostic and Statistical Manual of Mental Disorders* (5th edition (DSM-5); American Psychiatric Association, 2013), APA [2]).

The *DSM–5* [2] defines borderline personality disorder in terms of nine symptoms that span affective, interpersonal, and intrapersonal disturbances. Because borderline personality disorder is a polythetic disorder in which five of nine criteria are needed for the diagnosis, there are 256 different ways to meet criteria. This variety of potential combinations raises the possibility that there are different dimensions or forms of borderline personality disorder, which might have different etiologies, follow different paths of change, and respond to different treatments [37].

For the remainder of this chapter, we will discuss in more detail borderline, narcissistic, and antisocial personality disorders in adolescence. Our contention is that severe character pathology is associated with insecure forms of attachment, difficult temperaments, and cognitive vulnerabilities (see Chaps. 3 and 4). Conventionally, the affective symptoms and maladaptive behavior patterns are emphasized, despite extensive literature demonstrating a wide array of cognitive concerns, especially executive functioning deficits, in these individuals. Consider, for example, that in the context of insecure attachment and environment, overt weaknesses in working memory, fluid reasoning, and cognitive flexibility (theory of mind) can compromise a person's moral compass. Though these associations, in general, do not indicate causality, on a case-by-case basis, they can help illuminate individual factors for what often are viewed as difficult and refractory cases.

There is no question that work with patients with personality disorders can be challenging; however, these patients also have brief periods of lucidity, tempered social engagement, and vocational success [67]. There is also likely some selection bias in our perception of patients with personality disorders as they primarily interact with the healthcare system when they are in crisis [23].

Current research suggests that personality disorders have a multifactorial etiology including epigenetic, genetic, developmental, and psychosocial factors. To date, no specific genes have been identified, although some temperamental traits (see Chap. 3) have been correlated with borderline personality disorders [33]. Increasing knowledge from neurobiology has expanded the discussion of the etiology of personality disorders outside of dysfunctional families or early childhood trauma. We now recognize that certain genetic polymorphisms and nonshared environmental factors are at the root of personality disorders [55].

For many years, personality disorders have been tied primarily to dysfunctional families or early childhood trauma. In our perspective, this view developed primarily from a selection bias of clinical populations of youth, eventually diagnosed with personality disorders, who engage in high-risk behaviors. In addition, case studies in traditional psychodynamic literature appear to overrepresent youth with dysfunctional families and underrepresent youth with personally disorders raised in healthy and well-functioning families [12, 40]. This misunderstanding was not entirely dissimilar to the early historical perception that autistic children were raised only by emotionally cold, distant parents. To clarify, maladaptive parenting is an important risk factor for the development of borderline personality disorder (and likely character pathologies), but no evidence suggests that it is broadly causative [70]. Especially given new research on the prevalence of resilience in youth, it may be that youth who develop severe personally disorders have similar genetic vulnerabilities as their parents. Further, high-risk-taking behaviors, difficulties with emotional regulation, and poor decision-making can be the main contributing factors for youth who find themselves in situations that can be traumatic.

Given that our knowledge of personally disorders, especially at the biological level, remains incomplete, we recommend that clinicians think broadly of multiple risk factors. We are aware that some youth are unfortunately raised in very dysfunctional and traumatic environments, but this should not be considered to be the single contributing factor of personality disorders, as some of these youths have proven to be resilient, with successful psychosocial outcomes. Stable families can provide a nurturing and growth-promoting environment, but there remains the risk of underlying medical or mental health illnesses. In the case of a youth with a personality disorder who was raised in a high-functioning and securely attached family (especially with otherwise healthy siblings), it is essential to incorporate the results of psychological testing, including personality testing, to capture a view of the patient's neurobiological systems. In doing so, we can avoid assuming the parents and their behavior are at the root of their child's condition.

Although it is agreed that the precursors of personality disorders occur in childhood and that the clinical presentation during adolescence is similar to that in adults, there continues to be a great deal of reluctance in diagnosing a personality disorder in adolescence. Kaess et al. [38] aptly capture the main reasons for this reluctance: symptoms are normative in adolescence, as an individual's development is in flux, and to be labeled with a personality disorder can feel pejorative and stigmatizing. Diagnosis of personality disorders during adolescence, however, can lead to early practical and effective nonpharmacological approaches that can help promote new and more adaptive behaviors (e.g., Dialectical Behavior Therapy-Adolescent (DBT-A), Interpersonal Therapy-Adolescent (IPT-A), and Mentalization-Based Therapy-Adolescent (MBT-A); see Chap. 7). Further, a clinician's avoiding diagnosing a personality disorder can increase the likelihood of an adolescent being diagnosed with a disease-based model condition, with increased risk in polypharmacy—with often limited results.

Personality Testing

The widespread depiction of personality testing (e.g., inkblot tests) by popular media has fostered the perception that personality assessments are highly biased or enigmatic. From a clinical standpoint, however, modern personality testing is a specialized field used reliably in high-value situations such as clinical, forensic, and vocational domains.

We can more easily understand personality tests if we conceptually divide them into "projective" and "objective" tests (described in the following sections). Next, we should consider tests based on their appropriateness for age (or developmental level) and cultural validity.

Validity and Reliability of Personality Testing

When considering personality tests, clinicians should consider both validity and reliability. Validity is the degree to which the test is measuring the quality of interest; reliability is how well the test can provide reproducible results. Both objective and projective tests have limitations, which should be considered carefully.

Though objective tests are considered to have greater validity, it is highly dependent on the participant's willingness and ability to report their "true" personality. For example, a patient with narcissistic personality may describe himself or herself as a caring person and wonderful friend, when the informed clinician may conclude the opposite.

Commonly Used Personality Tests

To assist the clinician, we provide a list of the most known tests used in personality assessment of youths.

Projective Tests

- Rorschach Test (ages 6+)
- Children's Apperception Test (CAT) (ages 3–10)
- Thematic Apperception Test (TAT) (ages 10+)
- Human Figure-Drawing (House-Tree-Person, Draw-A-Person) (ages 6–17)

Objective (Self-Report) Tests

- Millon Adolescent Personality Inventory (MAPI)
- Millon Adolescent Clinical Inventory, Second Edition (MACI-II)
- Millon Pre-Adolescent Clinical Inventory (M-PACI)
- Minnesota Multiphasic Personality Inventory-2 (MMPI-2)
- Minnesota Multiphasic Personality Inventory–Adolescent (MMPI-A)
- Personality Inventory for Children, Second Edition (PIC-2)
- Personality Inventory for Youth (PIY)
- The Shedler-Westen Assessment Procedure (SWAP-II)

Projective Personality Tests

Projective tests rely on the person administering the test to interpret the patient's responses to ambiguous stimuli and, in general, tend to be grounded within a psychoanalytic framework [60]. In this regard, projective tests can assess aspects of personality that may be impossible to measure by self-report. The most common projective measures include the Rorschach inkblot technique, in which individuals describe what they see in a standard inkblot (Chap. 5); the Thematic Apperception Test (TAT), in which children imagine stories about standard pictures depicting people interacting; the Human Figure-Drawing assessment, in which children are asked to draw a person or a family, or, for a younger patient, a house, tree, and person together; and the Children's Apperception Test (CAT) a series of 10 quasiambiguous pictures about which the child is asked to create a story. Though there is no escaping the subjective nature of these tests, they are well established and have systematic approaches for administration and interpretation. Compared to other psychometrics, projective testing is highly dependent on the experience, perspective, and skill of the psychologist giving the test.

Projective testing suffers from rater bias and may be less reproducible. Individuals tend to agree with vague generalizations about themselves, and, in research studies, when a random group of individuals are unknowingly given the same results on a personality test, they feel the results are highly applicable to them. This phenomenon is known as the Forer effect and is a significant weakness in projective testing [47].

Projective Testing

Rorschach Test | Ages 6+

The Rorschach, a projective test, consists of a series of black-and-white and color "inkblots" that have been used to assess personality, emotional functioning, unconscious conflict, and psychopathology. It was widely used in the psychoanalytic circles to assess intrapsychic functioning, for example, ego functioning, quality of object relations, sublimation abilities, superego integration, motivation for treatment, etc. [15, 16]. The test involves showing an individual five black-and-white inkblots and five color inkblots. The person is asked to describe what he or she sees (projects) in each inkblot. The Rorschach test is perhaps the most controversial projective psychological test [32]. Further Wood et al. [77] observed that when the Rorschach was administered to "healthy" individuals, almost half had Rorschach interpretations that suggested distorted thinking. Thus, false positives are common with the Rorschach and it should be used cautiously.

Children's Apperception Test (CAT) | Ages 3–10

The Children's Apperception Test (CAT) is a projective measure of a child's personality and psychological processes. The test includes a series of 10 quasiambiguous pictures, about which the child is asked to create a story. This assessment technique was developed from psychoanalytic theory and was designed to obtain information about psychological functioning through the specific mechanism of projection. The CAT is used to assess a youth's personality and level of maturity. The test consists of pictures of animals (CAT-A) or humans (CAT-H) in common social situations. A supplement to the CAT, the CAT-S, includes pictures of children in common family situations such as prolonged illnesses, births, deaths, and separations from parental figures [30].

Thematic Apperception Test (TAT) | Ages 10+

Developed by the American psychologist Henry Murray and psychoanalyst Christiana Morgan in the 1930s, this test uses what is known as a picture interpretation technique [54]. The TAT consists of 31 cards (30 with pictures and one blank card) with drawings of human figures in ambiguous situations. Subjects are asked to interpret the pictures by creating a story describing the situation of the person shown on each card. When shown the blank card, subjects are asked to create their own scene or story. The test is used to reveal a person's self, view of the world, and attitudes toward others to help identify their personality [44].

Human Figure Drawing (House-Tree-Person; Draw-A-Person) | Ages 3–17

This test consists of asking a child to draw a house, a tree, and the figure of a person on three separate sheets of paper. The youth is then asked to describe the drawings, which is believed to capture their inner world. The examiner asks a series of questions related to the drawings. For example, when viewing the house, the examiner might ask: Who lives in the house? What goes on inside the house? Is it a happy house? When viewing the tree, the examiner might inquire: What kind of tree is it? Who waters the tree? What season is it? Is the tree old?

While somewhat controversial, the house has been considered to represent family and family values with different elements of the drawing reflecting different values (e.g., windows and doors represent social connectedness and integration). The tree has been formulated to represent unconscious aspects of personality, and the person has been suggested to be a symbolic representation of the ideal self. Generally, the House-Tree-Person test is administered as part of a series of personality and intelligence tests, like the Rorschach, TAT or CAT [17].

Objective Personality Tests

Objective (Self-Report) Personality Tests

Objective tests take an "inventory" approach to querying an individual's characteristics; answers are then compared to a large, standardized sample. These tests are largely self-report in style, written in a question format with a graded scale as a response. Today, objective tests are more commonly used than projective tests.

Millon's Theory of Personality

Theodore Millon (1928–2014) was an American psychologist known for being a leader in the field of personality and personality disorders. He viewed personality as the evolutionary adaptation to life and personality disorders as a problem in adaptation. He believed in three essential goals of life: existential survival (avoiding death or pain and enhancing life and pleasure), ecological adaptation (passive environmental accommodation and active environmental modification), and species replication (maximizing reproduction and self-focus and nurturing progeny). Millon derived 15 core personality styles associated with adaptive and maladaptive expressions of personality [53] (Table 6.2).

Millon defined personality pathology as conflict, deficiency, or overinvestment in one or more of the basic principles of evolutionary adaptation. He viewed people as having eight domains, four functional and four structural, representing the expression of personality in facets aligned with the traditional psychodynamic schools of thought expressed in Table 6.3 [58, 59].

Table 6.2 The Millon 15 normal and abnormal personality styles

Retiring/Schizoid
Eccentric/Schizotypal
Shy/Avoidant
Cooperative/Dependent
Sociable/Histrionic
Confident/Narcissistic
Suspicious/Paranoid
Assertive/Sadistic
Pessimistic/Melancholic
Aggrieved/Masochistic
Skeptical/Negativistic
Capricious/Borderline
Conscientious/Compulsive
Exuberant/Turbulent

Table 6.3 Expression of personality in domains

Functional Domains
Expressive Emotion
Interpersonal Conduct
Cognitive Style
Intrapsychic Dynamics
Structural Domains
Self-Image
Intrapsychic Content
Intrapsychic Architecture
Mood/Temperament

Millon Adolescent Personality Inventory (MAPI) | Ages 13–19

The MAPI was initially published in 1982 and is a 150-question self-report personality inventory that assesses personality styles based on Millon's theory of personality types. The test was written at a sixth-grade reading level and can be completed in less than 30 minutes [52]. Unlike the Millon Adolescent Clinical Inventory (MACI), the MAPI was designed for use with both "normal" adolescents and adolescents involved in clinical settings [18].

Millon Adolescent Clinical Inventory, Second Edition (MACI-II) | Ages 13–19

The MACI-II was designed to evaluate adolescents with clinical symptoms in a variety of clinical settings [51]. The test, a self-report measure, contains twelve personality patterns scales, based on Millon's theory of personality and parallels the criteria for personality disorders (originally Axis II of the *Diagnostic and Statistical Manual of Mental Disorders 4th ed., DSM–IV-TR,* APA 2000) [1]. The MACI offers eight scales representing potential areas of concern for adolescents, such as peer insecurity and identity diffusion.

Millon Pre-Adolescent Clinical Inventory (M-PACI) | Ages 9–12

The M-PACI was developed by Millon [52]. The M-PACI is specifically designed to identify psychological problems in children ages 9–12. It provides an integrated view that synthesizes emerging personality styles and clinical syndromes as well as a summary of treatment strategies, tailored to each patient. The normative population of the M-PACI consisted of 292 pre-adolescents, ages 9–12, from 53 sites across the United States. The test consists of fewer than 100 questions and takes most pre-adolescents only 15–20 minutes to complete.

Minnesota Multiphasic Personality Inventory-2 (MMPI-2) | Ages 17–64

The MMPI was one of the first tests to use an empirical approach for personality testing. The MMPI assesses the degree to which an individual expresses atypical behavior relative to a normative sample (age- and sex-matched). Since its inception in 1943, the MMPI has undergone many revisions, with the most recent edition entitled the MMPI-2 [5]. The MMPI-2 provides clinical measures that can be effective in delineating mental health symptoms and personality traits.

Minnesota Multiphasic Personality Inventory–Adolescent (MMPI-A) | Ages 14–18

The Minnesota Multiphasic Personality Inventory–Adolescent (MMPI-A; [6]) is an adolescent-specific revision of the original, broadband personality instrument, the Minnesota Multiphasic Personality Inventory (MMPI; [64]). The original MMPI, designed primarily for adult clinical assessment, had been applied to evaluate adolescents from the time of its release. The revision to the MMPI-A was prompted by several considerations. First, the passage of nearly five decades since the original test's release made it necessary to develop contemporary adolescent norms. Second, it was apparent that MMPI items did not provide sufficient information about the adolescents' experiences. Adolescent response patterns were quite distinct from those of adults, warranting a developmentally appropriate instrument to achieve interpretive accuracy. The revision effort was undertaken with the goals of updating and refining item content, reducing test length and reading-level demands, developing a uniform set of contemporary adolescent norms, and developing scales to measure adolescent-relevant difficulties such as school- and family-related problems [3, 4, 6].

Personality Inventory for Children, Second Edition (PIC-2) | Ages 3–16

The Personality Inventory for Children (PIC-R) was developed in 1956 by Robert D. Wilt, who was influenced by the MMPI; his test is known as the "Children's MMPI" [68]. The PIC is based on a pool of 600 items; hence, its length is similar to the MMPI; however, the PIC is not a self-report measure. Instead, the parent rates their child's behavior.

Personality Inventory for Youth (PIY) | Ages 9–18

The PIY was developed in 1994 by David Lachar and Rex Kline as a self-report measure; it consists of 270 items [41]. It was written at a third-grade reading level and can be completed in 45 minutes. It was designed as a diagnostic tool to assess youths' emotional and behavioral adjustment, family interaction, and attention-related academic functioning. The PIY has four validity scales to help determine whether a youth is uncooperative, exaggerating, malingering, responding defensively, carelessly, or without adequate comprehension.

The Shedler-Westen Assessment Procedure (SWAP)

The Shedler-Westen Assessment Procedure (SWAP) is a personality assessment instrument. It diagnoses personality styles and disorders and provides clinical case formulations to guide treatment and decision-making. The psychologist scores 200 personality-descriptive items. It relies on psychometric and statistical methods to optimize reliability, validity, and predictive accuracy. SWAP-II is the latest edition of the instrument [66] followed by a second edition of the Shedler-Westen Assessment Procedure for Adolescents (SWAP-A) [22].

Cases

As it is beyond the scope of this book to provide a full description of all the cognitive functions and processes of youths with character pathology and insecure attachment, we have focused on the main personality disorders affecting youths for which parents request help. We have concentrated our energy on the most relevant clinical contributions of weaknesses in cognitive functioning in borderline, narcissistic, and antisocial personality disorders (e.g., working memory, fluid reasoning, and cognitive flexibility), as these serve as the foundation of a person's moral compass within the context of his or her environment and culture.

Borderline Personality Disorder in Adolescence

The diagnosis of borderline personality disorder in youths remains controversial. Some fear that diagnosing borderline personality disorder might stigmatize and undermine self-esteem during maturation. However, there is accumulating evidence that borderline personality disorder in adolescents represents a reliable and valid diagnosis [38]. Moreover, for these adolescents, early intervention improves regulation of emotional states and social interactions. Beyond that, several psychotherapies have been developed for youths with borderline personality disorder [13, 42].

Nearly 2% of American youths meet the criteria for borderline personality disorder by the age of 16, which rises to 3.2% by the age of 22. Importantly, the incidence of borderline personality disorder has an estimated prevalence of 11% in youths treated in outpatient psychiatric clinics [19] and up to 50% in inpatient settings [34]. Some people with borderline personality disorder respond well to outpatient treatment and are never hospitalized, while others have a more tumultuous course. However, a small percentage of patients spontaneously recover and no longer require treatment.

Adolescents with borderline personality disorder often engage in risk-taking behaviors, act impulsively, struggle with emotional regulation, and have increased suicidal ideation with nonsuicidal self-injurious (NSSI) behaviors and suicidal attempts in response to conflicted social interactions in which they experience people as criticizing or abandoning them. The presence of nonsuicidal self-injurious behaviors is generally associated with a more complex set of maladaptive behaviors and portends a more difficult course [21, 72]. Despite our understanding of environmental risks, the etiology of borderline personality disorder remains poorly understood. To date, no specific genes have been identified [20] although there seems to be some genetic vulnerability linked to temperamental traits [39].

Too often, deferment or avoidance of this diagnosis has led to inappropriate and ineffective conceptualization and treatment of this disorder, to parents' dismay. It is not unusual to have a parent, to whom the diagnosis and treatment plan is clearly described, exclaim, "I wish we had known about this sooner." Paris [57] asserts that "all too many adolescents with a classical picture of BPD are receiving aggressive pharmacotherapy based on faddishly unjustified diagnoses of bipolar disorder." Given this, it is not surprising that the high prevalence of borderline personality disorder in adolescents who are treated in psychiatric settings—both outpatient and inpatient—is often not captured in our electronic medical record systems. We submit that borderline personality disorder diagnosis and treatment, as needed, should be considered routine practice in youths' mental health. Doing so will improve well-being and long-term prognosis, with improved emotional regulation and quality-of-life outcomes [38, 48].

As described in Chap. 4, youths with weaknesses in working memory and fluid reasoning unknowingly push family or friends away because they feel social norms are unrealistic or rigid and defy them (e.g., bully others, laugh at other people's mishaps, defy adults' expectations, etc.) although they commonly experience others as bullying them. Frequently, they misinterpret the intent of others and feel unfairly treated due to their impairments in cognitive flexibility/ToM (see Chap. 5).

Cognitive Profile of Adolescent with Borderline Personality Disorder: A Storm Chaser

The notion of a Storm Chaser described in Chap. 4 reflects the unknowing efforts adolescents with borderline personality disorder use to seek others with similar emotional and cognitive weaknesses: "Enough like me to become my role model and I your interpreter," as Meltzoff [49] puts it. As a group, individuals with borderline personality disorder are in conflict with others that do not agree with their view of social norms and with their perception of situations. They lack the ability to successfully register, maintain, and manipulate visual and auditory information for accurate discrimination of the facts needed for adaptive behaviors. Although the criteria for borderline personality disorder are the same for adolescents as for adults, emotional dysregulation is a prominent symptom that leads to maladaptive behaviors, which may mimic symptoms of mood disorders (e.g., depression, bipolar disorder, disruptive mood dysregulation disorder). Substance use disorders can also be a serious problem in adolescents with borderline personality disorder.

Olivia

Synopsis: Olivia, a 15-year-old female, was referred for a next-day emergent psychiatric evaluation after having suicidal thoughts and a plan to overdose on her medications.

DSM–5 Relevant History

The night before the evaluation, Olivia's parents asked her to turn over her smartphone to them after they found her posting provocative photos of herself on social media as a desperate way to seek friends. Although she relinquished her smartphone, Olivia later snuck into her parents' bedroom and took her smartphone back in order to post more pictures. When confronted, Olivia became increasingly agitated, threatened suicide, and took her medication to her room. Her mother called the police, who came and talked with Olivia for an hour and told her mother that Olivia was no longer feeling suicidal and should be taken for an urgent, same-day psychiatric evaluation at the local hospital emergency department. Olivia had minimal insight about the severity of the consequences of her risk-taking behaviors.

Olivia began to have explosive and aggressive episodes when she was nine years old. Her parents were frustrated by Olivia's "lack of any remorse" after her violent outbursts. The episodes had become more frequent and more intense despite regular outpatient psychiatric services that included individual, family, and pharmacologic therapies. Her parents began to feel hopeless about Olivia's progress and feared for their well-being. They began to consider a residential facility for their daughter, stating, "Medications and therapy do not work. She is not fixable."

Contributing Family, Social, and Educational History

Olivia had a history of impulsive behavior. Despite going to psychotherapy and being on medication for several years, her behaviors had worsened. Her mother was overwhelmed and did not know how else to help her and medication was "not working." Her mother reported that Olivia did well most days but would escalate when she was told "no" or when limits were set as a result of her poor decision-making behaviors. Her parents were exasperated by Olivia's confusing behavior. "It's hard to know how she really feels, because she will say she is fine and loves us; other days she is angry and feels we don't like her and hates us and goes to her room to engage in self-harming behaviors. It's like Jekyll and Hyde," her mother stated. Her mother was concerned with Olivia's lack of remorse when hurting other people's feelings. The parents' narrative was consistent with what is called "splitting" in borderline personality disorder. The same person is admired one day and devalued the next, with difficulties integrating that people can have both good and bad qualities. Splitting represents a deficit in cognitive flexibility/ToM and mentalization abilities (See Chap. 5).

Olivia was in tenth grade at a local high school at the time of her evaluation. She was in honors classes, with her teachers noting that her grades fluctuated depending on her mood. When she was in a negative mood and engaged in peer conflict, it increased her maladaptive behaviors, Olivia was allowed to leave the classroom and seek help from school counselors.

Olivia had caring and attentive parents who were consistent and provided her the extensive psychiatric treatment needed. They took Olivia regularly to her dialectical behavioral therapy group and individual sessions and attended the family component. Olivia had three brief psychiatric hospitalizations because of suicidal ideation and on three all occasions she asked to be discharged the following day, saying she was feeling better. She added that her parents and others overreacted to her comments and demanded that her attending child psychiatrist understand she was never suicidal, and that the hospitalizations were not helpful to her in learning new coping skills.

Formulation

Olivia's medical record noted diagnoses of adjustment disorder with mixed disturbance of emotions and conduct, disruptive mood dysregulation disorder, and impulse control disorder. During her last inpatient psychiatric hospitalization, the treatment team considered changing her primary diagnosis to borderline personality disorder as she met the *DSM–5* criteria for the disorder, but her child psychiatrist disagreed with this assessment, believing she had a treatment-resistant form of bipolar disorder. The psychiatrist changed her medications and increased her mood stabilizer.

Contemporary Diagnostic Interview

In the first interview during of the urgent outpatient evaluation, it became apparent to the clinician, who used a Contemporary Diagnostic Interview (CDI), that Olivia had cognitive weaknesses. She had concrete thinking, poor working memory (devaluing social norms), and limited cognitive flexibility when processing emotions, with frequent examples of splitting that came to light when she described how she experienced her parents and friends. She also presented as having difficult/feisty temperament style using the criteria set forth by Thomas and Chess [71]. Olivia was referred for a psychological assessment that included personality testing to better understand the nature of her functioning.

Olivia's parents—happily married professionals—both had easy/flexible temperaments (Chap. 3), good cognitive flexibility (Chap. 5), and a secure attachment with Olivia and her two siblings.

Session (moral compass) pearls
Olivia was upset at her parents for setting limits around her smartphone and social media. She failed to recognize that sending provocative pictures was a dangerous, risk-taking behavior. "My phone is my life. What's the point of living if I can't use it?"
Olivia had suggestive weakness in working memory: "My parents are out of touch with teenagers. All my friends have parents that let them do whatever they want."
She showed evidence of splitting: "If you (psychiatrist) can tell my parents to give my phone back, I will go to DBT groups again. If you can't, then I want to go to the hospital. I like the teenagers there."

Results of Psychological Testing

FSIQ	VCI	FR	VS	WM	PS
89 (23%) Low Avg.	98 (45%) Average	88 (21%) Low Avg.	84 (14%) Low Avg.	86 (18%) Low Avg.	89 (23%) Low Avg.

Summary of Psychological Testing: WISC-V

Primary Drivers

Low average full scale IQ and low average working memory.

Secondary Drivers

Low average fluid reasoning, visual-spatial, and processing speed.

Information from Olivia's psychological assessment revealed difficulties with emotional and behavioral functioning. She had cognitive skills in fluid reasoning, visual-spatial, working memory and processing speed that were in the low average range. As discussed earlier (Chap. 4), weaknesses in working memory, when accompanied by a difficult/feisty temperament, and rigid cognitive flexibility can produce symptoms that are consistent with a borderline personality disorder profile (Storm Chaser). Further, Olivia's weaknesses in fluid reasoning contribute to difficulties understanding emotionally arousing situations with limited ability to understand how other people feel and think. Taken together, her deficits make it difficult for her to predict the social consequences of her maladaptive behaviors.

The fact that, upon initial assessment, Olivia was in tenth grade and in honors classes can suggest several possibilities. First, her teachers may have placed her in classes that were inappropriate and based their decision on past academic history rather than current academic performance. Second, as with other youths with average to above average verbal comprehension abilities, she may have communicated well verbally with her teachers and they assumed that her grades "fluctuated" because of her mental health issues and did not carefully attend to her broad academic deficits. As discussed earlier (Chap. 4), asking youths or their parents about academic abilities often fails to capture the full picture. Olivia would not have been identified as struggling cognitively if her placement in honors classes was accepted as accurate and appropriate.

Results of Personality Testing

The MACI revealed that Olivia had a personality structure characterized by intense and frequent unpredictable changing moods. Further, there are periods where she feels sad and rejected, as well as stretches of time where she feels angry and alone. Her long-held expectation that people will reject her or be unkind to her leads to feelings of disappointment and resignation. Although she wishes for closeness and acceptance by family and friends, she protectively moves further away from them. Despite her tendency to put herself down, Olivia feels bitter toward the people she allows to take advantage of her. She may even convince herself that being embarrassed and degraded is what she deserves, and that unhealthy and abusive relationships are normal. Further, there may be suicidal gestures and she may take the role of the victim when interacting with others. Her vacillation between being self-sacrificing, pouty, self-destructive, and disparaging leads to frequent fights with and disappointment in the people who are close to her. Suffering from low self-esteem, Olivia exaggerates the smallest of insults from others and turns them into episodes of major rejection.

Summary of Personality Testing: MACI

Personality structure characterized by intense and frequent unpredictable changing moods.

Formulation After Psychological Testing

Diagnostically, Olivia can be understood as having borderline personality disorder. As this case demonstrates, adolescents with borderline personality disorder have poor social competence that stem from difficult/feisty temperamental, cognitive weaknesses, rigid cognitive flexibility, and dismissive attachment schemas that will not dissipate with age or educational achievement. Her multiple cognitive weaknesses explain the origin of her character pathology and her maladaptive emotional and behavioral problems (Fig. 6.3).

Maladaptive Manifestation

- Expects that people will not be available to support her.
- Develops intense and unstable relationships that alternate between extremes of idealization and devaluation.
- Breaks up close relationships in anticipation of being rejected. This leads to feeling abandoned.
- Feels empty, with fluctuations in self-image, and feels dependent on specific negative relationships to maintain her sense of identity.
- Experiences intense instability, irritability, or anxiety that may last for several days.
- Projects blame onto others for her mishaps.
- Displays recurrent self-injurious and suicidal behaviors.

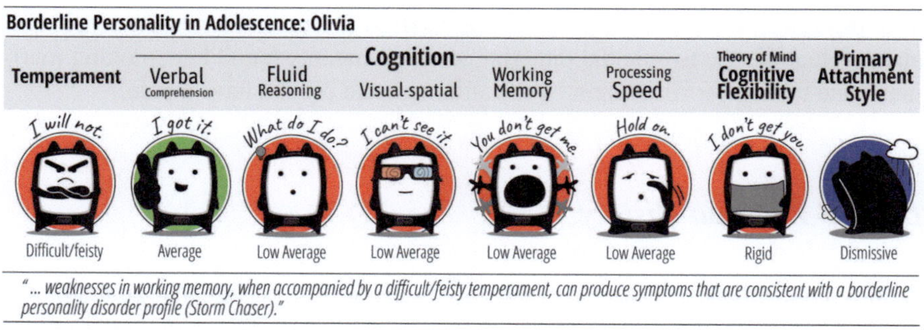

Fig. 6.3 Borderline personality in adolescence: Olivia

Treatment and Intervention Recommendations

Olivia can benefit from individual psychotherapy, a key component of early intervention for borderline personality disorder. The type of therapy is less relevant than the experience of the therapist with youths like Olivia. She may need a mix of elements from Dialectical Behavior Therapy-Adolescent (DBT-A), Interpersonal Therapy-Adolescent (IPT-A), and Mentalization-Based Therapy-Adolescent (MBT-A) according to her emotional states. The therapist should remember that the use of a workbook is not recommended as her cognitive skills are in low average range and her reading comprehension is in the sixth-grade range in spite of her proficiency in oral reading fluency. As stated before, there is no current evidence for any specific pharmacotherapy as a first-line treatment for adolescents with borderline personality disorder.

It is essential to engage Olivia's parents in a therapeutic process so that they can educate themselves about the biological underpinnings of her personality disorder and alleviate any anxiety and self-blame (see Chap. 7). Parent and family therapy can help recalibrate how family members interact with each other under distress.

Cross-References

- Working memory, fluid reasoning, processing speed: Chap. 4
- Cognitive flexibility: Chap. 5

Cognitive Profile of Adolescent with Borderline Personality Disorder: Not a Storm Chaser

Jade

Synopsis: Jade, a 15-year-old female, was referred for a next-day emergent psychiatric evaluation due to suicidal thoughts after her parents found her smoking marijuana and taking her smartphone away, although she did not have a plan.

DSM–5 Relevant History

Before the evaluation, Jade was ostensibly doing well academically, although she disliked virtual learning during the COVID-19 pandemic. She earns good grades and her teachers like her. When confronted by her parents about her marijuana use, Jade became agitated, expressed felt as though she wanted to kill herself and her mother called the local Children's Hospital for an urgent evaluation.

When Jade was 12 years of age, she was diagnosed with generalized anxiety disorder and an antidepressant medication was started by a local mental health advance practice nurse. She was seen every 4 months by her clinician and Jade liked working with her clinician.

As she began high school, Jade's parents began to notice that Jade had difficulties getting along with her friends whom she had been close to since elementary and middle school. She gravitated to peers who had difficulties getting along with their parents. She also began to oscillate between feeling she had good friends who understood her and, at times, became angry at her friends "because they were rude and two faced." Her arguments with her parents became more frequent and more intense. Her parents initially thought her difficulties were "typical adolescent stuff" and when they set firm limits on her behaviors, family conflict increased. To help with her upheaval, Jade began to see a psychotherapist weekly.

Contributing Family, Social, and Educational History

Despite psychotherapy and being on medication for several years, her behaviors worsened. Her father believed that Jade needed firm limits on her maladaptive behaviors and her mother was overwhelmed and did not know how to help her. Her mother reported that Jade did well academically but that, at home, she would escalate when told "no" or when limits were set as a result of her poor decision-making behaviors. Jade's behavior perplexed her parents. "She does well academically but is unhappy when we praise her. She then feels we don't like her and says she hates us." The parents' narrative was consistent with what is called "splitting" in borderline personality disorder. Splitting represents a deficit in cognitive flexibility/ToM and mentalization abilities (See Chap. 5).

Jade had caring and attentive parents who were consistent and provided her the outpatient psychiatric treatment needed.

Formulation

Jade's medical record noted diagnoses of generalized anxiety disorder that had responded well with use of an SSRI. Her therapist considered her diagnosis regarding her recent maladaptive behaviors and difficulties with others to be more in line with a borderline personality disorder and her psychiatrist agreed with this assessment,

Contemporary Diagnostic Interview

In the urgent outpatient evaluation, it became apparent to the psychiatrist, who used a Contemporary Diagnostic Interview (CDI), that Jade was bright but had deficits in cognitive flexibility. She was articulate in describing her experience of her parents as being overbearing and overreacting to her marijuana use (devaluing social norms). However, her psychiatrist noted her limited cognitive flexibility when processing emotions, with frequent examples of splitting. She also presented as having difficult/feisty temperament style (Chap. 3). Jade was referred for a psychological assessment to better understand the impact of her psychological functioning on her current symptoms and difficulties.

Jade's parents—married professionals—had easy/flexible temperaments (Chap. 3), good cognitive flexibility (Chap. 5), and a secure attachment with Jade and her sister.

Session (moral compass) pearls
Jade was upset at her parents for setting limits around smartphone, social media, and marijuana use. However, she failed to understand that her parents were worried about others taking advantage of Jade, including those who supplied her marijuana. She reflected: "I would like to see my mom and dad not have their phone and see if they don't become suicidal."
Jade had demonstrated above average cognitive abilities "My parents should be happy I am getting very good grades."
She showed evidence of splitting: "If you (psychiatrist) can tell my parents to back off and not be so stressed, I would feel better."

Results of Psychological Testing

FSIQ	VCI	FR	VS	WM	PS
118 (88%) High Average	121 (92%) Very High Average	112 (79%) High Average	114 (82%) High Average	112 (79%) High Average.	105 (63%) Average

Summary of Psychological Testing: WISC-V

Primary Drivers

Deficits in cognitive flexibility/ToM.

Secondary Drivers

Mixed temperamental styles, predominantly difficult/feisty

Formulation After Psychological Testing

Information from Jade's psychological assessment revealed significant strengths in her cognitive skills. Thus, her difficulties with emotional and behavioral functioning are due to her deficits in cognitive flexibility/ToM that, when accompanied by a difficult/feisty temperament, can produce symptoms consistent with a borderline personality disorder profile, although it is distinct from a Storm Chaser profile with working memory weaknesses as in the case of Olivia (Fig. 6.4).

Diagnostically, Jade can be understood as having borderline personality disorder. As this case demonstrates, adolescents with borderline personality disorder have poor social competence that stem from difficult/feisty temperamental, cognitive flexibility deficits, and dismissive attachment schemas that will not dissipate with age or educational achievement. Her multiple deficits explain the origin of her character pathology and her maladaptive emotional and behavioral problems.

Maladaptive Manifestation

- Expects that people will not be available to support her.
- Develops intense and unstable relationships that alternate between extremes of idealization and devaluation.
- Breaks up close relationships in anticipation of being rejected. This leads to feeling abandoned.
- Feels empty, with fluctuations in self-image, and feels dependent on specific negative relationships to maintain her sense of identity.
- Experiences intense instability, irritability, or anxiety that may last for several days.
- Projects blame onto others for mishaps.
- Displays recurrent self-injurious and suicidal behaviors.

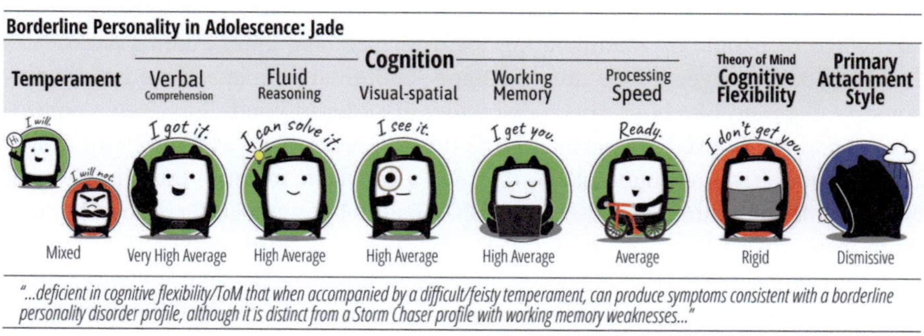

Fig. 6.4 Borderline personality in adolescence: Jade

Treatment and Intervention Recommendations

Jade can benefit from individual psychotherapy, a key component of early intervention for borderline personality disorder. She may need a mix of elements from Dialectical Behavior Therapy-Adolescent (DBT-A), Interpersonal Therapy-Adolescent (IPT-A), and Mentalization-Based Therapy-Adolescent (MBT-A) according to her emotional states. The use of a workbook is highly recommended as her cognitive skills are mostly in the above average range. As stated before, there is no current evidence for any specific pharmacotherapy as a first-line treatment for adolescents with borderline personality disorder.

It is essential to engage Jade's parents in a therapeutic process so that they can educate themselves about the biological underpinnings of her personality disorder and alleviate any anxiety and self-blame (see Chap. 7). Parent and family therapy can help recalibrate how family members interact with each other under distress.

Cross-References

- Difficult/feisty temperament: Chap. 3
- Cognitive flexibility: Chap. 5

Narcissistic Personality Disorder in Adolescence

Youths often have brief periods of self-centeredness before they eventually return to their normal adaptive state of getting along with others. When the periods of self-centeredness are persistent and accompanied by grandiose beliefs of superiority and uniqueness, limited ability for empathy, and need for admiration, it suggests the presence of narcissistic personality disorder of adolescence. Such youths are often arrogant and preoccupied with success and power. They exploit or take advantage of people by manipulating them for personal gain. Parents and others fear the youth's anger if they do not comply with their demands. Narcissistic personality disorder, like borderline personality disorder in youth, has been a controversial and rarely used diagnosis despite it being recognized as having precursors in childhood. It was thought that giving such a diagnosis to youth was stigmatizing and detrimental to their self-esteem, as they had not completed their developmental process.

Research on narcissism in adolescents has predominantly focused on differentiating normal and pathological narcissism, often limiting the latter to its grandiose presentation [9]. Adolescent narcissism has been associated with aggression and delinquency [10], conduct problems [7, 35]. No specific genes have been identified; there seems to be some genetic vulnerability linked to temperamental traits.

Youths with narcissistic personality disorder, like adults with narcissistic personality disorder, do not see the need for change or treatment. They come to the clinician's attention when their family finds their demanding and maladaptive behaviors to reach a threshold that negatively affects their family system. Although there are limited effective and practical interventions available to improve such youths' ability to regulate their emotional state and social interactions, having a diagnostic formulation that makes sense to parents and helps them understand the neurobiology of the disorder is valuable.

Cognitive Profile of Adolescent with Narcissistic Personality Disorder: A Demanding Youth

The hallmarks of the prototypical narcissistic personality in youths are grandiose fantasies, excessive demands, intense self-absorption, grandiosity that defensively reverses overwhelming feelings of inadequacy and helplessness, and inability to experience genuine attachment, trust, and interest in others [12].

Harrison

Synopsis: Harrison, a 15-year-old male, was taken to the emergency department by the police due to aggression toward his parents. Harrison stated that he had been in an argument with his parents, "because they are stupid. They got mad at me for mowing the yard and getting grass all over their driveway. I tried sweeping it off, but I guess it was not good enough." In anger, Harrison shoved a broom down the driveway toward his mother and, in haste, said he hated her and wanted to kill her. During the conflict, he hit his mother's arm when she tried to block him from throwing the broom. Harrison stated, "It's her fault; she should have known better. I wasn't going to hit her." He demanded the psychiatric clinician understand why he had been screaming and cursing at his parents, adding that he acted that way "because they are not good parents. I am helping them know what I need, if they really care." During the interview, Harrison was calm and superficially stated, "I guess I feel bad about what happened tonight. I hope they apologize too." He denied suicidal or homicidal ideation and psychosis. Harrison was easily frustrated when asked questions about his behavior and was evasive in answering further questions.

His parents shared that Harrison had always been a very bright although demanding child. When asked to complete his chores, he would refuse and become argumentative, demanding his parents explain why they thought completing chores was good for a child. Although he got in trouble at school for correcting and arguing with his teachers, he was a straight-A student and told his parents that he was not being challenged enough. At family gatherings, he flaunted how bright he was by monopolizing conversations and talking about science or math facts.

Harrison's history of defiance and anger had led to several unsuccessful trials of Dialectical Behavior Therapy-A to help him use more adaptive coping skills and get along with parents and peers, but he became disruptive to the group and was asked to leave each program he enrolled in. He also had two admissions to day-treatment programs and one inpatient psychiatry hospitalization after damaging his parents' antique objects after becoming angry that they had not bought him the latest smartphone model. His parents were frustrated with the treatment interventions, feeling they were not helpful. Further, his parents felt they had done everything they could to help him, stating, "We don't want to take him to the hospital if he wants a break from us. He enjoys being there because they believe him—that everything is our fault—and that is not true."

Harrison had two siblings that were well mannered and doing well emotionally, socially, and academically. The only area of concern for the siblings was feeling upset at how their brother was mistreating their parents.

DSM–5 Relevant History

Harrison was diagnosed at age 10 with oppositional defiant disorder, disruptive mood dysregulation disorder, depression, anxiety disorder, and intermittent explosive disorder. His first psychiatrist diagnosed Harrison with a depressive disorder and started him on an antidepressant because of a family history of depression in his maternal grandfather, who had committed suicide, and a maternal uncle diagnosed with a bipolar disorder. The antidepressant was stopped, because it was thought to have caused some activation, as Harrison became more irritable. A later trial of aripiprazole for mood stability and irritability was not effective. His parents were frustrated at the multiple diagnoses, even though they felt at the time that they "were somewhat accurate, but nobody seems to know how to help us. He is getting worse with age."

Formulation

Harrison was seen the next day at an urgent outpatient appointment as he had contracted for safety the evening before and was not hospitalized. In the clinician's office, he was defiant and oppositional. He blamed his parents for overreacting and for not knowing how to help him "even though I tell them what I need." He had a noticeable difficult/feisty temperamental style. Although he was bright cognitively, conveyed by his knowledge and sentence structure, he had rigid cognitive flexibility with prominent traits of a narcissistic style. He noticed the clinician's car keys

(Toyota) and remarked, "They must not pay you very much if you drive that car … so sad. I already convinced my father to buy me a BMW, and I will definitely have a better-paying job than you when I am older."

Contemporary Diagnostic Interview

In the first interview during the emergency outpatient evaluation, the clinician, using the CDI, noted that Harrison had a difficult/feisty temperament, above average to superior intelligence, poor cognitive flexibility, and was dismissive of attachment, a common trait in narcissistic personality disorders of adolescence. The clinician requested a psychological assessment in order to support his diagnostic formulation and provide Harrison's parents with a written report about his condition. In the interview, Harrison displayed an exaggerated sense of self-importance, entitlement, and need for excessive admiration without being manic or psychotic.

Session (moral compass) pearls
Harrison was exceptionally good at making fun of adults and peers by highlighting their faults or defects (e.g., "You've never been good at math," "You look terrible in that outfit," or "You are a bad teacher; that's why you don't get paid very much.")
The interactions suggested weaknesses in working memory (poor moral compass).
Although Harrison did not use illegal substances, he argued that marijuana should be legal as he had vast knowledge that marijuana did not affect neurodevelopment, adding, "Stupid doctors think it is bad. Ridiculous."
Harrison was expelled from high school after making menacing remarks to a teacher who challenged him.

Results of Psychological Testing

FSIQ	VCI	FR	VS	WM	PS
117 (87%) High Average	124 (95%) Very High Average	109 (73%) Average	114 (82%) High Average	82 (12%) Low Average.	90 (23%) Average

Summary of Psychological Testing: WISC-V

Primary Driver

Low average working memory

Personality Test (MACI)

Harrison's deep-felt conflict between being dependent on or independent from others and his frustrating search for his identity characterizes his emerging personality profile. He displays significant conflicting feelings and behaviors about his reliance on others and being overly confident and independent. He is beginning to push for increased independence and self-reliance, which becomes apparent in his challenging behaviors and intensely volatile feelings. He has learned that the affective tone he uses in his interactions may be more powerful than the words he chooses. Although he can be quite evocative, he maintains the expectation that others be understanding and tolerant of his outbursts. Afterward he may appear to be remorseful, seek forgiveness, and promise to change, which does not occur.

Summary of Personality Testing: MACI

Primary Drivers

Harrison can be impulsive, manipulative, and vindictive. This makes it difficult for the people around him to be comfortable, since they never know what to expect. Harrison's capriciousness and manipulative nature frequently evoke the rejection he tries to avoid.

Formulation

Harrison can be best helped when he is understood as having a narcissistic personality disorder of adolescence. Although he has high average intelligence, he will have difficulties following social norms and participating in day-to-day interactions

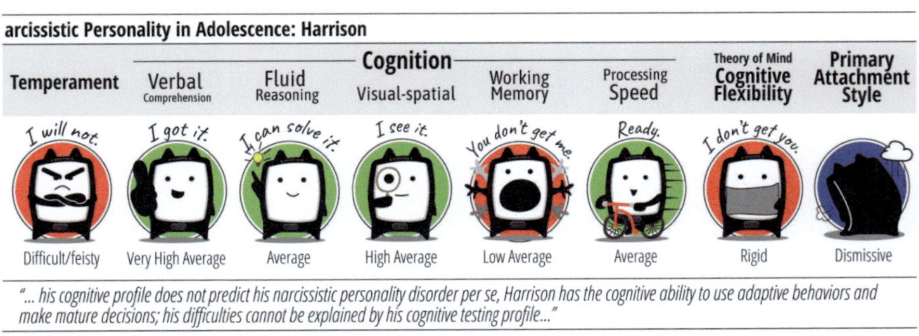

Fig. 6.5 Narcissistic personality in adolescence: Harrison

because of his low average working memory and rigid cognitive flexibility, skills necessary to translate visual and auditory information, verbal dialogue, and facial expressions within the context of a conversation. Surprisingly, Harrison's parents were relieved when this diagnosis was shared. After reviewing the criteria, they felt "this makes more sense that what other people have told us." It would be appropriate to add parent-child relational conflict as a secondary diagnosis. Harrison's socio-emotional dysfunction was reinforced by the negative patterns of interaction with his parents, even as they did their best to help him. Systems theory posits that relationships among family members should be considered dynamic processes that can change over time with treatment rather than static traits [75] (Fig. 6.5).

Discussion

In the case of a narcissistic personality disorder of adolescence, cognitive assessments may be of limited diagnostic use, unlike with patients with borderline personality disorder. Harrison had a high average full-scale IQ of 117, and subtest indices revealed a wide range of scores: very high verbal comprehension and visual-spatial abilities, average fluid reasoning and processing speed, and low average working memory. While his cognitive profile does not predict his narcissistic personality disorder per se, Harrison has the cognitive ability to use adaptive behaviors and make mature decisions; his difficulties cannot be explained by his cognitive testing profile. Thus, he has the capacity to learn information verbally and accurately categorize the information to solve his social and academic problems, but he lacks the cognitive flexibility to know how other people feel and think in regard to his actions.

Treatment and Intervention Recommendations

Harrison's parents were appreciative of the multifaceted treatment recommendations that helped them prepare for the possibility of small changes over time (see Chap. 7). Most adolescents with narcissistic personality disorders have a positive start to their individual therapy, hoping to be recognized for real or perceived achievements. The therapist will need to know how to validate the patient's feelings and carefully point out how other people feel and think in regard to his actions. (Chap. 7). The family therapist will benefit from helping the patient's parents understand the slow nature of change and that therapy will likely include frequent setbacks.

Although Harrison may have a positive start to individual therapy, he will more than likely fight any real attempts to become more self-sufficient. He may feel more comfortable keeping things the way they are than risk the discomfort and disappointment that can come with having higher expectations and will want to end treatment early and before any real improvement has been made. Attempts to explore the conflict between his feelings and attitudes may result in slow and inconsistent progress, although he may temporarily make improvement in some areas followed by periods where he will backslide. Long-term improvements will take time and intense work, as well as a gradual building of trust in the therapist and therapeutic process.

Antisocial Personality Disorder in Adolescence

It is understood that the roots of personality disorders are evident in childhood and adolescence. Most individuals with antisocial personality disorder have histories of disruptive behaviors and conduct disorders with a pervasive pattern of violating the rights of others, often without feelings of remorse as early as the age of 13 [31, 63, 76]. The hallmarks of the prototypical antisocial personality of adolescence in the *DSM–5* include deceitfulness, callousness, hostility, irresponsibility, impulsivity, and risk taking. The prevalence of conduct disorders is 1.8–16% [45]. Antisocial personality disorder is a complex and serious disorder that occurs more frequently in males. The prevalence is approximately 4% of the general population, although it is more common among the prison population, where studies have found a high incidence of temperamental and cognitive problems, two of the four pillars [46, 74].

In adolescents with antisocial personality disorder, there are often impairments in all pillars. There is an overrepresentation in juvenile and adult recurrent offenders with difficult/feisty temperament, poor cognitive abilities, impaired cognitive flexibility, and a history of being raised under a disorganized, environment-insecure attachment pattern. These individuals' maladaptive behaviors are characterized by impulsiveness, poor planning, a short time horizon, meanness, anger, and hostility. DeLisi and Vaughn [25] suggest that temperament theory is central to the etiological study of antisocial behavior over the life-course, adding that temperament theory is basic to the study of behavioral and emotional regulation facets of human behavior. As expected, an above average IQ was found to be the best-replicated protective factor from antisocial personality disorder [61]. Although there is compelling evidence from behavioral genetic research that heritable influences are of importance in the development of antisocial behavior, there is also evidence of nonshared environmental influences [73].

Treatment

Unfortunately, the evidence for psychological and pharmacological treatments for antisocial personality disorder is limited [27, 28]. Youths with antisocial personality disorder, like adults with antisocial personality disorder, do not seek treatment unless mandated through juvenile judicial services, when their maladaptive behaviors have reached a threshold that negatively affects society. Although there are limited effective and practical interventions to improve these youths' ability to regulate emotional states and social interactions, having a diagnostic formulation that makes sense to the parents and helps them understand the neurobiology of the disorder is valuable.

References

1. American Psychiatric Association. Diagnostic and statistical manual of mental disorders. 4th ed. Text Revision. DSM-IV-TR. Washington, DC: American Psychiatric Association; 2000.
2. American Psychiatric Association. Diagnostic and statistical manual of mental disorders. 5th ed DSM-5. Washington, DC: American Psychiatric Association; 2013.
3. Archer RP. MMPI-A: assessing adolescent psychopathology. 3rd ed. New York: Routledge; 2005.
4. Archer RP. Assessing adolescent psychopathology: MMPI-A/MMPI-A-RF. 4th ed. New York: Routledge; 2016.
5. Archer RP, Handel RH, Ben-Porath YS, et al. Minnesota Multiphasic Personality Inventory-Adolescent-Restructured Form (MMPI-ARF): administration, scoring, interpretation, and technical manual. Minneapolis: University of Minnesota Press; 2016.
6. Butcher JN, Williams CL, Graham JR, et al. MMPI-A (Minnesota Multiphasic Personality Inventory-Adolescent): manual for administration, scoring and interpretation. Minneapolis: University of Minnesota Press; 1992.
7. Barry CT, Frick PJ, Killian AL. The relation of narcissism and self-esteem to conduct problems in children: a preliminary investigation. J Clin Child Adolesc Psychol. 2003;32:139–52.
8. Barry CT, Kauten R, Lui JHL. Self-perceptions of social support and empathy as potential moderators in the relation between adolescent narcissism and aggression. Individ Differ Res. 2014;12:170–9.
9. Barr CT, Kerig PK, Stellwagen KK, et al. Narcissism and Machiavellianism in youth: implications for the development of adaptive and maladaptive behavior. Washington, DC: American Psychological Association; 2011.
10. Barry CT, Pickard JD, Ansel LL. The associations of adolescent invulnerability and narcissism with problem behaviors. Personal Individ Differ. 2009;47:577–82.
11. Benoit D. Infant-parent attachment: definition, types, antecedents, measurement and outcome. Paediatr Child Health. 2004;9(8):541–5.
12. Bleiberg E. Treating personality disorders in children and adolescents: a relational approach. New York: Guilford Press; 2004.
13. Biskin RS. Treatment of borderline personality disorder in youth. J Can Acad Child Adolesc Psychiatry. 2013;22(3):230–4.
14. Bowlby J. Attachment, 2nd edition, Attachment and loss, vol. 1. New York: Basic Books; 1999.
15. Bram AD. The relevance of the Rorschach and patient-examiner relationship in treatment planning and outcome assessment. J Pers Assess. 2010;92(2):91–115. https://doi.org/10.1080/00223890903508112.
16. Bram AD, Peebles MJ. Psychological testing that matters: creating a road map for effective treatment. American Psychological Association. 2014. https://doi.org/10.1037/14340-000.
17. Buck JN, Hammer EF, editors. Advances in house-tree-person techniques: variations and applications. Los Angeles: Western Psychological Services; 1969.
18. Cansler D. Review of the Millon adolescent personality inventory. J Couns Dev. 1986;64(7):469–71. https://doi.org/10.1002/j.1556-6676.1986.tb01168.x.
19. Chanen AM, Jovev M, Djaja D, et al. Screening for borderline personality disorder in outpatient youth. J Pers Disord. 2008;4(353–364):18.
20. Chanen AM, Kaess M. Developmental pathways to borderline personality disorder. Curr Psychiatry Rep. 2012;14(1):45–53.
21. Colle L, Hilviu D, Rossi R, et al. Self-harming and sense of agency in patients with borderline personality disorder. Front Psych. 2020;11:449. https://doi.org/10.3389/fpsyt.2020.00449.
22. DeFife J, Malone J, Dilallo J et al. Assessing adolescent personality disorders with the Shedler-Westen Assessment Procedure for Adolescents (SWAP-II-A). Clin Psychol Sci Pract. 2013;20. https://doi.org/10.1111/cpsp.12049.
23. Delgado SV, Songer D. Personality disorders and behavioral disturbances. In: More than medication: incorporating psychotherapy into community psychiatry appointments. Edgemont: Matrix Medical Communications; 2009. p. 65–76.

24. Delgado SV, Strawn JR, Pedapati EV. Contemporary psychodynamic psychotherapy for children and adolescents: integrating intersubjectivity and neuroscience. Berlin, Heidelberg: Springer; 2015.
25. DeLisi M, Vaughn M. Foundation for a temperament-based theory of antisocial behavior and criminal justice system involvement. J Crim Justice, Elsevier. 2014;42(1):10–25.
26. Dozier M, Bernard K. Attachment and biobehavioral catch-up: addressing the needs of infants and toddlers exposed to inadequate or problematic caregiving. Curr Opin Psychol. 2017;15:111–7. https://doi.org/10.1016/j.copsyc.2017.03.003. Epub 2017 Mar 8. PMID: 28649582; PMCID: PMC5477793.
27. Duggan C, Huband N, Smailagic N, et al. The use of psychological treatments for people with personality disorder: a systematic review of randomized controlled trials. Personal Ment Health. 2007;1:95–125.
28. Duggan C, Huband N, Smailagic N, et al. The use of pharmacological treatments for people with personality disorder: a systematic review of randomized controlled trials. Personal Ment Health. 2008;2:119–70.
29. Ellis EE, Yilanli M, Saadabadi A. Reactive attachment disorder. [Updated 2020 Nov 19]. In: StatPearls [Internet]. Treasure Island: StatPearls Publishing; 2020. Available from: https://www.ncbi.nlm.nih.gov/books/NBK537155/.
30. Faust J, Ehrich S. Children's apperception test (C.A.T.). In: Dorfman WI, Hersen M, editors. Understanding psychological assessment. Perspectives on individual differences. Boston: Springer; 2001.
31. Fergusson DM, Horwood LJ, Ridder EM. Show me the child at seven: the consequences of conduct problems in childhood for psychosocial functioning in adulthood. J Child Psychol Psychiatry. 2005;46:837–49. https://doi.org/10.1111/j.1469-7610.2004.00387.x.
32. Garb HN, Wood JM, Lilienfeld SO et al. Roots of the Rorschach controversy. Clin Psychol Rev. 2005;(1):97–118. https://doi.org/10.1016/j.cpr.2004.09.002.
33. Goodman M, Mascitelli K, Triebwasser J. The neurobiological basis of adolescent-onset borderline personality disorder. J Can Acad Child Adolesc Psychiatry. 2013;22(3):212–9.
34. Grilo CM, Becker DF, Fehon DC, et al. Gender differences in personality disorders in psychiatrically hospitalized adolescents. Am J Psychiatry. 1996;153(8):1089–91.
35. Ha C, Petersen N, Sharp C. Narcissism, self-esteem, and conduct problems. Eur Child Adolesc Psychiatry. 2008;17:406–13. https://doi.org/10.1007/s00787-008-0682-z.
36. Hathaway SR, Monachesi ED. Adolescent personality and behavior. Minneapolis: University of Minnesota Press. 1963.
37. Hawkins AA, Furr RM, Arnold EM, et al. The structure of borderline personality disorder symptoms: a multi-method, multi-sample examination. Personal Disord. 2014;5(4):380–9. https://doi.org/10.1037/per0000086.
38. Kaess M, Brunner R, Chanen A. Borderline personality disorder in adolescence. Pediatrics. 2014;134(4):782–93. https://doi.org/10.1542/peds.2013-3677.
39. Kendler KS, Aggen SH, Czajkowski N, et al. The structure of genetic and environmental risk factors for DSM-IV personality disorders: a multivariate twin study. Arch Gen Psychiatry. 2008;65(12):1438–46.
40. Kernberg O. Borderline conditions and pathological narcissism. New York: Aronson; 2000.
41. Lachar D, Boyd J. Personality inventory for children, second edition; personality inventory for youth; and student behavior survey. In: Grisso T, Vincent G, Seagrave D, editors. Mental health screening and assessment in juvenile justice. New York: Guilford Press; 2005. p. 205–23.
42. Larrivée MP. Borderline personality disorder in adolescents: the He-who-must-not-be-named of psychiatry. Dialogues Clin Neurosci. 2013;15(2):171–9.
43. Levy KN. The implications of attachment theory and research for under-standing borderline personality disorder. Dev Psychopathol. 2005;17:959–86. https://doi.org/10.1017/S0954579405050455.
44. Lilienfeld S, Wood J, Garb H. The scientific status of projective techniques. Psychol Sci Public Interest. 2000;1:27–66.
45. Loeber R, Burke JD, Lahey BB, et al. Oppositional defiant and conduct disorder: a review of the past 10 years, part I. J Am Acad Child Adolesc Psychiatry. 2000;39(12):1468–84.

46. Loeber R, Burke JD, Lahey BB. What are adolescent antecedents to antisocial personality disorder? Crim Behav Ment Health. 2002;12:24–36. https://doi.org/10.1002/cbm.484.
47. MacDonald DJ, Standing LG. Does self-serving bias cancel the Barnum effect? Soc Behav Pers. 2002;30(6):625–30. https://doi.org/10.2224/sbp.2002.30.6.625.
48. Mehlum L, Tørmoen AJ, Ramberg M, et al. Dialectical behavior therapy for adolescents with repeated suicidal and self-harming behavior: a randomized trial. J Am Acad Child Adolesc Psychiatry. 2014;53(10):1082–91. https://doi.org/10.1016/j.jaac.2014.07.003.
49. Meltzoff AN. 'Like me': a foundation for social cognition. Dev Sci. 2007;10(1):126–34.
50. Meltzoff AN. Social cognition and the origins of imitation, empathy, and theory of mind. In: Goswami U, editor. The Wiley-Blackwell handbook of childhood cognitive development. 2nd ed. Malden: Wiley-Blackwell; 2011. p. 49–75.
51. Millon T, Davis RD. The millon adolescent personality inventory and the millon adolescent clinical inventory. J Couns Dev. 1993;71:570–4. opinion in psychiatry 26(1);84–89.
52. Millon T, Tringone R, Millon C, et al. Millon pre-adolescent clinical inventory manual. Minneapolis: Pearson; 2005.
53. Millon T. Disorders of personality. In: Introducing a DSM/ICD spectrum from normal to abnormal. 3rd ed. Hoboken: Wiley; 2011.
54. Murray HA. Thematic apperception test manual. Cambridge, MA: Harvard University Press; 1943.
55. Nasrallah HA. Borderline personality disorder is a heritable brain disease. Curr Psychiatry. 2014;13(4):19.
56. Parkes CM, Stevenson-Hinde J, Marris P. Attachment across the lifecycle. London: Tavistock/Routledge; 1991.
57. Paris J. Personality disorders begin in adolescence. J Can Acad Child Adolesc Psychiatry. 2013;22(3):195–6. https://doi.org/10.1007/s00787-013-0389-7.
58. Pincus A, Krueger R. Theodore Millon's contributions to conceptualizing personality disorders. J Pers Assess. 2015;97:1–4. https://doi.org/10.1080/00223891.2015.1031376.
59. Pinto M, Grillo CM. Reliability, diagnostic efficiency, and validity of the Millon adolescent clinical inventory: examination of selected scales in psychiatrically hospitalized adolescents. Behav Res Ther. 2004;42(12):1505–19.
60. Piotrowski C. On the decline of projective techniques in professional psychology training. N Am J Psychol. 2015;17:259.
61. Portnoy J, Chen FR, Raine A. Biological protective factors for antisocial and criminal behavior. J Crim Justice. 2013 (special issue).
62. Roberts BW, Caspi A, Moffitt T. The kids are alright: growth and stability in personality development from adolescence to adult. J Pers Soc Psychol. 2001;81:670–83.
63. Rutter M, Kim-Cohen J, Maughan B. Continuities and discontinuities in psychopathology between childhood and adult life. J Child Psychol Psychiatry. 2006;47:276–95.
64. Schiele BC, Baker AB, Hathaway SR. The Minnesota multiphasic personality inventory. J Lancet. 1943;63:292–7.
65. Shaver PR, Hazan C. A biased overview of the study of love. J Soc Pers Relat. 1988;5: 473–501.
66. Shedler J, Westen D. The Shedler-Westen Assessment Procedure (SWAP): making personality diagnosis clinically meaningful. J Pers Assess. 2007;89:41–55.
67. Skodol AE, Bender DS, Oldham JM. Personality pathology and personality disorders. In: Roberts LW, editor. American Psychiatric Association publishing textbook of psychiatry. 7th ed. American Psychiatric Association, Washington, DC; 2019. p. 711–48.
68. Slade N. Personality inventory for children. In: Volkmar FR, editor. Encyclopedia of autism spectrum disorders. New York: Springer; 2013.
69. Spratt EG, Friedenberg SL, Swenson CC, et al. The effects of early neglect on cognitive, language, and behavioral functioning in childhood. Psychology. 2012;3(2):175–82.
70. Steel P, Schmidt J, Shultz J. Refining the relationship between personality and subjective well-being. Psychol Bull. 2008;134:138–61. https://doi.org/10.1037/0033-2909.134.1.138.
71. Thomas A, Chess S. Goodness of fit: clinical applications from infancy through adult life. New York: Routledge; 1999. p. 39–52.

72. Turner BJ, Dixon-Gordon KL, Austin SB, et al. Non-suicidal self-injury with and without borderline personality disorder: differences in self-injury and diagnostic comorbidity. Psychiatry Res. 2015;230:2835.
73. Tuvblad C, Beaver KM. Genetic and environmental influences on antisocial behavior. J Crim Just. 2013;41(5):273–6. https://doi.org/10.1016/j.jcrimjus.2013.07.007.
74. Washburn JJ, Romero EG, Welty LJ, et al. Development of antisocial personality disorder in detained youths: the predictive value of mental disorders. J Consult Clin Psychol. 2007;75:221–31. https://doi.org/10.1037/0022-006X.75.2.221.
75. Weaver CM, Shaw DS, Crossan JL, et al. Parent-child conflict and early childhood adjustment in two-parent low-income families: parallel developmental processes. Child Psychiatry Hum Dev. 2015;46(1):94–107. https://doi.org/10.1007/s10578-014-0455-5.
76. Whipp AM, Korhonen T, Raevuori A, et al. Early adolescent aggression predicts antisocial personality disorder in young adults: a population-based study. Eur Child Adolesc Psychiatry. 2019;28(3):341–50. https://doi.org/10.1007/s00787-018-1198-9.
77. Wood JM, Nezworski MT, Lilienfeld SO, Garb HN. What's wrong with the Rorschach?: science confronts the controversial inkblot test. San Francisco: Jossey-Bass; 2003.

Chapter 7
Putting it all Together: Adapting to Youths' Strengths and Weaknesses

As a child in school, things were very hard for me to understand often, and I developed a knack, I think ... I developed a process to simplify things so I would understand them.
—*Eric Carle (1929–2021) illustrator and author of The Very Hungry Caterpillar.*

The title of this book, *Promoting the Emotional and Behavioral Success of Youths*, represents the parents' wishes for their children. In the midst of the excitement of the infant's arrival, parents notice that their infant actively engages in his or her care—implicitly signaling to the parents whether his or her needs are met and when they are not. When the parents "get it right," the infant signals approval by smiling, waving with excitement, cuddling, etc. Consequently, parents, *if they are able*, quickly learn how the infant's temperament, activity level, rhythmicity, adaptability, sensory threshold, intensity of reactions, and mood influence his or her needs, and they increasingly appreciate the complexity in meeting these needs. When parents successfully attune to their child's temperament and needs, the "goodness of fit" that was described by Thomas, Chess, and Birch [45] develops (see Chap. 3).

Emphasis on Two-Person Psychology

The variation among different children's physical and emotional needs is a reminder that a one-size-fits-all in parenting is rarely a preferred approach. We all remember friends sharing stories of their babies. Some friends had "easy" babies who were "always happy," interested in new people, and slept well. Other friends shared stories of their babies being difficult to soothe, anxious of new people, and having difficulty sleeping. To comfort these "not so easy" babies, some parents had to rock them for long periods of time, while other parents would drive their baby around in her car seat until she fell asleep.

S. V. Delgado et al., *Promoting the Emotional and Behavioral Success of Youths*,
https://doi.org/10.1007/978-3-030-88075-0_7

Table 7.1 Characteristics of parent-youth relational difficulties

Parent weaknesses in four pillars
Youth weaknesses in four pillars
Psychiatric disorder in parent or youth
Medical or neurological illness in parent or youth
Social factors (e.g., poverty, access to support)
Cultural factors (e.g., beliefs related to mental illness)

These stories of two very different babies illustrate how pediatrician and psychoanalyst John Bowlby observed that "the baby shapes the parent" more than a half century ago [8]. However, we now know this view was incomplete. The qualities of the parent, including their four pillars, greatly influence how they observe and care for their infant and to what extent the parent can adapt to a baby's needs. This perspective is more consistent with "two-person" psychology. We define two-person psychology as a rich and complex process that involves a child and his parents, who through a process of mutual understanding of here-and-now moments of intersubjectivity cocreate experiences that are stored in nonconscious, nondeclarative memory systems as implicit relational schemas, which are needed for successful adaptive growth-promoting behaviors [16]. Indeed, a parent can only "rise" to the level of his or her strengths and may fall short of what an infant may need through his or her own weaknesses in the four pillars. In situations where parents do not "get it right," a careful review of the possible causes for the problem is important (Table 7.1). Thus, helping parents recognize the reasons for relational "mismatches" can help ensure the clinician is able to work in a productive and sufficiently individualized approach for each family.

How to Use this Chapter

We have stressed the importance for clinicians in identifying a youth's strengths and weaknesses by using the concept of the four pillars: temperament, intelligence, cognitive flexibility, and personality (internal working models of attachment). The reasons youths are brought to mental health clinicians vary widely, from inhibitions (social and academic) to disinhibitions (verbal or behavioral). In this chapter, we use the four pillars as the guiding principle to develop practical interventions tailored to address a youth's strengths and weaknesses as identified in the Contemporary Diagnostic Interview and by way of detailed psychological assessments.

In this chapter, we focus on practical interventions to ensure youths' emotional, behavioral, social, and academic success. We take special care to outline interventions that consider the youth's four pillars and focus on nontraditional, nonintuitive parenting approaches to work around his weaknesses and enhance his strengths in order to improve a youth's competencies and employment opportunities. Additionally, we illustrate how these interventions need to be modified according to parents' four-pillar profiles in order to promote healthy, adaptive parenting skills. This is the "art" of giving practical parenting advice that uniquely fits the individuals involved. However, we emphasize that the practical interventions described in this book are not exhaustive but rather serve as guardrails that clinicians can use to help parents support their youths. We also provide several resources that can help clinicians further improve their understanding of the complexities of youths and parents with four-pillar weaknesses; these sources will also help clinicians choose resources to share with parents.

However, the strategies described in this chapter are not intended to replace programmatic therapies such as family-focused therapy (FFT) for youth with bipolar disorder disorders [36], cognitive behavior therapy (CBT) for obsessive compulsive disorders [24] and fear-based anxiety disorders [43], interpersonal therapy for adolescents with depression (IPT-A, [37]), etc. Rather, the relational strategies outlined in this chapter are intended to provide practical help in day-to-day social and emotional functioning within the context of family and friends, regardless of whether a disease-based disorder is present. Indeed, any disease-based disorder may coexist with concerns captured by the four pillars. With this in mind, consider that a refractory mental illness may actually represent the persistence of these underlying "constitutional" concerns. For example, youths with weaknesses in the four pillars will have maladaptive patterns of behavior and emotional processing regardless of whether a disease-based disorder is present. For example, it is expected that depressed youths who respond well to antidepressants will continue to struggle with existing fluid-reasoning weaknesses; they may argue with parents by misinterpreting their good intentions, such as setting limits to help their child organize his or her daily schedule. Indeed, any *Diagnostic and Statistical Manual of Mental Disorders* (5th edition (DSM-5); American Psychiatric Association, 2013) [2] disorder including anxiety and attentional difficulties may coexist with concerns captured by the four pillars. Accordingly, we emphasize relational strategies to facilitate emotional and social functioning independent of whether or not a *DSM–5* disorder is present.

Additionally, it is outside the scope of this book to review educational interventions for youth with formal learning disabilities (e.g., dyslexia, dysgraphia) or moderate-to-severe intellectual disability disorders. Rather, we would encourage readers to communicate with our colleague psychologists or educational specialists to identify academic interventions [21].

Integration of Four Pillar Concerns with Psychiatric Diagnosis

For better or worse, youths with severe behavioral challenges are often met with an equally severe, authoritarian style of parenting. This often includes harsh punishments and unrealistic limit setting, and all too often, these prove to be ineffective interventions and contribute to escalating conflict and arguments. Moreover, even traditional advice given by mental health clinicians often misses the mark. The problem stems from the fact that the root of the issue is often the complex interplay of many factors, including four-pillar weaknesses. By classifying a youth's problems with self-regulation and behavior as solely part of a disease-based psychiatric disorder, the prognosis is often guarded. This can greatly discourage parents who may then consider their youth "broken" and "unfixable." In contrast, when the maladaptive emotional and behavioral problems in youths are understood as influenced by the interplay of weaknesses in their four pillars in addition to disease-based disorders, it allows the clinician to provide individualized interventions to help improve youths' growth and employment opportunities.

This doesn't negate the important role of diagnosing and treating psychiatric conditions; rather, it enhances the clinician's ability to understand specific "symptoms" beyond those under the rubric of a disorder.

Working Alongside Parents: Successes and Struggles

The goal of every mental health clinician is to help parents develop the ability to provide ongoing growth-promoting behaviors for their youth. But, as we have reiterated too often, clinicians tend to provide a one-size-fits-all psychoeducational approach to parents. But how often do we consider a parent whose difficult/feisty temperament makes her unable to offer a calm, neutral response when provoked by her youth's defiance and angry outbursts? Or a parent who struggles with working memory and fluid reasoning when asked to follow through with a complex behavioral plan for his youth? Furthermore, how often does a clinician, with excellent fluid reasoning or verbal communication skills, present information and create expectations that lead parents with four-pillar weaknesses to feel inadequate and defeated?

So how do we practically help parents possessing a wide range of four-pillar profiles provide practical, growth-promoting interventions for their youths' success? First, we start with a conversation about what strategies they typically employ. This information provides a window into their beliefs and opinions, as well as a glimpse of interactions that the youth has experienced throughout his or her life. Further, it provides insight about what the parents expect from their youth, and, more importantly, it alerts the clinician as to whether the parents have the ability to make the needed changes in their own four pillars. Similar to questions asked during the CDI, this discussion reveals aspects of the parents' abilities and characteristics of their four pillars. With this knowledge, the clinician can strategically influence parenting styles to better fit the youth's strengths and weaknesses. By considering both the parent and youth (and the four pillars of the clinician), we construct a therapeutic frame that is positioned for success. In doing so, we give a voice to youth and advocate on their behalf for best-fit expectations and individualized interventions.

Understanding the cultural models parents use to evaluate whether their youth is meeting development skills is crucial, as what they consider healthy can vary in profound ways. For example, research regarding parental perceptions of their young children's temperament suggests that individual variability is culturally structured. Some parents experience youths as difficult if they have temperamentally low adaptability and negative mood. In contrast, Italian parents associate reactive mood as an example of the infant being expressive, and express concern if the infant has a slow-to-warm-up temperament in new social situations, considering it a negative trait [23, 44]. Similarly, some cultures give importance to their youth's academic cognitive abilities, while others to their social and creative skills. In essence, a youth's cultural environment will have significant impact on the development of his or her four pillars.

It is not unusual for clinicians to work with parents who are challenging due to weaknesses in their four pillars. Occasionally, parents with four-pillar weaknesses, maladaptive temperamental traits (difficult/feisty), weakness in cognitive abilities, limited cognitive flexibility, or personality disorders may unknowingly be the main contributor to the youth's emotional and behavioral problems. We are not dismissing that there are parents that openly defy the clinician's interventions; rather, we posit that when we understand the rejection of our efforts from a neurobiological standpoint (four pillars), we can make inroads in appealing to the strengths in their pillars rather that reacting to the weaknesses that contribute to their minimally effective parenting style. In our experience, this approach leads to partnerships with parents who feel supported to implement growth-promoting interventions in their youth's lives.

> We recall a father with strong authoritarian views on parenting who became angry when asked to attempt to ignore the provocative behavior from his son rather than harshly punish him. We should have known better and anticipated his sharp negative reaction based on his difficult/feisty temperament when we "sprang" this new idea with little warning in session. Several sessions later, however, after the clinician had met with both parents alone to explain their son's weaknesses in verbal comprehension and the impact it had in his behavior, they agreed that ignoring his provocative behavior was effective by decreasing negative attention-seeking behaviors, allowing for redirection.

Parents with four-pillar weaknesses may, after conflicts with their youth, continue to interact negatively with their child, a behavior that exposes youths to maladaptive patterns that do not to help resolve conflicts. Youths with four-pillar limitations will implicitly learn that conflict is the norm and will repeat this maladaptive pattern with others.

A harsh, punitive approach by parents serves as a model for aggressive behavior and contributes to coercive parent-child interactions [38]. Furthermore, youths internalize standards for behavior and cognitive and emotional modulating through exposure to parents' harsh interactions, for example, yelling, arguing, and threatening. Thus, punitive and negative discipline from parents leads to cognitive and emotional dysregulation in youths, who will learn to display anger and defiance [17]. Further, contributing to youths' behavioral and emotional dysregulation are the failure of parents to form a warm, supportive relationship, which hampers youths' ability to share and consider the feelings of others [40].

A child with good four pillars may avoid conflict with caregivers with limitations in their pillars by distancing themselves from their parents when in conflict and find support from other people with good pillars in their life (family, teachers, friends, etc.) to model the use of adaptive behaviors.

It is important to learn what youths like—playing a musical instrument, math, or reading, for example—as these interests serve as indicators of their strengths. A youth who is confronted with difficulties in accomplishing a task or school assignment due to cognitive weaknesses may withdraw or act out when a task or assignment is too demanding. He or she may claim to hate a specific task, but may like another task he or she can master. For example, a youth who loves dance, art, and music but hates drama, or becomes agitated only when asked to work on math assignments, may have a weakness in verbal comprehension, fluid reasoning, or speech/language. Further, when youths experience academic frustration, it can lead to behavioral and emotional problems that further interfere with learning and increase the likelihood of failure. Such youths will benefit from individual psychotherapy to learn to identify their weaknesses as well as the strengths they can rely on for success.

Clinicians working with youths with complex problems and multiple four-pillar weaknesses should consider requesting speech/language and occupational evaluations to help determine if the four-pillar weaknesses have affected processes that may interfere with the youth's ability to perform daily activities. The speech/language therapist will tailor interventions to improve difficulties speaking and communicating. The occupational therapist will focus on physical, sensory, or cognitive problems to help the youth gain skills for everyday activities and learn adaptive behaviors and social skills to manage frustration and anger stemming from their weaknesses.

The "Art" of Giving Practical Parenting Strategies to Parents of at-Risk Youths

> Why do I have to tiptoe around my child, providing attention and praise? He or she is not grateful for what I have done for him or her. He or she is acting like Dr. Jekyll and Mr. Hyde.

We will now provide the reader a variety of practical and easy-to-understand interventions to help youths ensure the development of their emotional and behavioral success. We consolidated the practical strategies and interventions for easy reference. The intervention strategies are outlined in the same sequence as previous chapters, starting with difficulties in temperament (Chap. 3), intelligence (Chap. 4), cognitive flexibility (Chap. 5), and ending with personality (Chap. 6).

The reader will understand that it is not always easy to delineate where one four-pillar weakness ends and another begins. Thus, there will be some degree of overlap regarding interventions between areas of weakness and strategies. In our experience, youths rarely present with a single four-pillar concern; so to some degree, this overlap is reflective of real-world practice. For example, youths with temperamental problems can resemble youths with cognitive weakness in verbal comprehension, fluid reasoning, or working memory. Youths with poor working memory will often also have poor cognitive flexibility (rigidity in certain contexts or poor ability to perspective-share). Externalizing problems were associated with low levels of academic competence and high levels of internalizing psychopathology (Moilane et al. 2010).

One parent, a veterinarian and mother of a youth with difficulties in working memory, said: "You've reminded me of what I tell my clients: you can't treat all dogs the same. Not all dogs respond well to firmly being reprimanded. You need to learn what works for each dog."

Below we provide the reader examples of interventions best suited to help youths with specific weaknesses in their four pillars. We also provide examples in which youths may display better four pillars than their parents, and how the clinician can intervene in a useful manner to improve the outcome in such cases.

Temperament

Temperamentally "difficult" children, or those high in negativity or irritability, were rated greater on externalizing problems when parents used negative discipline strategies, whereas those whose parents employed more positive discipline techniques were rated with fewer problems [48]. Further, temperamentally difficult children showed larger decreases in externalizing problems over time when their parents were more sensitive [9, 35].

Youth with Difficult/Feisty Temperament

Briefly, difficult/feisty temperament describes youths with regular patterns of angry, irritable, or distraught moods and behaviors. Though they can be occasionally happy and well adjusted, they unknowingly find it easier to be difficult/feisty as it is familiar to them, and they know to expect a negative reaction from others. Herein, being patient and empathizing with them can be difficult. Difficult/feisty temperament moods can worsen due to family conflict, poor eating habits, poor sleep, loud sounds, and environmental stress. See Chap. 3 for more details on difficult/feisty temperament.

Youths with difficult/feisty temperament have similar maladaptive behaviors to those with poor working memory, poor fluid reasoning, or borderline personality disorder. Clinically, using a *DSM–5* model, they may meet criteria for disruptive behavior disorders, oppositional defiant disorders, disruptive mood dysregulation disorder, impulse control disorders, and mood disorders. Moreover, some youths with difficult/feisty temperament can developmentally improve and are more adaptable in adolescence, although the reasons for this are not fully understood.

Parents of youths with a difficult/feisty temperament initially believe these youths are aware of their negative attitude and that it is intentional. Accordingly, they feel compelled to "fix" the youth's attitude by taking an authoritarian approach. Instead of helping, this often escalates the youth's irritability and defiance. Often, these interactions will evolve into family arguments, which can lead to severe tantrums, physical aggression, or threats of self-harm. This is especially true if either parent also has difficult/feisty temperament.

Conversely, parents with strengths across all four pillars may initially remain patient and empathizing, although these parents may feel frustrated that the tone of the household mood is set by the youth, who needs excessive attention. However, in our experience, these parents eventually become frustrated and are pulled into conflict with their youth. These parents may regret their actions during a conflict, especially if they were excessively harsh, and feel they were pulled "out of character" by the behaviors of the troubled child.

We illustrate this with a case in which a clinician reacts out of character with a youth with difficult/feisty temperament; the parents recognize the clinician's struggle. The reaction begins at the implicit level until it reaches the clinician's consciousness; he or she should then modify the approach.

A 9-Year-Old Boy with a Difficult/Feisty temperament Elicits a Reaction in an Experienced Clinician

Clinician: I am sorry, Jake; this is my space. [*Jake is reaching behind the clinician's desk to open a file cabinet.*] You can use anything that is in your space [*Points to section of games and books.*]

Jake: Why? [*Proceeds trying to open file cabinet*] I just want to see what is in here.

Clinician: [*In a firm voice*] No!

Clinician: [*Looking at parents*] Wow, I am asking you to use a calm voice and I just raised mine. Sorry.

Clinician: [*In a calm voice*] Sorry, Jake, I keep my file cabinet closed, because I have important papers. Does that make sense?

Jake: No. I don't want to see what's in it anymore, anyway. [*Proceeds to play with his electronic game and ignores clinician.*]

Parents: Now you know how difficult he can be. We deal with this almost every day. We feel you now understand our struggle.

Interventions for Youths with Difficult/Feisty Temperament

As the example demonstrates, some youths have lived out years of implicit patterns of interactions that have trained their parents to anticipate fierce confrontations.

For some parents, the approaches below will initially be very difficult! Thus, some parents may report, "We tried to help her, but she became even more upset!" In this situation, we remind parents that the strength of these interventions is not how they work in the moment, but rather their effect when used routinely, which is to familiarize children with the cadence of how the family operates.

Behavior: Is Defiant and Resistant to Reason; Creates Negative Interactions with Others

Intervention

It is important to help parents avoid the natural inclination to address a youth's negative attitude with an authoritarian approach so that their child can "learn who is in charge." This approach reinforces negative behavior and does not allow time to model positive behavior (offering to help them understand why they are upset).

When at an impasse, it is best to redirect youth to a neutral, conflict-free topic, as there will be other less emotionally charged times that can be used as teachable moments. To help them conceptualize this, we ask parents how they would approach asking their spouse to complete a pending task (e.g., mowing lawn, getting the bicycles ready, etc.). Would they do it immediately after the spouse arrived home from work, and in an unhappy mood? Most individuals would inherently understand the benefit of giving their spouse time to settle in before bringing up the task.

The goal of this intervention is to reduce the likelihood that both parties will end in conflict. Herein, parents should be encouraged to meet the youth's yelling with a soft, calm voice to help the youth listen and calm down, and to provide space for de-escalation. It is expected that the youth will forcefully disagree with his parents' point of view. The parent, or parents, should calmly share why they disagree with the youth's point of view and engage their child about what he or she doesn't like about their point of view. This allows for dialogue. Youths may initially become angry if they feel misunderstood by their parents. When at an impasse, consider comments like, "It's hard for me to listen when you are angry. What can I do to help you? Let us figure out what will help you." Parents should take the lead and model moving on to another topic or activity, or, in some cases, disengaging entirely to promote de-escalation.

Some parents, especially those with difficult/feisty temperaments of their own, are at a higher risk to be emotionally swept into the conflict. In these situations, it can be helpful to remind parents that to remain in charge, they must resist the temptation to engage in the "same level" behaviors as the youth. The louder the parent's voice, the louder the youth's will be.

Behavior: Blames Misunderstandings and Mishaps on Siblings or Peers; Encourages Parents to Collude with their Point of View that they Were Treated Unfairly

Intervention

Parents should not assume that their troubled youth knows intuitively that he or she is in the wrong. Youth with difficult/feisty temperament have lifelong patterns of difficult reciprocal interactions. In severe cases, their presence can make other children wary and proactively avoid them. A sibling with good four pillars has years of implicit knowledge of how the troubled youth behaves and may be reluctant to share toys, knowing that getting the toys back will foster conflict. Parents should understand that concentrating on "who started it" will escalate the situation; it is more productive to focus on how the sibling can "end it" constructively. For example, remaining somewhat detached from the conflict and asking in a calm voice how each sibling understands the mishap can redirect the emotional energy of the interaction without leading the youths involved to place blame on each other. Deferring discussion of consequences to a later time will avoid escalating the situation further.

Behavior: Reacts Negatively to Planned or Unplanned Transitions

Intervention

Parents should be counseled to provide ample warning about nonroutine transitions. They should clearly explain the purpose of the new unplanned activity (e.g., "We need to go visit your uncle for his birthday tomorrow.") Proficient parents often remind children of these transitions several days ahead of time or maintain a visual calendar. On the day of the activity, provide verbal reminders ("Let's get ready to go to soccer—we leave in 15 minutes") and add a casual encouragement: "You'll have fun!" Share verbally any temporary changes in the family routine for the day or the week (e.g., "You'll need to take the bus to school this month since I'll be home late from work. It's okay for you to play video games until I get home.") Add a visual component such as a reminder on a whiteboard: "Bus week! Love, Dad."

Some parents who themselves struggle with transition may report that their child became even more upset when given advance warning. It is important to remember that the strength of these interventions is not in how they work in the moment, but rather in how they familiarize youths with the cadence of how the family operates—and set a foundation of expectation for the future.

Behavior: Becomes Oppositional when Asked to Complete Chores or Tasks

Intervention

Parents are not always aware of the environmental circumstances that lead youths to feel angry and distraught. Unhappy youths do not easily accept parents' attempts to help them feel better. When parents sense the emergence of oppositional or hostile emotions, we recommend they take a "wait, watch, and wonder" approach, a nonconfrontational strategy to engage their child (see Chap. 8).

For a younger child, this may mean sitting and playing with them without talking. For an older child, asking what would make them feel happy could offer clues on what is troubling them. This is also an opportunity to gently remind youths of any daily accomplishments or reflections on happy moments (e.g., "Remember when you were happy while skateboarding yesterday?") For some parents, this will be very difficult! (Table 7.2).

Table 7.2 Interventions for youths with difficult/feisty temperament

Behavior	Interventions
• Is defiant; resists reasoning with others, e.g., becomes angry when parents do not agree to buy a requested item or when losing a game to peers. • Experiences negative interactions with others (e.g., parents, friends, and teachers), which perpetuates the maladaptive behaviors and reinforces his or her negative attitude.	• Use a calm and reassuring voice. During conflicts, it is difficult for these youths to accept help from parents, so modeling a calm demeanor is crucial. • Keep in mind that the louder your voice is, the louder your youth's will be. Using a soft,calm voice will help him or her listen. • Model positive behavior by offering to understand what drives your youth's anger. "It's hard when you are angry. What can I do to help you? Let me know what you need, and I will write it down, so we can figure out what happened." • When it isn't possible to discuss the cause of the youth's anger, redirect him or her to a different, conflict-free topic. There will be other opportunities for teachable moments.
• Becomes angry when asked to complete chores. • May loudly declare "No!" or "I don't want to!" when asked. This may stem from difficulties processing information related to the chore or task.	• During better moods, invite her to create a list of chores they find reasonable. Together, make a list of rewards he can expect upon completion. • Do not give lengthy lists of tasks or chores. "Brush your teeth, take a bath, and then get your clothes ready for tomorrow." Rather, ask for completion of one chore at a time and praise his or her efforts: "Good job for brushing your teeth." • For example, If the youth escalate, it is not the time to "win" and demand shecomplete the tasks. Instead,redirectherto a neutral activity.
• Is angry and distraught. • Does not easily accept parents' attempts to help them feel better.	• Inform him that you notice he isnot happy. • Remember that parents are not always aware of the circumstances that lead youths to feel distraught; a friendly question about what would make them feel happy could provide clues on what is troubling them.

Table 7.2 (continued

	• Praise daily accomplishments. • Reflect often about times when she was happy. For example: "Remember yesterday? You were happy playing video games with your friends." • Consider sitting or playing with him without talking. • Use the Wait Watch and Wonder approach (Chapter 8).
• Blames misunderstandings and mishaps on siblings or peers; requests parents collude with their point of view.	• Remain detached from the conflict. In a calm voice, ask how the mishap occurred; this will redirect the emotional energy without placing blame. • Defer discussion of consequences to a later time to avoid escalating the situation.
• Reacts negatively to planned or unplanned transitions.	• Remember that youths need ample advance knowledge of nonroutine transitions. • To prevent "You never told me!" accusations, share multiple times—verbally and in written form—any upcoming changes in the family routine for the day or week, so no one is caught off guard. For example: "…I will be late from work this week.You will take the bus home; it is okay to play until I get there." • Share the purpose of the new activity: " "We need to go visit your aunt this week because it is her birthday." • Before it is time to leave for an activity, give a reminder about expectations: "Let's get ready to go to the park in 15 minutes. We'll have fun on the swings!"

Employment Opportunities

Adolescents with difficult/feisty temperament will perform better in activities that do not require frequent dialogue with people, which will help them avoid conflict. They are often hardworking adolescents if they feel interested in the activity and their work environment is predictable, for example, competitive sports, construction work, vehicle service, landscaping, etc. Their success will vary according to strengths in other aspects of their four pillars. They have similar needs as those with weakness in working memory or borderline personality disorder.

Interventions for Youth with Slow-to-Warm-up Temperament

Review

Youth with a slow-to-warm-up temperament often feel anxious and withdraw from interactions with others when faced with some degree of uncertainty in situations that involve complex reasoning. They generally rely on family or friends to help them know how to make decisions, and this may be frustrating to others who may mistakenly think that the youth is limited.

Youth with slow-to-warm-up temperamental style have similar characteristics as youth with low average to below average processing speed. They should also be carefully assessed for a formal cognitive disability or formal mental health disorders: generalized anxiety disorder, autistic spectrum disorders, etc.

Behavior: Displays Reluctance to Participate in Activities, Even though he or she Wishes to Engage

Intervention

In a nonjudgmental manner, encourage youths to choose activities (with family or peers) that do not require complex reasoning and are not fast-paced. Encourage group activities that do not require active communication with others, like bicycling, golf, swimming, hiking, horseback riding, singing, etc.

In helping a youth prepare to attend a chosen activity, it is important to provide time for them to get ready and not to rush them. They will need time to gather things needed for the activities and, upon arrival, they will need time to acclimate to peers. It is important for them to know in advance the activity rules. After activities, parents can help by encouraging them to engage in dialogue with peers that may have a similar temperamental style.

Behavior: Displays Low Self-Esteem

Intervention

Often, youths with slow-to-warm-up temperament have much to share, but quickly shut down and become anxious when pressured by others to talk ("Come on, tell us what you are thinking!" or "Why aren't you answering the question? You know the answer.") When possible, others should be made aware that the youth will need time to share his or her thoughts. It is helpful to educate others in using encouraging, patient comments: "Take your time; let us know when you are ready to share your thoughts."

Although many parents are anxious about the use of electronic devices and social media, for youths with slow-to-warm-up temperament, these methods can promote competency and self-esteem. For example, they may be more adept at communicating with the use of drawings or text-messaging (Table 7.3).

Table 7.3 Interventions for youths with slow-to-warm-up temperament

Behavior	Interventions
▪ May have much to share but shuts down and becomes anxious when pressured by others: "Come on, tell us what you're thinking." ▪ Experiences low self-esteem when others misinterpret the need for more time to feel safe and speak as defiance.	▪ Giving these youths time to share their thoughts is essential. ▪ Make encouraging, patient comments: "Take your time. Let us know when you are ready to share your thoughts." ▪ Consider communicating through drawings or text-messaging.
▪ Is reluctant to participate in activities, even though he or she wishes to engage.	▪ In a nonjudgmental way, encourage the youth to choose activities (with family or peers) that are not rule-bound, fast-paced,or of high energy level. ▪ Encourage bicycling, swimming, hiking, horseback riding, singing, etc. ▪ Allow the youth ample time to gather things needed for activities, as well as time to acclimate once she arrives.

Employment Opportunities

Adolescents with slow-to-warm-up temperament can do well in activities that do not require fast-paced activities or interactions with many people, for example, teaching music young children, one-on-one tutoring, financial and data management, graphic design, department stores office work, etc. Their success will vary according to strengths in other aspects of their four pillars. They have similar needs as adolescents with slow processing speed.

Cognition

Broadly, cognition—or intelligence—includes the cognitive processes needed to develop an understanding of nonverbal and verbal communications, which means learning from experience and then using this information to make decisions. Cognition helps individuals adapt to environmental demands, develop successful relationships, and achieve academic or career success. Importantly, intelligence is not simply knowing when to act, but also learning to successfully use inhibitory mechanisms to prevent poor decision-making and avoid negative consequences. Further, cognitive development is an ongoing and fluid process. Children must layer cognitive and social skills to best match their developmental cohort and remain competitive.

Interventions for Youths with Verbal Comprehension Weakness

Review

Verbal comprehension, or verbal reasoning, is the ability to access and apply acquired word knowledge. It assumes long-term retrieval functions and the ability to verbalize meaningful concepts, think about verbal information, and express that knowledge by using words. When verbal comprehension is in the low average to below average range, youths have limited abilities to access and apply acquired word knowledge.

Youths with verbal comprehension weakness have similar maladaptive behaviors as those with low to below average fluid reasoning and working memory, as well as those with a cognitive profile of a borderline personality disorder. Using a *DSM–5* model, they may meet criteria for disruptive behavior disorders, oppositional defiant disorders, disruptive mood dysregulation disorder, impulse control disorders, and mood disorders.

Behavior: In Preschool and Elementary Years, Fails to Understand Others: "What do you mean?"

Intervention

Parents' natural inclination is to expect their child to learn useful skills by observing and listening to others. Youths who struggle with verbal comprehension often have more willingness and capacity to understand others—even when difficult—early in the day, since they are more alert and have forgotten difficulties from prior days. As the day goes on, however, they may become overwhelmed with the amount of verbal information they have failed to process; thus, their willingness to give maximum effort to understanding others fades. Further, they may also notice others' frustration with them for not understanding.

Parents should be helped in noticing signs of verbal comprehension weakness. Does their youth expression look bored or otherwise occupied during verbal exchanges? Does the child feel overwhelmed or argue when given complex instructions, or say they are confused about what to do?

These symptoms are often initially interpreted as a negative attitude, with parents believing that an authoritarian approach is needed "so that he or she can learn to pay attention to me." However, as stated before, this approach does not model positive behavior by demonstrating willingness to understand what is making the child upset. Rather, this approach models and reinforces negative behavior.

To help parents conceptualize this, we often use the following example. How would you react, we ask parents, if after a poor night's sleep, your child asked you to help them with an intense task, such as practicing for a final exam by reading questions and checking answers for accuracy? Even a loving, caring parent would likely find herself or himself wishing to delay the task or mentally drifting while attempting to complete it. We emphasize to parents that the negative feelings evoked by participating in such difficult activities are something youths with verbal comprehension weakness feel daily. This helps parents understand the root of the oppositional behaviors regarding complex verbal interactions, as well as why their child's behavior is healthier in areas of competency, for example, reading or visual-spatial abilities.

Behavior: In Middle- and High-School Years, Reacts with Anger when Given Complex Verbal Directions

Intervention

In adolescence, there is an increased need for complex verbal interactions with family, friends, and teachers. As one youth shared, "Yeah, exactly. The more you explain, the more I complain." It is important to help parents recognize that when they engage in a lengthy conversation, they may notice their youth demonstrating signs of frustration due to lack of understanding. When the parents notice this, it is beneficial to apologize and reduce the complexity of the verbal dialogue by talking about one topic at a time. For example, "Can you please tell me what I can help you with? You look frustrated," or "How was your baseball practice?"

Without being too obvious, communication can be improved by writing or drawing daily chores on a whiteboard, and checking them off when completed. As youths grow, text messages can be helpful: "Can you take the trash out? Text me when done" followed by "Thank you for helping" can help promote healthy communication.

Behavior: Misinterprets Verbal Information and Experiences the Frustration of Others as Rejection

Intervention

For children of preschool and elementary school age, ask youths to repeat back directions to show comprehension. If they do not understand the instructions, rephrase, and reduce complexity of the sentence.

In adolescence, youths may feel infantilized by this approach. By then, parents will likely have practiced reducing verbal complexity and learned other tools for confirming comprehension, such as via text: "Sound good?" (Table 7.4).

Table 7.4 Interventions for youths with verbal comprehension weakness

BEHAVIOR	INTERVENTIONS
▪ In preschool and elementary years, when interacting with parents, friends, and teachers, fails to understand interactions. May say, "What?" or "What do you mean? I don't know what you are saying."	▪ Keep language and directions clear and simple: "Please help me put the groceries [on the counter/in the pantry/etc.]." ▪ Avoid repeating questions and statements if she does not understand the first time. ▪ Share information that the youth can conceptualize as a visual image: "Put you coat on because it is [raining/snowing/etc.]. ▪ Point to what he needs: "There's your book," or "The trash can is right there." ▪ Model behaviors through action: "Pick up your clothes like this."
▪ During middle and high school years, may become angry when verbally given complex or multiple directions. ▪ Becomes angry when adults attempt to verbally engage and reason with him or her; this is due to difficulties accessing and applying acquired word knowledge. May say, "You talk too much," or "You always give me long sermons that I don't even understand." Also, "The more you explain, the more I complain."	▪ Reduce background noise when engaged in conversations. ▪ If, during a lengthy conversation, the youth's frustration becomes apparent, stop. Apologize. ▪ Model language with vocabulary and sentence structure that is age appropriate. ▪ Ask the youth to repeat back directions. If he does not understand the instructions, rephrase, reducing the complexity of the sentence(s). ▪ Encourage youth to seek activities she can master (art, animal care, etc.).
▪ May feel left behind. Conversations are more complex in adolescence, and he or she may be surprised by how difficult it is to understand conversations with friends, compared to elementary or middle school years. ▪ Misinterprets information and experiences people's frustration as rejection. ▪ When frustrated, can display regressive and immature behaviors.	▪ Talk about one topic at a time: "How was baseball practice?" ▪ Write or draw daily chores on a dry erase board. Leave space for tasks to be checked off when completed. ▪ Send text messages, even at home: "Can you help take the trash out? Text me when you are done." Follow up with, "Thank you for helping." ▪
▪ Finds learning difficult if not accompanied by visual explanation. ▪ During the COVID-19 pandemic, youth with verbal comprehension weakness had more difficulties with virtual learning that relied on verbal directions.	▪ Remind youths engaged in virtual learning that they can ask for help from their teachers through messaging platforms. ▪ Encourage her to study; give space and ample time for homework. Remain available if she needs help with certain concepts.

Employment Opportunities

Adolescents with verbal comprehension weakness can do well in activities that do not involve fast-paced activities requiring verbal commands, or situations with frequent verbal interactions with customers. They perform better in activities that require visual-spatial reasoning, for example, musical activities, lighting crew, graphic design, bicycle or vehicle repair, etc. Their success will vary according to strengths in other aspects of their four pillars.

Interventions in Youths with Visual-Spatial Weakness

Review

Visual-spatial index measures the ability to evaluate visual details and to understand the details within the context of visual-spatial relationships. It requires visual-spatial reasoning, attention to visual details, and visual-motor integration (e.g., remembering where their next classroom and locker is, etc.). Visual-spatial processing is the ability to mentally manipulate and tell where objects are in two-dimensional and three-dimensional space. Youths with weakness in visual-spatial abilities struggle to evaluate visual details and consequently struggle in visual-spatial reasoning and visual-motor integration. In reading, for example, similar-looking symbols may have different meanings depending on how they are oriented or ordered; youths may misinterpret these if they have trouble what's up, down, left, right, etc. Consider the many common situations that require these skills of youth, such as navigating to their next class, locating their locker, or driving to a new friend's house.

Youth with visual-spatial weakness have similar maladaptive behaviors as those with poor fluid reasoning or nonverbal learning disorders. Using a *DSM–5* disease-based model, they may meet criteria for impulse control disorder and generalized anxiety disorder.

Behavior: Struggles to Evaluate Visual Details

Intervention

Children's struggles with visual-spatial reasoning and visual-motor integration can be noticed when, for example, a child plays with a pegboard and does not know which way to move their peg. Such youths also have difficulties when looking at symbols that have different meanings depending on how they are oriented or ordered in a word.

In later years, they have difficulties knowing which direction to take when walking down school hallways or shopping in large stores. They may also struggle to recognize the meanings of different facial expressions, and later may avoid sports or driving lessons.

To promote competencies, provide examples of constructive solutions and avoid punitive measures. There is evidence that training in perceptual learning can strengthen visual-neural circuits to enhance functioning over time [32].

10-Year-Old Boy with Visual-Spatial Weakness Playing with LEGOs

Parent: Jeff, try putting the LEGO on the other side. [*Parent wants Jeff to move piece to the left side of the tower they are building]* You can see that in the picture, it goes on the other side [*Points to picture of the tower on the box*].

Jeff: Oh yeah [*Proceeds to turn the LEGO on its side and does not move it to the opposite side, where it belongs.*]

Parent: [*Recognizes Jeff does not understand*] Jeff, let me point to where I think it should be.

Jeff: [*Looking at parents*] Wow, it worked. I figured it out.

Behavior: Becomes Frustrated when Following Directions in Complex or Competitive Activity

Intervention

Provide explicit step-by-step verbal and written directions, make cause-effect relationships, and give several examples.

Ask youths to repeat directions or salient information being introduced. Teach youths how to recognize facial expressions, body language, and emotions by role-playing different perspectives (Table 7.5).

Table 7.5 Interventions for youths with visual-spatial weakness

Behavior	Interventions
▪ Displays poor ability to make use of visual images quickly and accurately (for example, while playing complex games that require strategy). ▪ Struggles to evaluate visual details (knowing which direction to go when walking down school hallways, shopping in large stores, etc.).	▪ Provide examples of constructive solutions. Avoid negative comments. ▪ Teach the youth how to recognize facial expressions, body language, and emotions through role-playing different perspectives. ▪ Visit school when not in session to practice walking around to important spaces he will be using (classrooms, gym, cafeteria). ▪ Engage collaboratively in activities designed to enhance visual discrimination skills. ▪ Practice opening a combination lock. ▪ Load (fit) dishes into a dishwasher. ▪ Organize and search a backpack for assignments. ▪ Practice visual (typing in phone) or auditory (recorded memo) of to-do chores: take out trash, etc. ▪ Have a "buddy" assigned during the first two weeks of school to help him learn how to get around. ▪ Enhance navigation skills. In the car, ask him to read street signs out loud. ▪ Count the exit ramps on the way home. ▪ Give examples of important details in visual information: "That car is parked incorrectly; it's taking up two spaces." ▪ When assembling a game or project, read directions aloud and point at what is needed. "The small parts go in the front, like this," or "You will need the pliers and screwdriver here (pointing to the objects)." ▪ Break tasks down into manageable parts and remove time constraints.
▪ Becomes overwhelmed, anxious, and worried when she feels she is not meeting parents', peers',or teachers' expectations. ▪ Has difficulty understanding humor.	▪ Reassure her. Help with tasks. ▪ Point out cause-effect relationships and explain why a given joke or conversation is funny: "When you hear 'Don't let the door hit you on your way out,' it means they are glad you are leaving."

(continued)

Table 7.5 (continued)

▪ Has difficulties remembering where he placed personal items (textbooks, shoes, coat, etc.).	▪ Allow the youth time to gather personal items forfamily activities.
▪ Has difficulties remembering orientation of numbers, letters, and written symbols. ▪ Has difficulty identifying information from clocks (poor sense of time), maps, and charts.	▪ Provide concept maps or charts with important information highlighted. ▪ Use digital clocks. ▪ Ask him to repeat directions or new information.
▪ Becomes frustrated when friends ask her to follow directions in games or competitive activities. ▪ May be clumsy (during bike riding, skipping, use of household tools, etc.).	▪ Practice sports and activities with family members or neighborhood friends.
▪ In adolescence, may delay driving and/or pursuing team sports.	▪ Practice driving in empty parking lots.

Employment Opportunities

Adolescents with visual-spatial weakness can do well in activities with written language or mathematical tasks. Many have very strong verbal skills and can use these to compensate well for their visual-spatial weakness. They do well when interested in the activity, for example, editors, tutors in math or reading, data managers, etc. Their success will vary according to strengths in other aspects of their four pillars.

Interventions in Youths with Fluid Reasoning Weakness

Review

Youths with fluid reasoning weakness demonstrate difficulty in comprehending nuances of instruction or directives when trying to find solutions to unexpected problems in day-to-day activities, for example, spilling their drink, knowing where to look after losing an important object: smartphone, jacket, car keys, etc. At home, they do not grasp the rewards and increase in self-esteem that come from completing chores.

Youths with fluid reasoning weakness have similar maladaptive behaviors as those with low to below average working memory or borderline personality disorder. Clinically, using a *DSM–5* model, they may meet criteria for disruptive behavior disorders, oppositional defiant disorders, disruptive mood dysregulation disorder, impulse control disorder, and mood disorder.

Behavior: Becomes Frustrated in Situations in which he or she can't Identify Solutions; Demands Answers from Others

Intervention

In preschool and elementary years, teach problem-solving strategies by sequencing questions that need to be asked when approaching a problem, and slowly teach multiple approaches to solving problems. Provide analogies and examples they can relate to in daily life.

Role-play with a think-out-loud step followed by guided practice with feedback.

Visually explain the benefits of completing an activity or chore: "You will be able to keep your bike ready to ride if you put it in the garage [pointing] every day and don't leave it outside.

In adolescence, when youths become frustrated trying how to solve complex problems, share out loud possible solutions and reasons why it may work. "It might help if you write the things you need to do this week; after that, you can rearrange them to prioritize by importance or deadline."

Behavior: Has Difficulty Generalizing Past to New Experiences

Intervention

Youths may have difficulties making use of the information obtained from one experience as it may apply to others. In these situations, the use of graphic organizers can help visualize and organize this approach (much like a storyboard seen in TV crime dramas, in which police look at characters on the board to solve the crime). At home, use activity maps that categorize and sequence typical daily and weekend activities. Allow space to write down praise after a youth completes daily/weekly chores (Table 7.6).

Table 7.6 Interventions for youths with fluid reasoning weakness

Behavior	Interventions
▪ Has difficulty retrieving from memory information necessary to solve new problems (e.g., running late and missing the school bus, setting up for virtual learning, etc.). ▪ Has difficulties identifying and applying rules of conceptual relationships and abstract thinking to day-to-day obstacles.	▪ Teach problem-solving strategies by sequencing questions when approaching a problem. Gradually teach multiple approaches to solving problems. "When you miss the bus, walk back home and tell us. We'll drive you to school." ▪ Provide analogies they can relate to in daily life. "Just like you text your friends, you can text us at home when you need help with your schoolwork." ▪ Role-play with a think-aloud step followed by guided practice with feedback.
▪ Has difficulties understanding and evaluating the opinions and views of others.	▪ Share out loud your opinion of others' views, as well as the reasons behind your opinion. ▪ Ask clear, concise questions versus open-ended questions Do not say "How did it go?"
▪ Worries about how he will perform on new tasks and may be resistant to learning new strategies or approaches.	▪ Use a graphic organizer to help him organize his thoughts. ▪ Make home activity maps. Categorize and sequence typical daily and weekend activities. ▪ Praise him when completed chores/tasks leadto good outcomes.
▪ Becomes easily frustrated in situations where shecan't identify solutions. Demands others tell her how to solve the problem.	▪ Teach hands on problem-solving strategies. ▪ Sequence questions that need to be asked when approaching a problem. ▪ Role-play with a think-aloud step followed by guided practice with feedback.
▪ Experiences the suggestion to slow down and consider the options as an attack on his intelligence.	▪ Break chores or schoolwork into smaller parts and time frames; do not hesitate to help him directly.
▪ May develop generalized anxiety; uncertainty and learning something new may be intimidating, because she feels something bad may happen in unpredictable situations.	▪ Consider psychiatric evaluation for anxiety and possible use of psychotherapy and medication.

Employment Opportunities

Fluid reasoning, in youth, accurately predicts performance in school, university, and cognitively demanding occupations [19]. Adolescents with fluid reasoning weakness do well in activities that do not require a significant amount of complex reasoning. Many have strong visual-spatial skills and can use these to compensate well for their weakness. They are hardworking adolescents if they feel interested in the activity, for example, tutoring in math or reading, data management, etc. Their success will vary according to strengths in other aspects of their four pillars.

Interventions for Youths with Processing Speed Weakness

Review
The processing speed index measures the ability to rapidly identify, register, and make decisions about visual information. It requires the ability to visually scan, discriminate, and use short-term visual memory. Processing speed is key to being able to process relevant information between brain regions. Youths with processing speed weakness require longer to reason and integrate social information in their daily fast-paced activities. Nearly every activity at home and school comes with the implicit expectation that youths will complete the activity within a standard period of time. In that sense, youths with processing speed weakness will be frequently challenged. As a result, they require extra time to articulate what they hope to say to others. Sadly, their delay in response is often experienced by others as being defiant or as a sign of severe cognitive impairment. Further, youths with superior (gifted) or above average intelligence who also have slow processing speed are often thought as having attention-deficit/hyperactivity disorder, predominantly inattentive, but do not improve with the use of medication. Youths with processing speed weakness have similar maladaptive behaviors as those with slow-to-warm-up temperament.

As we illustrated with the brave turtle (Chap. 3), the term "lazy" is not appropriate to use with these youths, considering they may be exerting considerably more effort to complete a task on time compared to their peers.

Clinicians should consider processing speed weakness as a possible reason for youth's "symptoms" when using a disease-based model, as they often are given the diagnoses of oppositional defiant disorders, attention-deficit/hyperactivity disorder, and anxiety disorders and may not improve even if medication helps the comorbid disorder.

Behavior: Is Reluctant to Participate in Activities, Even though he or she Wishes to Engage

Intervention

In elementary-, middle-, and high-school years, parents can expect to see their youth become reluctant to participate in activities with other peers, as they intuitively know participating will be difficult, even though emotionally, they wish to engage. In a nonjudgmental way, parents should encourage these youths to choose activities (with family or peers) in which they are more likely to succeed and enjoy. These activities should not be rule-bound, fast-paced, or require a high energy level. Suitable activities include bicycling, swimming, hiking, horseback riding, singing, etc.

Parents should also be mindful that their youths will need more time than is common to gather things needed for activities and to acclimate once they arrive.

Behavior: Takes Longer than Others to Reason and Integrate Social Information

Intervention

Often youths with processing speed difficulties have much to share but shut down and become anxious when pressured by others to speak up: "Come on, tell us what you are thinking!" or "Why aren't you answering the question? You know the answer." Parents can help by learning about what can be expected from their youth and helping them not feel ashamed to share with peers and teachers that they need extra time to share their thoughts.

Encouraging comments can be helpful: "Take your time; let us know when you are ready to share your thoughts."

Additionally, communication can be facilitated with the use of drawings or text messaging (Table 7.7).

Table 7.7 Interventions for youths with processing speed weakness

BEHAVIOR	INTERVENTIONS
▪ Is reluctant to participate in activities even he or she wishes to engage.	▪ In a nonjudgmental way, encourage the youth to choose activities (with family or peers) that are not rule-bound, fast-paced, or of high energy level. ▪ Encourage bicycling, swimming, hiking, horseback riding, singing, etc.
▪ Takes longer than usual to reason and integrate social information in fast-paced activities.	▪ Allow him ample time to respond to questions, make decisions, and complete schoolwork. ▪ Reduce environmental distractions. ▪ Teach the youth how to monitor time (use an hourglass or digital timers).
▪ Is socially awkward, due to slow processing of conversations. ▪ Has difficulties processing nonverbal behavior (e.g., facial expressions, object-related gestures).	▪ Parents should share with family and friends the reasons for the youth's slow responses: "Please give him time to explain what he means." ▪ Maximize verbal components of instructions.
▪ Experience's feelingsof depression and anxiety. ▪ Feels inadequate or like a slow learner.	▪ Encourage him to develop coping skills to reduce feelings of depression, demoralization and anxiety when challenged. ▪ Acknowledge the youths' distress by repeating what seems to be bothering them. ▪ If behavior escalates, re-direct emotions by reflecting understanding of their distress and feelings of being overwhelmed. ▪ Encourage youth to think about solutions when they are in a place that has fewer time constraints/time pressures.
▪ Struggles to work under pressure from time constraints.	▪ Do not require the youth to work under time constraints.
▪ Is slow to understand and follow directions. ▪ May be slower to make decisions.	▪ For lengthy tasks or assignments , teach her to monitor time and provide short breaks.
▪ Is often bullied or ostracized for being slow,with a negative impact on his self-esteem.	▪ Consider psychotherapy or a medication evaluation.

Employment Opportunities

Adolescents with processing speed weakness, similar to those with slow-to-warm-up temperament, are successful in slow-paced work environments. Although they may have trouble coming up with quick verbal responses, they can be very good in graphic design, writing, research, or in the analysis of sports teams' statistics, financial records, data management, etc. Their success will vary according to strengths in other aspects of their four pillars.

Interventions for Youths with Working Memory Weakness

Review

Working memory is essential for interactions with others within the context of social norms and culture. This index measures the ability to register, maintain, and manipulate visual and auditory information in conscious awareness. Working memory requires attention and concentration in order to accurately discriminate information. Day-to-day verbal conversations are influenced by one's ability to translate visual and auditory information, verbal dialogue, and facial expressions within the context of the conversation. Likewise, games that require long periods of play with many alternatives require a significant amount of working memory.

Youths with working memory weakness have significant difficulties interacting with others. They struggle in situations that require the use of simultaneous processing and storing information and may fail to understand implicit meaning in the ebb and flow of conversations with others. These difficulties lead them to unknowingly push family and friends away due to the inability to stay on topic for resolution of day-to-day conflicts. They feel social norms are unrealistic or rigid and defy them (e.g., bully others, laugh at mishaps of others, defy adults' expectations, etc.). They commonly experience others as bullying *them* and lack insight about their own bullying behaviors toward others who have difficulty being around them. Consequently, they have problems with the internal moral compass needed for understanding and respecting the intent and thoughts of others as different than their own. The notion of a Storm Chaser (Chap. 3) captures their unconscious efforts to seek relationships with youths that think and act like them. Moreover, they are in constant conflict with others, believing their own perceptions to be correct. These youths are at particular risk of misusing social media, with behaviors including cyberbullying, "sexting," or over-disclosure. Consequently, they have problems assimilating traditional views of morality and societal norms, including respecting the intent and thoughts of others. Working memory weakness contributes to the neurobiology of borderline personality disorder in adolescence. Relevant cases are described in more detail in Chap. 5.

Youths with working memory weakness have similar maladaptive behaviors as those with poor fluid reasoning or borderline personality disorder. Clinically, using a *DSM–5* model, they may meet criteria for disruptive behavior disorders, oppositional defiant disorders, disruptive mood dysregulation disorder, impulse control disorder, and mood disorder.

Behavior: Fails to Develop Adaptive Ways of Managing Complex Social Situations

Intervention

Encourage youths to process maladaptive behaviors with their dialectical behavior therapist. Parents should be active participants in their children's treatment and should learn how to use mindfulness and dialectics to provide growth-promoting comments and to reward and reinforce positive behavior: "I hear what you said. What if we look at the situation in another way?"

Use DBT skills (see below). Praise a youth when he or she uses positive coping skills.

Behavior: Unknowingly Pushes Family or Friends Away Due to an Inability to Resolve Day-to-Day Conflicts

Intervention

Parents who find themselves in conflict with their youth because of his or her maladaptive behaviors will find it helpful to describe how he or she—the parent—feels, and to provide possible solutions: "I feel (sad/upset), but I will use my coping skills to help us get along. Okay?" Avoid arguments and engage in problem-solving skills: "I heard what you said. What if we look at the situation in a different way?" Encourage processing conflicts with the youth's dialectical behavior therapist. Praise the youth for using positive coping skills.

Behavior: Feels Social Norms Are Unrealistic or Rigid and Defies them

Intervention

Parents will find that youths with working memory weakness think of social norms as unrealistic and do not have the insight needed to understand their value. During arguments about social norms, use a calm and reassuring voice to model regulation (mindfulness). This can be followed by a brief explanation of the benefits in following norms; for example, completing chores/assignments will give them more time with friends, use of car, etc. Use DBT skills (see below). Praise youths when they use positive coping skills (Table 7.8).

Table 7.8 Interventions for youths with working memory weakness

Behavior	Interventions
▪ Does not follow directions due to short-term memory deficits. ▪ Has trouble learning to read, reading efficiently, and comprehending material. ▪ Has poor attention and concentration.	▪ Break directions down into individual, numbered steps (checklists). ▪ Reduce environmental distractions. ▪ Encourage the use of external memory aids for home or extracurricular activities (chore lists, electronic calendar entries, and digital alarms). ▪ Consider evaluating for formal attention-deficit/hyperactivity disorder or formal learning disability.
▪ Has difficulty interacting with others because he or she has problems grasping the implicit meaning of conversations. ▪ Fails to remember how to make use of adaptive ways of managing complex, emotionally laden social situations. ▪ Displays disruptive behavior at home and school when limits are set. ▪ When upset, demonstrates frustration, anger, and mood swings. Can be impulsive.	▪ Use a calm voice to model regulation of affect (mindfulness). ▪ Provide brief explanations of the benefit in completing the chore/assignment. ▪ Ask her to repeat back your request; praise her for accuracy. "Call me when you get to your friend's house and when you leave. Got it?" ▪ Limit comments and keep them to the point.
▪ Feel unfairly treated or rejected. Unknowingly pushes family or friends away due to his inability to discern the intent of others. ▪ Has poor self-care coping strategies. ▪ Uses self-harm to manage emotional dysregulation. ▪ Is at risk for substance use disorder.	▪ Praise the youth when he uses positive or DBT coping skills.
• Feels social norms are unrealistic or rigid and defies them.	• Use a calm and reassuring voice to model regulation (mindfulness). This can be followed by a brief explanation of the benefits in following the norms: e.g., completing their chores/assignments will give them more time with friends, use of the car, etc. • Use DBT skills (see below).

Employment Opportunities

Adolescents with working memory weakness do well in activities that do not require complex decision-making or frequent customer interaction. Like adolescents with difficult/feisty temperament or borderline personality disorder, they must have interest in the activity to be successful, for example, retail, construction work, vehicle service, landscaping, etc. Their success will vary according to strengths in other aspects of their four pillars.

Personality

Interventions in Youths with Borderline Personality Traits or Disorder

Review

Borderline personality disorder is not only a reliable and valid diagnosis among adolescents; having an early diagnosis can also lead to beneficial early interventions to improve regulation of their emotional state as well as social interactions. Evaluating for borderline personality disorder should be routine practice in youth mental health care in order to provide tailored treatment interventions to improve well-being and long-term prognosis [28]. No specific genes have been linked to this disorder, but there seems to be some genetic vulnerability linked to temperamental traits [29]). In Chap. 3, we defined the "Storm Chaser" as the archetype of a youth with borderline personality disorder by highlighting specific patterns of weakness in his or her four pillars: difficult/feisty temperament and low to below average working memory.

In contrast to conventional thought, borderline personality disorder is increasingly viewed as a neurobiological disorder that may emerge in children in stable, secure families with no history of traumatic or adverse events. The clinician may find that youths with borderline personality disorder can have caring parents with good four pillars who may feel guilty and responsible for their child's problems even though they have raised other children successfully. In some cases, the emergence of severe behavioral symptoms may result in a caustic and chaotic environment that contributes to the higher likelihood of adverse childhood events. Parents will benefit from understanding the biology of borderline personality disorder and should receive help in managing their guilt and learning adaptive interventions.

In adolescence, these youths gravitate to peers with similar weaknesses and, thus, their risk for secondary traumatic events increases. However, they may also face familial biological vulnerabilities: some parents of youths with borderline personality disorder also have personality disorders themselves and may demand the clinician use specific medications even if not indicated (medical marijuana or other high-risk drugs like benzodiazepines). These parents may also reject the clinician's interventions.

Classification in the *DSM–5* disease-based model often will include co-occurring disorders or capture specific contextual/reactive symptoms such as for oppositional defiant disorders, disruptive dysregulation mood disorder, nonsuicidal self-injury disorder, impulse control disorder, substance use disorders, and bipolar disorders.

Behavior: Develops Unstable Relationships (Becomes Overly Attached and Quickly Disappointed for Not Having Undivided Attention and Emotional Needs Met)

Intervention

Parents who find themselves in a conflict with their youth should use mindfulness to avoid engaging in verbal conflict. Avoid arguments; instead, engage in problem-solving skills: "I like what you said. What if we look at the situation in a different way?"

Encourage the youth to process conflicts with their dialectical behavior therapist.

Behavior: Displays Impulsive Risk-Taking behaviors (Substance Use, Sexual Activity, Runaway Activity, Nonsuicidal Self-Injury [NSSI], or Suicidal Attempts)

Intervention

Encourage youths to process risk-taking behaviors with their dialectical behavior therapist. Parents should be active participants in the treatment of their youth to learn how to provide growth-promoting comments as well as to learn to validate the adolescent's emotional experience. For example, parents should reward and reinforce positive actions and show empathy: "Thank you for ... ;" "I can tell this is difficult; I'm sorry things are so tough right now," etc. (Table 7.9).

Table 7.9 Interventions for youths with borderline personality traits or disorder

Behavior	Interventions
▪ Has a tendency toward unstable relationships; becomes overly attached and quickly disappointed for not having undivided attention and emotional needs met. ▪ Idealizes and later devalues family members or others: "I love you, I hate you." This is commonly known as "splitting."	▪ Provide possible solutions to their disappointments: "I hope you can use your coping skills to help you with your disappointment about what happened in chorus today. Things will get better. I am proud of you." ▪ Encourage the youth to process conflicts with his therapist. ▪ Avoid sharing negative feelings about his difficulties in the moment, as he feels abandoned at such times.
▪ Engages in impulsive risk-taking behaviors when angry (substance use, sexual activity, running away, non-suicidal self-injury (NSSI) or suicidal attempts).	▪ Reward and reinforce positive actions: "Thank you for remaining calm and using coping skills." ▪ When she is calmer, reflect on the dangers of risk-taking behaviors and describe/remind her of DBT skills she can use when she has the urge toward risky behaviors.
▪ Displays low or inflated self-esteem.	▪ Show interest by listening without interrupting.
▪ Displays verbal and physical aggression toward family and peers for not meeting his or her expectations (common with difficult/feisty temperament).	▪ Avoid arguments and engage in problem-solving skills: "I heard what you said. What if we look at the situation in a different way?" ▪ Acknowledge the youth's distress by repeating back what seems to be bothering them. Encourage her to think about solutions in which the parent can give his or her opinion. ▪ If behavior escalates, redirect emotions by using DBT skills.

Employment Opportunities

Like adolescents with working memory weakness, these youths do well in activities that do not require complex decision making or direct contact with customers; this allows them to avoid conflict. They often are hardworking adolescents if they feel interested in the activity and find the work environment supportive, for example, elder care, animal care, data management, filing, etc. Their success will vary according to strengths in other aspects of their four pillars.

Treatment for Borderline Personality Disorder in Youth

When developing treatment interventions for adolescents with borderline personality disorder, an important goal is to decrease maladaptive behaviors and improve psychological and social functioning. To do so, treatment planning should include psychotherapies, family therapy, pharmacology, and hospitalization when in crisis.

Two evidence-based psychotherapeutic interventions most often used for borderline personality in adolescents are Dialectical Behavior Therapy (DBT-A) and Mentalization-Based Therapy (MBT-A).

Dialectical Behavior Therapy (DBT) Skills and Techniques

Dialectical behavior Therapy (DBT) is a cognitive behavioral treatment program developed to treat suicidal patients who meet criteria for borderline personality disorder. It targets suicidal behavior, behaviors that interfere with treatment, and dangerous, severe, or destabilizing behaviors. Standard DBT addresses the following five functions: increasing behavioral capabilities, improving motivation for skillful behavior (through contingency management and reduction of interfering emotions and cognitions), assuring generalization of gains to the natural environment, structuring the treatment environment to reinforce functional rather than dysfunctional behaviors, and enhancing therapist capabilities and motivation to treat patients effectively. Treatment includes four interventions: weekly individual psychotherapy (one hour per week), group skills training (two and a half hours per week), telephone consultation (as needed within the therapist's limits to ensure generalization), and weekly therapist consultation team meetings to enhance therapist motivation and skills and to provide therapy for the therapists [33] (Table 7.10).

Mentalization-Based Therapy for Adolescents with BPD

Mentalization-based therapy (MBT) is a treatment model rooted in a psychodynamic framework and in attachment theory. MBT for adolescents (MBT-A) is based on the view that a core problem for adolescents with borderline personality disorder is a breakdown of their mentalizing capacity in emotional and interpersonal situations. The aim of MBT-A is to promote skills through a transference-based approach to establish mentalizing abilities to allow uncomfortable affective states to become manageable [5, 6].

Table 7.10 Practical DBT Social Skills for Adolescents

DIALECTICAL BEHAVIORAL THERAPY

Treatment Interventions for Adolescents with Borderline Personality Disorder

MINDFULNESS "RADICAL ACCEPTANCE"

Letting go of the illusion of control, and a willingness to notice and accept things as they are, without judging.

INTERPERSONAL EFFECTIVENESS

Learning to get along with others while also asserting your own needs is essential to healthy relationships.

- objective effectiveness, relationship effectiveness, and self-respect effectiveness

EMOTIONAL REGULATION

Appreciate the importance of emotions and work toward having greater control to identify emotions, how they affect behaviors, and process of intense emotional reactions.

DISTRESS TOLERANCE

Becoming aware of internal emotional states and its effect on thought patterns or actions

Interpersonal Effective Skills adapted from Marsha M. Linehan's book, Skills Training Manual for Treating Borderline Personality Disorder 1993, The Guilford Press, New York, NY

(continued)

Table 7.10 (continued)

"DEAR MAN" SKILL

Interpersonal Effectiveness from Dialectic Behavioral Therapy

How to make an effective request.

PURPOSE

How to effectively ask for what you want.

Describe

Describe the situation in terms of facts.
Seek mutual starting point.

Express

Express your understanding & feelings.
Use "I", not "you" statements.

Assert

Assert yourself by asking for what you want or do not want. Avoid others "mind reading" you.

Reinforce

Reinforce to others the positive effects of getting what you want.

Mindful

Focus on the current issue.
Avoid distractions and past grievances.

Appear Confident

Make eye contact and convey your seriousness with a confident tone of voice.

Negotiate

Make the situation a "win win".
Make your position more appealing.

A successful process does not always mean you will get what you want. Being able to hear "no" and keep communication open will foster healthy and growing relationships.

Interpersonal Effective Skills adapted from Marsha M. Linehan's book, Skills Training Manual for Treating Borderline Personality Disorder 1993, The Guilford Press, New York, NY

(continued)

Table 7.10 (continued)

"WHAT" AND "HOW" SKILLS

Mindfulness Skills from Dialectic Behavioral Therapy

PURPOSE

Once you decide to be mindful, these skills are "what" to do and "how" to do it.

WHAT?

Observe	Describe	Participate
Pay attention to events, and emotions.	Use words to describe events and label emotions.	give attention to the activity and be present

HOW?

Non-judgmentally	One-mindfully	Effectively
Let go of thinking in terms of good and bad, right and wrong.	One-thing at a time with full awareness.	Do what works, rather than inaction and wishing reality was different

Interpersonal Effective Skills adapted from Marsha M. Linehan's book, Skills Training Manual for Treating Borderline Personality Disorder 1993, The Guilford Press, New York, NY

(continued)

Table 7.10 (continued)

"GIVE" AND "FAST" SKILLS

Interpersonal Skills from Dialectic Behavioral Therapy

Valuing self and others.

"GIVE" PURPOSE:

Foster positive interactions.

Gentle

Stay tempered in conversations.
Don't judge, name call, or threaten.

Interested

Listen and appreciate for the point of view of others.

Validate

Acknowledge the feelings, wishes, difficulties, and opinions of others.

Easy manner

Have an easy attitude, smile, and be light hearted.

The "GIVE" skills communicate respect for the feelings, opinions, and thoughts of others. They promote growth in relationships.

"FAST" PURPOSE:

Foster value in yourself.

Fair

Focus on the current issue.
Avoid distractions and past grievances.

Apologies

Apologize only when needed.
Do not apologize for disagreement.

Stick

Stick to your values and morals.
Be clear in your way of thinking and acting.

Truthful

Avoid lies and exaggeration.
Make observations and be factual.

The four "FAST" skills develop self-respect and develop a foundation of trust in your own actions.

Interpersonal Effective Skills adapted from Marsha M. Linehan's book, Skills Training Manual for Treating Borderline Personality Disorder 1993, The Guilford Press, New York, NY

(continued)

Table 7.10 (continued)

"PLEASE, MASTER" SKILLS

Emotional Regulation Skills from Dialectic Behavioral Therapy

Resilience to Negative Emotions

PURPOSE: STAYING OUT OF THE EMOTIONAL MIND

P L Physical Illness

Be aware of your body, keep healthy, and take prescribed medications.

Eating

Be aware of how certain types and quantites of food affect your emotions.

Avoid

Avoid mood altering drugs including alcohol.

Sleep

Have a sleep routine that helps you feel good.

Exercise

Engage in exercise daily, building up to at least 20 minutes daily.

PURPOSE: FOCUS ON BUILDING STRENGTH

MASTERy

Building mastery develops strengths that enhance self-respect and interpersonal interactions.

Example:

- enhance an existing skill or hobby
- build positive experiences with others
- concentrate on what you enjoy
- be mindful of current emotions
- give yourself credit for what you accomplished
- seek opportunities to practice and gain experience

Together PLEASE MASTER skills can reduce emotional vulnerability and enhance control over emotional decision making.

Interpersonal Effective Skills adapted from Marsha M. Linehan's book, Skills Training Manual for Treating Borderline Personality Disorder 1993, The Guilford Press, New York, NY

Bleiberg emphasizes a fundamental division in mentalizing processes: they can be either fast and implicit (automatic/implicit) or slow and regulated (controlled/explicit). Automatic/implicit mentalizing involves the parallel and visceral activation of thoughts and actions, which require little effort, attention, or intention. On the other hand, controlled/explicit mentalizing involves a more sequential and intentional process of balancing an awareness of one's own mental states while also incorporating that of others.

Stress is a key regulator of mentalizing states. Often, as Bleiberg writes, controlled/explicit mentalizing will be inhibited at a certain "switch point" of stress. In this model, disruptions in mentalizing are central to the adolescents' psychopathology, especially involving borderline personality signs and symptoms. Indeed, there is substantial neurobiological evidence that patients with borderline personally disorder have a lower threshold for activating the sympathetic ("fight or flight") nervous system and preferentially deactivate regions of the brain involved in controlled/explicit mentalizing in neuroimaging studies [20].

MBT for adolescents and their families provides a systematic approach that shifts misunderstanding and mistrust (nonmentalizing) to understanding (mentalizing) of self and others, which is particularly important to practice in the contexts in which it becomes impaired. Promoting mentalizing helps families shift from coercion or impasse to mentalizing interactions by creating a "scaffolding" that supports effective communication and problem solving. The core components of MBT include psychoeducation for parents and adolescents, the development of a mentalizing formulation, adopting a mentalizing stance, and a structured approach to individual and family sessions. A mentalizing approach can reduce epistemic mistrust by techniques such as (1) nonjudgmental listening; (2) acknowledging that trust needs to be earned; (3) appreciating others' feelings; and 4) checking to be sure they feel understood.

Thus, MBT-A seeks to develop a mentalizing stance through skill training, insight, and encouragement, which includes the following:

(a) An actively curious, inquisitive demeanor.
(b) Emphasis on uncertainty and plurality of individual perspectives.
(c) Efforts to stop and rewind misunderstandings.
(d) Self-disclosure about one's own thoughts and feelings in ordinary language (to model sound mentalizing).
(e) Attention to comprehending highly charged emotions, especially in the context of the therapeutic relationship.

MBT-A sits as an evidence-based alternative to DBT-A. Compared to DBT-A, MBT-A approaches require less formal training. However, in practice, the two techniques share similarities in terms of overall treatment goals. The adolescent format has been empirically validated and used to treat eating disorders, depression, posttraumatic stress disorder, and antisocial personality disorder [42] (Table 7.11).

Table 7.11 Components of mentalizing the transference

Validation of experience
Exploration in the current relationship
Accepting and exploring enactment (therapist's contribution)
Collaborating in arriving at understanding
Presenting alternative perspective
Monitoring patient's reaction
Exploring patient's reaction to new perspective

Adapted from Bleiberg E [6]

Interventions for Youths with Narcissistic Personality Traits or Disorder

Review

Narcissistic personality disorder in youths has been a controversial and rarely used diagnosis. Despite the presence of the disorder's precursors in childhood, many clinicians believe that diagnosing a youth with narcissistic personality disorder was stigmatizing and detrimental [15].

Narcissistic personality disorder in youths best describes a pathological pattern of behavior including persistent periods of limited empathy, self-centeredness, a desperate need for admiration, and grandiose beliefs of superiority. Importantly, most teenagers are, to some degree, self-centered and insecure—and may demonstrate an inflated view of their abilities. Children are expected to have narcissistic traits during typical development and will increasingly develop empathy as they socially integrate. In determining the diagnosis, the clinician should broaden the context of the history, including the youth's behaviors with neighbors, teachers, relatives, and peers to best identify *pervasive* and *pathological* narcissistic behaviors. The term "narcissist" holds an especially harsh connotation in popular media and should not be used lightly by clinicians, especially when dealing with youths.

In pathological narcissism, the core symptoms are expected to cause significant functional impairment in multiple domains. These youths are often dominating and preoccupied with success and power. Others may be preoccupied with extreme hypersensitivity over rejection and criticisms, appearing condescending and arrogant. They exploit or take advantage of people by manipulating for personal gain. Parents, teachers, and siblings often fear the youth's anger and avoid setting limits for fear of verbal aggression. In these cases, though the youth may not see a need for treatment, a diagnosis may provide opportunities for early intervention or de-escalation.

The relationship of how narcissistic personality disorder develops, and how to parent a narcissistic youth, remains complex. A recent study of over 300 participants with narcissistic personality disorder, ages 17–25, found that participants recalled childhood experiences in which they felt overprotected, overvalued, and experiencing leniency in parental discipline—more so than maltreatment [47].

Youths with narcissistic personality disorder come to the clinician's attention when their demanding and maladaptive behaviors reach a threshold that negatively affects their family system. Parents may feel guilty and responsible for their youth's problems, even though they may have raised other children successfully.

Although there are limited effective and practical interventions to improve these youths' ability to regulate emotional states and social interactions, having a diagnostic formulation that helps parents understand the biological underpinnings of the cognitive flexibility deficit of the disorder is valuable.

Formalized, programmatic interventions for youth with NPD remain in their infancy. Therapy for narcissistic personality disorder remains the mainstay treatment as pharmacological interventions remain of limited effectiveness. Different styles of therapy seek to improve the ability to form relationships by addressing self-centered behaviors, realistic goal setting, and managing feelings. On a day-to-day basis, we have provided a number of techniques to help proactively manage common, expected behaviors of youths with narcissistic personality disorder. Habitual use of these techniques will orientate parents toward maintaining a healthy attachment with their youth and will limit the predilection toward escalation and crisis.

In our experience, parents with features of narcissistic personality disorder seek to minimize symptoms in affected youths and ultimately disagree with the diagnosis. This can be a difficult paradox, as the youth may be referred for therapeutic work following a request from an external source such as school, an athletic department, or summer camp.

Behavior: Displays a Strong Sense of Entitlement, Exaggerates Achievements, and Monopolizes Conversations

Intervention

Do not contradict individuals displaying this behavior, as they can feel they are being devalued and escalate their behavior. It is best to attempt redirecting conversations to areas of mutual agreement: "Let's talk about your thoughts on [the movie we saw last night, what we should eat tonight, etc.]."

When they are emotionally receptive to dialogue, share the importance in listening to others: "I really liked what Manny said. What did you think?"

Behavior: Takes Advantage of Others

Intervention

It is difficult for any parent to observe their youth purposely take advantage of others. Parents should try to inhibit their natural inclination of reacting with a firm approach to stop the process, and instead help the youth divert their negative actions toward others by asking them for reasoning without necessarily agreeing. Diffuse conflict further by steering conversation to a future event and, when possible, remove the youth from the situation. In most difficult situations, parents may need to ask the person being hurt to remove themselves from the situation.

Behavior: Displays Poor Cognitive Flexibility; Is Unable to Recognize the Feelings and Needs of Others

Intervention

Discuss and reflect on shared experiences to improve empathy.

Provide proactive opportunities for altruistic acts to others (e.g., helping a grand-parent take the trash out) rather than as a punishment or consequence (Table 7.12).

Table 7.12 Interventions for youths with narcissistic personality traits or disorder

Behavior	Interventions
▪ Believe she is superior to others. ▪ Has a grandiose sense of self and requires constant admiration. ▪ Exaggerates achievements and talents. ▪ Monopolizes conversations.	▪ Avoid contradicting the youth. ▪ When he makes negative or hostile comments, redirect conversations to areas of mutual agreement: "Let's talk about the movie we watched last night." ▪ Share the importance of listening to others: "I like what Ravi said. What did you think?" ▪ Emphasize the effort and enjoyment of an accomplishment rather than elements of skill or competition.
▪ Has a strong sense of entitlement and attention. ▪ Takes advantage of others to get what he or she wants (the best seating assign mentor cosmetics/apparel). ▪ Parents fear the youth's anger when setting limits and, as a result, minimize consequences or over indulge her.	▪ Listen to her reasoning without necessarily agreeing. ▪ Set aside scheduled individual time with the youth each week to develop a relationship without competing interests. ▪ Defuse conflict by asking about a future event. Consider phrases such as "Let me think about that" or "I'm not ready to decide."
▪ Does not value others' point of view in affect-laden situations. ▪ Is unable to recognize the feelings and needs of others.	▪ Incorporate role-playing of difficult situations. ▪ Encourage her to reflecton the opinions of others. "Why do you think your teacher asked you to talk to her first before making announcements to the class?" ▪ Discuss and reflect on shared experiences to improve empathy. ▪ Provide proactive opportunities for altruistic acts to others (e.g., helping grandparents take out the trash) rather than as a punishment or consequence.

Employment Opportunities

Adolescents with narcissistic personality disorders do well in activities that do not require much direct contact with customers. Like adolescents with difficult/feisty temperament or those with weakness in working memory, they do better in activities they can feel important in, for example, theatre, film, sales, journalism, etc. Their success will vary according to strengths in other aspects of their four pillars.

Special Issues

Bullies

Emerging research suggests that childhood bullying can have serious physical and psychological impacts into adulthood [4]. To date, it is poorly understood why certain youth engage in bullying. Recent literature on adolescents suggests that bullies may share traits of low empathy and lack sufficient skills to take the perspective of others [13]. Bullies often use moral disengagement (or believe that ethical standards do not apply to themselves in a particular context) to justify their aggressive behaviors. In the language of the four pillars, many bullies can be understood as youth with difficult/feisty temperament traits, weakness in working memory and fluid reasoning, and poor cognitive flexibility. There is overlap with this combination and what has been termed cluster-B personality traits.

Cross-References

- Difficult/feisty temperament: Chap. 3.
- Working memory, fluid reasoning: Chap. 4.
- Personality disorders: Chap. 6.

Bullying Victims

Victims of youth bullying may have complex presentations that are poorly understood. Victims of bullying can develop psychosomatic, depressive symptoms, anxiety, and self-harming behavior, and are at risk for substance abuse. Interventions for bullying and suicidal ideation should not be isolated to the individual being bullied [7]. Rather, interventions are needed for the prevention of bullying that require changes by those responsible for the youth's environment (parents, school administrators, sports coaches, work managers, etc.). A study from the Netherlands suggests that youths who are bullied develop psychosomatic and psychosocial problems and become depressed, while depressed youths are more likely to be bullied [18]. Additionally, social media complicates the victim's life further—bullying can occur at any time of day, even if the youth is physically separate from peers. Consequently, this type of bullying can occur outside of the jurisdiction of the school or place of employment, depending on who is involved [1]. In these cases, help may need to involve law enforcement. Parents should be aware that the U.S. Department of Health and Human Services has a resource website available (stopbullying.gov) that can provide various levels of support for different forms of bullying including cyberbullying, "revenge porn," and targeted bullying based on race, ethnicity, or sexual orientation.

When addressing bullying, it is helpful to understand how the victim's four pillars may contribute to adverse events. Consider, for example, that a youth with a slow-to-warm-up temperament may be at risk for bullying, because he or she typically withdraws in novel situations, struggles with adapting to change, and may be overly thoughtful and thus appear "slow" in decision making. Similarly, weakness in cognition can result in behaviors that may lead to teasing or ostracization. Youth with deficits in cognitive flexibility may have an additional challenge, including misinterpretation or overly rigid interpretations of teasing, even from friends. For these bullied youth, consider interventions that improve pragmatic language skills and role-playing scenarios as in trauma-focused cognitive behavior therapies.

Cross-References
- Verbal compression, visual-spatial, fluid reasoning: Chaps. 4 and 6.
- Cognitive flexibility: Chap. 5.

Suicidal Behaviors

We have tried to make a compelling case that difficult/feisty temperament and weaknesses in cognitive processes in children and adolescents are critical precursors to the development of maladaptive behaviors and psychological distress. However, the disease-based model of diagnostic classification rarely incorporates these complexities, even though they may be an important modifying factor.

The four-pillar information is extremely relevant to understand the complex issue of suicidal behaviors in youths. Often, we consider suicidal behavior in the context of a depressive disorder. However, in many youths and young adults, suicidal behavior has been linked to despair, loss of hope, and illicit drug use. These findings are consistent with evidence from other studies that suggest that suicidal behavior and drug use are a result of a period of diminished valuing of oneself and others [11]. In addition, despair and associated behaviors are more common among those with a low educational level or limited financial means. Despair, then, is an emotional and cognitive state experienced by many individuals that may further reflect socioeconomic disparities. Thus, clinicians need to be cognizant of suicidal behaviors not fitting into a traditional disease-based model; instead, they should consider a broader diagnostic formulation when a youth presents with suicidal behavior and weaknesses in their four pillars. Ideally, all treatments integrate consideration of biological, psychological, and social factors [16].

Substance Use in Adolescents

Substance use among adolescents can range from early experimentation to a severe substance use disorder. Parental substance abuse remains a key predictor of several adverse outcomes in children including maltreatment and later development of substance use disorder. Parents set the example to youth by their own amount, frequency, and location of the use of alcohol, tobacco, prescription drugs, and other substances. Parents do often convey clear expectations to their adolescent regarding substance use including how to set limits and how to monitor intake. Still, adolescents whose parents use substances excessively may assume this behavior is acceptable (or adaptive) and are at risk to later develop a substance use disorder themselves. Adolescents should be discouraged from using illegal substances.

Risk factors for adolescent substance use are the following:

- Parents who use illegal substances.
- Peers who use illegal substances.
- Poor school performance.
- Weaknesses in four pillars with poor problem-solving abilities.
- Family history of substance use.
- Family rejection of adolescent's difficulties (academic, emotional, interpersonal, sexual orientation, gender identity, etc.)
- Association with delinquent or substance-using peers.

Adolescents that use illegal substances generally use alcohol, nicotine (in tobacco or vaping products), and marijuana (THC). Both nicotine and marijuana are addictive. Recently, more potent and dangerous illegal substances have become available (opioids, high-potency marijuana products, and fentanyl). All substance use, even experimental use, puts adolescents at risk for emotional and behavioral problems and poor school performance.

Focus on Opioids

Overdose deaths attributed to opioids is a rising cause of mortality and morbidity in adolescents and adults. For example, over a seven-year period (1999–2016), the annual estimate mortality rate for adolescents in the United States grew from 0.78 to 2.75 per 100,000 [22]. Today, there is considerable evidence that office-based treatment of opioid use disorder (OUD) can be highly effective in the adolescent population, including retention in outpatient programming and reduction in overdose deaths. Typically, either buprenorphine or oral/injectable naltrexone can be prescribed. Since 2002, the Federal Drug Administration (FDA) has approved the use of buprenorphine in youth above 16-years of age by waiver-trained prescribers. The American Academy of Pediatrics (AAP) has released a comprehensive policy statement on Medication-Assisted Treatment of Adolescents with Opioid Use

Disorders, which summarizes the evidence and provides treatment recommendations (https://pediatrics.aappublications.org/content/pediatrics/early/2016/08/18/peds.2016-1893.full.pdf).

Given the high risk of death associated with opioid use disorder, clinicians who identify at risk behaviors should aggressively seek the appropriate diagnosis and treatment options. The strength of the parental relationship can also moderate substance use behavior in adolescents. Andrews et al. [3] found in a six-year longitudinal study that adolescents who had a "good" or "moderate" relationship with parents, who smoked either cigarettes or marijuana, would likely model this behavior. If the relationship was relatively poor, adolescents were less likely to model their parents' behavior. This example can be illustrative of how not all positive attachments may be protective, and clinicians should carefully consider other parental and youth factors when making a risk assessment.

Treatment for Substance Use in Adolescents

Substance use disorders are a complex issue, and it is best to involve a physician with expertise in this area to determine whether a drug screen is needed. Often parents demand a drug screen or demand information that may create an atmosphere of confrontation. In the United States, state-by-state laws regarding parental and adolescent decision making for substance abuse treatment vary [30]. These laws were created to recognize adolescent autonomy for sensitive issues such as pregnancy, sexually transmitted diseases, and mental/substance abuse treatment. However, outside of formal intellectual disability, the laws do not account for individual variations in youth's cognitive abilities to accurately understand and assess the risk of delaying or refusing treatment.

Treatment should be tailored to the youth's four pillars' strengths for success [31]. Clinicians should also attend to the youth's four pillars' weaknesses as they can prevent them from being able to make use of the treatment. In general, adolescents should not be treated in the same programs as adults. Adolescents should receive services from adolescent programs and therapists with expertise in treating adolescents with substance use disorders [12].

Resources

- Al-Anon Family Groups: Access to resources and support for families and friends of alcoholics.
- Alcoholics Anonymous (AA): An international fellowship of nonprofessional men and women who support each other to confront and overcome a drinking problem.

- American Lung Association: Resources about how to prevent children from smoking and how to help those that smoke to quit.
- Narcotics Anonymous (NA): Support resources and a recovery program for people who are addicted to drugs or alcohol.
- National Institutes on Drug Abuse: Agency within the U.S. National Institutes of Health that has information specific to children and adolescents about how drugs affect their brain, facts about widely used drugs, and links to related content.
- Substance Abuse and Mental Health Services Administration: Agency within the U.S. Department of Health and Human Services that leads public health efforts to reduce the impact of substance abuse and mental illness on America's communities.
- American Academy of Pediatrics: Resources to address substance use in children and adolescents. https://www.aap.org/en-us/advocacy-and-policy/aap-health-initiatives/Substance-Use-and-Prevention/Pages/opioid-epidemic-resources.aspx

Social Media and Technology

The "digital world" has offered new and unexpected concerns for parents. In our experience, there is an increasing number of youth crises (including those that lead to hospitalization) that involve social media. Consequently, there is rising public anxiety regarding youths' personal safety, well-being, and mental health in a digital world. Yet, for better or worse, social media is an essential component of everyday life for most youths, and helps maintain networks among family, peers, and teachers. The relationship between an individual's social media and mental health is best predicted by estimating a youth's personal characteristics (including their four pillars), social networks, and cultural factors. In addition, though parental supervision can be a mitigating force, parents often lack the knowledge to implement restrictive controls or even know which social media platforms their youth uses. Often, by the time parents discover their youth's social network, such as Facebook, the youth has already started migrating to another platform. Youths also have different levels of proficiency with different platforms. For example, though the platform Snapchat advertises that pictures or messages sent will only be available to the recipient for a short period of time, many youths know how to circumvent these limitations by capturing screenshots. Moreover, there remains no absolute way to confirm a person's identity on social media, so youths are also at significant risk for interacting with imposters, which is a danger not only in terms of significant criminal behavior, but also with peers posing as other peers.

Digital life is increasingly being required for many educational programs and increasingly used for social events. Thus, it's valuable to identify key protective or vulnerabilities that could lead to harm for susceptible youths. The evidence regarding vulnerability for aggressive and sexual behaviors through social media point to personality factors (thrill-seeking, low self-esteem, psychological difficulties), social factors (lack of parental support, peer norms), and digital factors (online practices, digital skills, specific online sites) [34, 39].

Though the research pool on this topic is still growing, several rigorous and large studies have reported small inverse associations between daily use of technology and an adolescent's sense of well-being [39]. While internet use is not necessarily linked to psychopathology, the overuse of the internet has been associated with impairments across various domains of functioning. Some have suggested that it can be viewed as a behavioral version of a substance use disorder, impulse-control disorder, or a subtype of obsessive-compulsive disorder, although empirical evidence for these designations is lacking [41].

During the COVID-19 pandemic, digital media was essential in providing youths with a virtual education and with mental health interventions that went beyond simply replicating traditional face-to-face interventions [10]. Despite the stated risks, there remains a great deal of hope that innovations across digital media could enhance education and therapy for some youths. Hybrid implementations of digital learning, such as online lectures from a master teacher combined with in-person behavioral support, may allow broader access to specialized learning. Further, telemedicine or virtual therapy may provide benefits to youths who suffer from conditions (severe anxiety or intellectual disability) that cause them to struggle with traditional, in-person visits.

Having a Digital Strategy at Home

The relationship between internet, digital life, social media, and mental health is best characterized by a complex mix of positive and negative influences varying over time based on a youth's personal characteristics (four pillars) and socioeconomic and cultural factors. One recommendation is clear: every parent should have a consistent digital strategy in their home [25]. This includes the use of technology, consumption of digital content, and communication on social networks.

Use of Technology

In contrast to previous generations, most households will expect to have hand-me-down smartphones and computers to give to younger family members. Thus, how this technology is regulated within the home will be an early and ongoing struggle for most parents and can be a major point of contention with their youths. In our opinion, an overly strict policy on technology is no longer helpful. Most children will have periods of unsupervised access to the internet through school, relatives, or peers, regardless of which personal devices they own. But more importantly, they are growing into a world, which will be more, not less, reliant on technology for daily living (e.g., grocery shopping, health care, and finances). Thus, there is a new onus on families to raise responsible digital citizens that can use technology productively and safely.

Consider the common advice to ban all electronics at the dinner table. For certain youths, especially those who have difficult/feisty temperaments or cognitive weaknesses, such instruction may be detrimental and cause severe tension, causing youths to race to finish dinner. We often remind parents that youths who engage in avid reading and bring a book to the dinner table are not frowned upon. For some youths, their electronic device should be considered as helpful as a good book. We see an increasingly troubling trend wherein children who view their parents as hostile toward technology may opt to "split" their digital life from their everyday activities rather than incorporating it into the family structure. On the other hand, a more lenient policy may allow for less confrontation, allowing parents to shape behaviors around technology (e.g., encouraging eye contact and focus) and to discuss more relevant matters. Since there will be no rush to get back to the book or screen, dinnertime can be extended, including conversation and cleaning up afterward.

We recommend parents regularly implement and revisit parental controls around technology. This is a rapidly developing area that is increasingly being taken seriously (to shield liability) by major device and service providers. Most major parent websites include information describing how to use parental controls. Parents are often unaware that they can block content at various levels, including the whole device, at the content level, or at the message level. In addition, for most devices, parents can set preplanned time limits. Also note that it's worthwhile for parents to search terms like "hack" or "bypass" for the parental control they wish to implement. Parents will quickly discover how innovative and resourceful the online community of youths can be! (Tables 7.13 and 7.14).

Table 7.13 Use of technology

Topic	Recommendations
Parent education and guidance on media	Internetmatters.org provides device- and content-specific guidance for parents. Use the drop-down menu to select your device and find customized tutorials. Commonsensemedia.org reviews digital content, including movies, TV, and video games, listing controversial content and age-range recommendations.
Structured settings for video games	Formal electronic sports (e-sports) leagues are a safe alternative to unrestricted video game play for children. In the United States, e-sports leagues are being adopted at the state level and include rigorous background checks to ensure player identity and age Check for compliance with the United States Center for Safesport (safesport.org), a federally sponsored, safe-harbor-certified digital platform Games in these programs are highly popular, but do not include games with explicit or realistic violence or games with a "mature" rating. They include sports titles, chess, noncompetitive building games, as well as more action-oriented games Children under 13 are not allowed to create online accounts. Thus, these programs allow for parent-supervised accounts with set permissions and time tracking

Table 7.14 Resources for behavioral interventions in youths with cognitive weaknesses (Table 7.15)

livesinthebalance.org
ldaamerica.org
khanacademy.org
understood.org
ldonline.org

Table 7.15 Resources for employment opportunities for youths with cognitive weaknesses

smartpolicyworks.com
abilityjobs.com
gettinghired.com

Medication Adherence in Youth

Although adherence to healthy lifestyle behaviors and treatment recommendations in youths is complex and multidimensional, a common frustration expressed by psychiatrists and advanced nurse practitioners is the ability to provide optimal care when patients are nonadherent with pharmacologic recommendations. Nonadherence is a common problem among patients, with some estimates suggesting that as many as 50% of patients are nonadherent to treatment. Among patients with a psychiatric disorder who were prescribed antidepressants, fewer than 30% took the medication at six months following the initiation of pharmacotherapy [46]. Importantly, nonadherence affects patients of all ages and socioeconomic levels. Furthermore, poor adherence to treatment recommendations leads to negative outcomes, including an increased risk of complications, hospitalizations, functional disability, and even premature death [26].

Although there is no one-size-fits-all solution to improve adherence, there is a pressing need for tailored approaches that attend to the various four-pillar factors for nonadherence in order to improve the patient's overall health [27]. Although there are many known reasons for nonadherence (intolerable side effects, plus numerous psychological, disease-specific, social, and financial factors), the foundation of most nonadherence is often likely due to weaknesses in both cognition and cognitive flexibilities, aspects that are unique to each patient. In essence, it confirms the clinical approach of different rules for different pillars [14]. Youths who are at more risk for nonadherence are those whose parents have weakness in verbal comprehension, fluid reasoning, or working memory, who often leave youths in charge of their own medication regimen. This is not optimal, as it increases missed or incorrect dosing or, even worse, leads to youths not taking their medication at all (Table 7.16).

Table 7.16 Practical strategies to promote treatment adherence in youth

Make visible, in EHR, information that can identify patients and families with weaknesses in cognition (e.g., colored notes or alerts). This allows the clinician or physician, in advance, to tailor how he or she communicates the treatment recommendations.
To promote understanding, ask for a repeat back of information by parents on medication and how it will be taken. Include patient if adolescent.
Provide handouts with visual cues to explain the diagnosis and how medication is to be taken.
Consider asking permission to send youths and/or parents text-message reminders for appointments, medication times, or pending lab work.
Provide parents updated information about the overall cost of medications most frequently prescribed. Affordable and once-daily medications should be considered.
Have awareness regarding the distance of the family's pharmacy in relation to their home—and whether transportation is needed and/or delivery services offered.
When liquid medication is prescribed, provide a syringe with markings or a visual handout outlining how to measure the prescribed amount with a household item.
Inquire about other household members that require medical or mental health care and their compliance with treatment. This provides a window on what to expect about the parents' ability to help with adherence.

Future Direction

This book represents a first step in understanding how temperament, attachment, and cognitive abilities contribute to personality. Understanding these connections will facilitate understanding developmental changes in the four pillars and, in the future, the contributions of molecular, genetic, and brain functions. We continue to discover clues about the brain functions that underlie developmental changes—and how these changes underlie the emotional regulation needed for success—and we expect that future research will provide better insight into how complex relationships between temperamental and cognitive abilities contribute to emotional and behavioral regulating abilities. A deeper understanding of the mechanisms underlying four-pillar development will enable us to develop more tailored and effective interventions for youths who struggle emotionally, behaviorally, and academically.

References

1. Alavi N, Reshetukha T, Prost E, et al. Relationship between bullying and suicidal behaviour in youth presenting to the emergency department. J Can Acad Child Adolesc Psychiatry. 2017;26(2):70–7.
2. American Psychiatric Association. Diagnostic and statistical manual of mental disorders. 5th ed. Washington, DC: DSM-5. American Psychiatric Association; 2013.
3. Andrews JA, Hops H, Duncan SC. Adolescent modeling of parent substance use: the moderating effect of the relationship with the parent. J Fam Psychol. 1997;11(3):259–70. https://doi.org/10.1037/0893-3200.11.3.259.
4. Arató N, Zsidó AN, Lénárd K, Lábadi B. Cybervictimization and cyberbullying: the role of socio-emotional skills. Front Psych. 2020;11:248. https://doi.org/10.3389/fpsyt.2020.00248.

5. Beck E, Bo S, Gondan M, et al. Mentalization-based treatment in groups for adolescents with borderline personality disorder (BPD) or subthreshold BPD versus treatment as usual (M-GAB): study protocol for a randomized controlled trial. Trials. 2016;17:314. https://doi.org/10.1186/s13063-016-1431-0.
6. Bleiberg E. Mentalizing-based treatment with adolescents and families. Child Adolesc Psychiatric Clin N Am. 2013;22:295–330. https://doi.org/10.1016/j.chc.2013.01.001.
7. Borowsky IW, Taliaferro LA, McMorris BJ. Suicidal thinking and behavior among youth involved in verbal and social bullying: risk and protective factors. J Adolesc Health. 2013;53:S4–S12.
8. Bowlby J. Attachment, 2nd edition, attachment and loss (vol. 1). New York: Basic books; 1999.
9. Cipriano-Essel E, Skowron EA, Stifter CA, Teti DM. Heterogeneity in maltreated and non-maltreated preschool Children's inhibitory control: the interplay between parenting quality and child temperament. Infant Child Dev. 2013;22(5):501–22. https://doi.org/10.1002/ICD.1801.
10. Cliffe B, Croker A, Denne M, et al. Clinicians' use of and attitudes towards technology to provide and support interventions in child and adolescent mental health services. Child Adolesc Mental Health. 2020;25(2):95–101.
11. Copeland WE, Gaydosh L, Hill SN, et al. Associations of despair with suicidality and substance misuse among young adults. JAMA Netw Open. 2020;3(6):e208627. https://doi.org/10.1001/jamanetworkopen.2020.8627.
12. Das JK, Salam RA, Arshad A, et al. Interventions for adolescent substance abuse: an overview of systematic reviews. J Adolesc Health. 2016;59(4S):S61–75. https://doi.org/10.1016/j.jadohealth.2016.06.021.
13. Del Rey R, Lazuras L, Casas JA, et al. Does empathy predict (cyber) bullying perpetration, and how do age, gender and nationality affect this relationship? Learn Individ Dif. 2016;45:275–81. https://doi.org/10.1016/j.lindif.2015.11.021.
14. Delgado SV. Non-adherence to treatment: different rules for different patients. Scientific Pages Fam Med. 2016;1:003.
15. Delgado SV, Strawn JR. Psychodynamic understandings. In: Levesque RJ, editor. Encyclopedia of adolescence. Springer; 2016. https://doi.org/10.1007/978-3-319-32132-5_8-2.
16. Delgado SV, Strawn JR, Pedapati EV. Contemporary psychodynamic psychotherapy for children and adolescents: integrating Intersubjectivity and neuroscience. Springer; 2015.
17. Dodge KA, Pettit GS. A biosocial model of development of chronic conduct problems in adolescence. Dev Psychol. 2003;39:349–71.
18. Fekkes M, Pijpers F, Fredriks AM, et al. Do bullied children get ill, or do ill children get bullied? A prospective cohort study on the relationship between bullying and health-related symptoms. Pediatrics. 2006;117:1568–74.
19. Ferrer E, O'Hare ED, Bunge SA. Fluid reasoning and the developing brain. Front Neurosci. 2009;3(1):46–51. https://doi.org/10.3389/neuro.01.003.2009.
20. Fonagy P, Luyten P. A developmental, mentalization-based approach to the understanding and treatment of borderline personality disorder. Dev Psychopathol. 2009;21(4):1355–81. https://doi.org/10.1017/S0954579409990198.
21. Franz C, Ascherman L, Shafiel J. A Clinician's guide to learning disabilities. Oxford: University Press; 2018.
22. Gaither JR, Shabanova V, Leventhal JM. US national trends in pediatric deaths from prescription and illicit opioids, 1999-2016. JAMA Netw Open. 2018;1:e186558.
23. Harkness S, Super CM, Ríos Bermúdez M, et al. Parental ethnotheories of children's learning. In: Lancy DF, Bock J, Gaskins S, editors. The anthropology of learning in childhood. Lanham, MD: Alta Mira Press; 2010. p. 65–81.
24. Harris E, Delgado SV. Managing treatment-resistant obsessive-compulsive disorder. Current Psychiatry. 2018;17(11):10–2,14-18,51.
25. Hollis C, Falconer CJ, Martin JL, et al. Annual research review: digital health interventions for children and young people with mental health problems: a systematic and meta-review. J Child Psychol Psychiatry. 2016;58:474–503.

26. Hubbard T, McNeill N. Thinking outside the pillbox: improving medication adherence and reducing readmissions. NEHI; 2012.
27. Hugtenburg JG, Timmers L, Elders PJ, et al. Definitions, variants, and causes of nonadherence with medication: a challenge for tailored interventions. Patient Prefer Adherence. 2013;7:675–82. https://doi.org/10.2147/PPA.S29549. Published 2013 Jul 10.
28. Kaess M, Brunner R, Chanen A. Borderline personality disorder in adolescence. Pediatrics. 2014;134(4):782–93. https://doi.org/10.1542/peds.2013-3677.
29. Kendler KS, Aggen SH, Czajkowski N, et al. The structure of genetic and environmental risk factors for DSM-IV personality disorders: a multivariate twin study. Arch Gen Psych. 2008;65(12):1438–46.
30. Kerwin ME, Kirby KC, Speziali D, et al. What can parents do? A review of state Laws regarding decision making for adolescent drug abuse and mental health treatment. J Child Adolesc Subst Abuse. 2015;24(3):166–76. https://doi.org/10.1080/1067828X.2013.777380.
31. Leslie K. Youth substance use and abuse: challenges and strategies for identification and intervention. CMAJ. 2008;178(2):145–8. https://doi.org/10.1503/cmaj.071410.
32. Lev M, Ludwi K, Gilaie-Dotan S, et al. Training improves visual processing speed and generalizes to untrained functions. Sci Rep. 2014;4:7251. https://doi.org/10.1038/srep07251.
33. Linehan MM, Comtois KA, Murray AM, et al. Two-year randomized controlled trial and follow-up of dialectical behavior therapy vs therapy by experts for suicidal behaviors and borderline personality disorder. Arch Gen Psychiatry. 2006;63:757–66. https://doi.org/10.1001/archpsyc.63.7.757.
34. Livingstone S, Smith P. Annual research review: children and young people in the digital age: the nature and prevalence of risks, harmful effects, and risk and protective factors, for mobile and internet usage. J Child Psychol Psychiatry. 2014;55:635–54.
35. Mesman J, Stoel R, Bakermans-Kranenbrug MJ, et al. Predicting growth curves of early childhood externalizing problems: differential susceptibility of children with difficult temperament. J Abnorm Child Psychol. 2009;37:625–36. https://doi.org/10.1007/s10802-009-9298-0.
36. Miklowitz DJ, Chung B. Family-focused therapy for bipolar disorder: reflections on 30 years of research. Fam Process. 2016;55(3):483–99. https://doi.org/10.1111/famp.12237.
37. Miller L, Hlastala SA, Mufson L, et al. Interpersonal psychotherapy for adolescents with mood and behavior dysregulation: evidence-based case study. Evid Based Pract Child Adolesc Ment Health. 2016;1(4):159–75. https://doi.org/10.1080/23794925.2016.1247679.
38. Miller S, Loeber R, Hipwell A. Peer deviance, parenting and disruptive behavior among young girls. J Abnorm Child Psychol. 2009;37(2):139–52. https://doi.org/10.1007/S10802-008-9265-1.
39. Odgers CL, Jensen M. Annual research review: adolescent mental health in the digital age: facts, fears, and future directions. J Child Psychol Psychiatry. 2020;61:336–48.
40. Olson SL, Sameroff AJ, Kerr DCR, et al. Developmental foundations of externalizing problems in young children: the role of effortful control. Dev Psychopathol. 2005;17:25–45.
41. Restrepo A, Scheininger T, Clucas J, et al. Problematic internet use in children and adolescents: associations with psychiatric disorders and impairment. BMC Psychiatry. 2020;20:252. https://doi.org/10.1186/s12888-020-02640-x.
42. Rossouw TI, Fonagy P. Mentalization-based treatment for self-harm in adolescents: a randomized controlled trial. J Am Acad Child Adolesc Psychiatry. 2012;51(12):1304–13.
43. Strawn JR, Lu L, Peris TS, et al. Research review: pediatric anxiety disorders - what have we learnt in the last 10 years? J Child Psychol Psychiatry. 2021;62(2):114–39. https://doi.org/10.1111/jcpp.13262.
44. Super CM, Axia G, Harkness S, et al. Culture, temperament, and the "difficult child" in seven Western cultures. Eur J Dev Sci. 2008;2(1–2):136–57.
45. Thomas A, Chess S, Birch HG. The origin of personality. Sci Am. 1970;223(2):102–9.
46. Tierney R, Melfi CA, Signa W, et al. Antidepressant use and use in naturalistic settings. Drug Benefit Trends. 2000;12:7BH–12BH.

47. van Schie CC, Jarman HL, Huxley E, et al. Narcissistic traits in young people: understanding the role of parenting and maltreatment bord personal disord emot dysregul. 2020;7:10. https://doi.org/10.1186/s40479-020-00125-7.
48. van Zeijl J, Mesman J, Stolk MN, et al. Differential susceptibility to discipline: the moderating effect of child temperament on the association between maternal discipline and early childhood externalizing problems. J Fam Psychol. 2007;22:626–36. https://doi.org/10.1037/0893-3200.21.4.626.

Chapter 8
Parenting Principles to Help Youths: Debunking Common Parenting Myths

Feelings of worth can flourish only in an atmosphere where individual differences are appreciated, mistakes are tolerated, communication is open, and rules are flexible: the kind of atmosphere that is found in a nurturing family.
—Virginia Satir (1916–1988).

Introduction

In earlier chapters, we reviewed detailed interventions for youths and parents with weaknesses in their four pillars. Although providing practical interventions for all difficult parenting situations is beyond the scope of this book, in this chapter, we provide interventions for the most common issues that arise from patients and parents with weaknesses in their four pillars. These examples are based on many of the reasons that patients seek help from mental health providers. The goal of providing these interventions is to give clinicians a go-to template to provide parents with practical, growth-promoting interventions to ensure the emotional and behavioral success of their youth.

In this chapter, we note that some clinicians, like some parents, believe that what his or her parents modeled, if effective, should work for most patients and their families. Unfortunately, handing down the same advice through generations without carefully assessing the best interest of a particular youth or family nidus increases the likelihood of conflict and failure. Further, giving parenting suggestions because they helped with a clinician's own children is problematic, because doing does not carefully attend to patients' and parents' abilities, needs, and four pillar weaknesses. As such, we hope that our clinical readers can make use of the practical interventions for parenting the most common issues that arise from patients and parents with weaknesses in their four pillars.

S. V. Delgado et al., *Promoting the Emotional and Behavioral Success of Youths*, https://doi.org/10.1007/978-3-030-88075-0_8

A Brief Review of the Four Pillars

The four pillars arise from innate and environmental processes and are a scaffold for the child's development and maintenance of self-regulation and implicit relational patterns, which guide successful interaction with others. The first three pillars—temperament, cognition, and cognitive flexibility—form the foundation of the fourth pillar, personality, the interpersonal expression of the internal working model of attachment (IWMA). By understanding each pillar's contribution, clinicians will gain understanding of the patient, his or her needs, and his or her parents from a biopsychosocial perspective.

The four pillars represent the foundation of adaptive behaviors (e.g., how to succeed in interpersonal relationships, play, and learning/working). When individuals can successfully love, play, work/learn, and tolerate distress, they generally have "good" pillars. Some individuals with weak pillars adapt to or work around their weaknesses, while others develop maladaptive emotional and behavioral patterns that undermine their ability to love, play, work/learn, and tolerate distress. For parents, strengths and weaknesses in the four pillars guide their parenting.

Understanding Parents

Youths learn about emotional regulation through observation, and incorporate social behaviors modeled by their parents. A youth's ability to emotionally regulate is affected by the emotional climate of the family, his or her quality of attachments, parenting style, family expressiveness, and the quality of the marital relationship. In essence, the development of emotional regulation is a bidirectional process in which children and families mutually influence each other [45].

To help parents learn how to provide practical, growth-promoting interventions for their youth's success, clinicians must begin by understanding the typical strategies a parent has used to manage day-to-day difficulties or conflict. Knowing the strategies used provides clinicians a window into the parents' beliefs and opinions, as well as their expectations for their child. More importantly, knowing which strategies parents use can alert the clinician to their ability to change in relation to their strengths and weaknesses, as well as the strengths and weaknesses of their children. With this knowledge, the clinician can strategically modify parenting interventions according to the patient's strengths and weaknesses. In doing so, the clinician can prevent the parents from feeling defeated when they cannot meet their child's emotional and social needs.

Four Pillar Parenting

Parents with difficult youths will find clinician's expertise helpful in learning the reasons behind their youth's maladaptive behaviors; this will help them adapt new interventions to promote adaptive behaviors. Common reasons behind maladaptive behaviors are temperamental difficulties, cognitive weaknesses, and emerging personality difficulties. We do not commonly recommend that parents use a firm, authoritarian approach. Of course, we acknowledge that some youth benefit from this approach, but many do not. Some youths respond well and comply to a parent's friendly and stern glance, implying "I will count to three and you know the consequence if I get there." However, we disagree with the assumption that (1) all youths can comply with firm limit setting, and (2) noncompliance represents manipulation and defiance. Further, some clinicians believe that if youths continue to be disrespectful, the parent is not effective because he or she is too lenient and not firm enough. But we posit that youths may react defiantly to firm parental approaches particularly if it is difficult for them (as a result of weaknesses in their four pillars) to understand the advantages of complying.

What Should Parents Do When their Child Is Defiant, Oppositional, or Disrespectful?

Limit-setting with youths with defiant, oppositional, and disrespectful behaviors cannot be a one-size-fits-all intervention. Parental interventions must be developmentally appropriate and must consider the youth's and parents' four pillar strengths and weaknesses. In this chapter, we provide suggestions for limit-setting by age for youths and parents with reasonably good four pillars. For a more detailed review of interventions for youths with four pillar weaknesses, see Chap. 7.

Divorce

The process of a divorce is never easy on children or adolescents. Although on some occasions the parents' divorce is in the best interest of the child, this does not necessarily make it easier. Fortunately, most youths recover from the shock and loss of the original family structure. The seminal work by Wallerstein and Blakeslee on the impact of divorce on youths, which was published more than three decades ago, remains one of the best references for clinicians and parents. Below, we review the psychological tasks needed for parents and youths as they process divorce (Table 8.1).

Table 8.1 The Psychological tasks of divorce

Parents	Youths
End the marriage	Understanding the parents' divorce
Mourn the relationship	Strategic withdrawal from the parents' divorce
Re-establish self-identity as single	Learn to accept the loss
Resolving grievances	Manage angry feelings
Seek new intimate relationship	Work through feelings of guilt for the parents' divorce
Support the children needs	Accept the divorce is permanent
Build a new family	Begin to seek intimate relationships

Adapted from Wallerstein and Blakeslee [59]

We emphasize that the process of overcoming a divorce and moving on in life will be strongly influenced by the four pillars of the parents and the youth.

Elsa and Julian React to their Parents' Divorce

Elsa and Julian are 9-year-old twins. They have always been close to their father and desired a closer relationship with their mother, who could be distant toward them and critical when they wanted her attention. Several months after their parents divorced, Elsa and Julian's father shared with the youths' therapist that "when they get back from a visit with their mother, they get angry with me over trivial things. Should I let them continue to see their mother?" In short, most of the time, the answer is yes. Prior to the divorce, Elsa and Julian's mother was distant; now Elsa and Julian recognize that they prefer to see her to avoid creating more distance. Their mother is important to them. However, Elsa and Julian may behave in a way to prevent their mother's criticism when they visit her, pleasing her with their behavior. Consequently, knowing implicitly that their father will always be supportive, upon returning from their mother's home they may be unconsciously releasing internal anger they may feel toward their mother. Helping their father understand this as a possibility will allow him to know that his children are seeking his support because they know he is consistent in his closeness to them.

Mental health clinicians should consider identifying the parents' four pillars. In this case, the youth's mother would be considered to have a difficult/feisty temperament, limited cognitive flexibility, and a dismissive style of attachment. Of course, there are many iterations of this example, and interventions must be individualized based on family dynamics and the specific needs of the family and the youth.

Divorced Parents

The reasons why some parents end marriages are complex. Many divorced parents overcome the failure of their marriage and provide home environments that ensure their youth's emotional success. However, in clinical settings, divorced parents who arrive in need of help for their youth are a select group with problems; they do not represent the general population of divorced couples with youths.

Divorced Parents Should be on the Same Page. Right?

We recall being told by experienced social workers that "if a couple could be on the same page regarding relationships, parenting, intimacy, and religious and cultural beliefs, they likely would not have divorced." Although this may be an overstatement, we acknowledge the fact that many divorced couples are helpful to their youths even when they disagree on certain aspects of their care. We have family and friends who have divorced, because they were unable to get on the same page on many issues. However, most of these people managed the divorce well and raised emotionally successful children despite different parenting styles. They had the temperament, cognition, and, above all, cognitive flexibility needed to provide what was in the best interest of their youth. Furthermore, the youths of these parents also had good four pillars and were able to adapt to the differences in their parents' approaches.

Newly minted clinicians in child and adolescent psychiatry, psychology, advanced practice nursing, and social work have recommended that divorced parents work together in parenting matters, as it is in the best interest of their children. Parents are asked to be on the same page regarding chores, limit setting, choice of medication, etc. But by emphasizing the necessity for agreement, clinicians may unwittingly sidestep understanding the reasons behind disagreement on certain parenting issues.

Sometimes It's Okay to Not be on the Same Page

For divorced couples who disagree on parenting approaches, these differences are not always detrimental, despite common belief (Table 8.2). What's more important is that parents support each other despite their differences. We are not dismissing that some parents who divorce become contentious and argumentative about how best to raise their children. But by understanding the strengths and weaknesses of

Table 8.2 Divorced parents on different pages with regard to their daughter with dyslexia, Sophie

Sophie's specific weakness or difficulties	Father	Mother
Sophie needs to read directions out loud or to hear directions read aloud to understand them. She has difficulty organizing ideas and planning assignments when instructions are presented in written form	Sets time aside to calmly help Sophie Reads the instructions on how to complete her homework When Sophie has large amounts of homework, her father encourages her to take brief breaks	Feels that Sophie's homework difficulties reflect avoiding the work. This often creates conflict When Sophie's mother sees her struggling with her homework, her mother becomes tense and worries about Sophie. This limits her mother's ability to understand how Sophie's disability affects her
When Sophie becomes overwhelmed by her homework, she cannot fully understand the directions.	Sophie's father checked in weekly with Sophie's teachers about her progress and areas of concern, which he conveyed to her mother and tutor Her father encouraged her to email her teachers about important information she did not understand	After taking Sophie to group activities with other learning-disabled youths, Sophie's mother met other parents and learned about the anxiety that youths with learning disabilities may have completing homework. This information helped her to understand Sophie's struggles with schoolwork. As a result, Sophie's mother was less anxious and more able to help Sophie
Sophie is socially awkward and struggles to process nonverbal behaviors (e.g., facial expressions, object-related gestures)	Sophie's father helps her by sharing what he thinks people's facial expressions mean. He allows her to share her thoughts about others	Sophie's mother helps her participate in and enjoy social interactions. Her mother encourages her to attend neighborhood and family events
Sophie struggles to complete homework or chores under pressure from time constraints	Sophie's father prepares her by giving her ample time to complete chores and provides reminders when needed	Due to her own anxiety and difficulties with cognitive flexibility, Sophie's mother sometimes rushes Sophie to complete chores or homework, especially when they are running late. This results in conflict

the parents' and youth's four pillars, the clinician can make great strides in knowing how to develop practical interventions for each household—rather than imposing interventions that a parent may not be able or willing to implement. The clinician will need to be familiar with different parenting interventions to facilitate collaboration and reduce conflict between parents, in the best interest of their child (Chap. 7).

Sophie, a 9-year-old fourth grader with dyslexia (Specified Learning Disorder, with impairment in reading), disliked going to school due to her delay in reading skills. She made good efforts at her father's home to complete her schoolwork because he had the temperament and cognitive flexibility needed to encourage her in a calm and reassuring manner to use the skills her tutor had suggested. Sophie had more difficulties at her mother's home, as her mother had an easy/flexible temperament but also an anxiety disorder—as well as limited cognitive flexibility—that caused her difficulty in grasping why Sophie needed extended periods of time to complete her homework due to her dyslexia. Sophie's mother often felt her daughter was being defiant, and conflict ensured.

Understanding the parents' strengths and weaknesses with regard to the four pillars (as well as those of their children) allows the clinician to develop practical interventions for each household rather than focusing on interventions that may be difficult for one parent to implement. By establishing rapport with the family, clinicians will generally find the families to be more receptive to the different interventions recommended.

In Sophie's case, both parents were caring and loving, despite their different strengths. The father's four pillars allowed him to discern Sophie's behavioral and academic difficulties. Because of this, he was able to modify how he approached his daughter (providing rewards for her efforts to learn). In contrast, her mother had weaknesses in her four pillars that contributed to her difficulties helping Sophie academically, although she was helpful to Sophie by helping her engage in family and peer activities in spite of her difficulties understanding the ebb and flow of conversations.

As such, possible recommendations may have included: (1) scheduling tutoring sessions during times when Sophie was with her father; (2) beginning a mother/daughter therapy to improve homework communication; (3) having Sophie's father send an email to Sophie's mother with information about important homework and school progress; (4) encouraging both parents to have Sophie attend group activities to meet peers with learning disabilities (Table 8.2). In short, clinicians need to be familiar with different parenting interventions to facilitate collaboration and reduce the conflict between parents, in the best interest of their child (Chap. 7).

Stepparents and Adoptive Parents

Stepparents are often portrayed as evil, much like the Cinderellian wicked stepmother. Mostly, this is far from the truth. Stepparents and adoptive parents come with many four pillar profiles. Some have the innate, intuitive abilities to accommodate the step/adopted child's needs and help her to adapt. Other stepparents may experience children as competitors for their partner's attention.

The role of a stepparent or adoptive parent is usually unclear and poorly defined for youths. The role is mostly defined by the biological parent's reasons for the new relationship. Scenarios are many, and a one-size-fits-all view for blended families can be detrimental. Parents, as well as stepparents and adoptive parents, should be assessed for their four pillar strengths and weaknesses to discover the best way, clinically, to help them understand and help their youth. Thus, clinicians should avoid making implicit negative assumptions of blended families' difficulties, as many live successfully (and do not step foot in our offices).

Parents and stepparents with Good Four Pillars (Adaptive Responses)

The following examples illustrate successful exchanges and interactions within blended families. These are provided to remind the reader of the many blended families who are functioning well and do not present to our clinics and consulting rooms.

Behavior: Youth Arrives Home from School and Wants to Play with Friends
"You may play after school and finish your homework after supper. We know your mother and stepfather prefer you finish your homework before you go out and play, but we have agreed it is fine to have different rules in each home."

Behavior: Youth Visits Maternal Grandmother and Becomes Hungry before Dinner Is Ready
"We can get something from McDonald's when we visit your grandma so that you don't get hungry (because she serves dinner later than we do). We spoke with your father and stepmother, and they agreed it is okay for you to eat early."

Behavior: Youth Stays out Late and Does Not Call Father and Stepmother
"You broke our trust by staying out late and not calling us to let us know you were going to be late returning home. We want you to think about what you can do to regain our trust, and we can talk about it later when you calm down. We already called your mother and stepfather, and they agree your behavior affects both homes. We will call them and let them know what you decide to do to regain the trust of all your parents."

Parents and Stepparents with Deficits in Cognitive Flexibility (Maladaptive Responses)

Behavior: Youth Arrives Home from School and Wants to Play with Friends
"Before you can go and play, you need to finish all of your homework. We know your father and stepmother let you go play first, but they are bad parents and don't know how to raise you."

Behavior: Youth Visits Maternal Grandmother and Becomes Hungry before Dinner Is Ready
"We are going to visit your grandma, and you better wait to eat until she says it is ready; do not make a scene. We can't believe your mother buys you McDonald's instead of teaching you to obey parents' rules."

Behavior: Youth Stays out Late and Does Not Call Mother and Stepfather
"You broke our trust by staying out late and not calling us. You are going to be grounded from your phone and friends for a month. You will stay in your room without internet access and think about what you did. We will not let you visit your father and stepmother until your punishment is over. We don't care if they call their lawyer about custody rights. You are grounded, period."

What Is a Clinician Supposed to Do?

As with youths who have weaknesses in their four pillars, clinicians should identify areas of strength in the four pillars of the parent, stepparent, or adoptive parent in order to understand their abilities to learn and modify their approaches and provide tailored interventions to help the youth they care for (Table 8.3). The clinician should consider seeing the conflicted parent more frequently to help him or her to gradually modify his or her parenting styles. The clinician may incorporate case management to provide in-home support for youths and parents or guardians.

Table 8.3 Stepparents and adoptive parents with different pillars

Adoptive/stepparent, good four pillars	Adoptive/stepparent, mild weaknesses in four pillars	Adoptive/stepparent, significant weaknesses in four pillars
Recognizes he or she is not the parent and gives the youth time to adjust to his or her presence Allows the child to communicate with the parent when in need of support	Recognizes he or she is not the parent, but may not allow youth to communicate with parent when in distress	Fails to recognize that his or her role differs from that of the parent May tell youth he or she has the same authority as the parent and can set limits when necessary; endorses harsh consequences if the youth has a negative attitude
When initially setting limits, recognizes that this is best done together with the youth's parent to demonstrate collaborative parenting and avoid eliciting disagreement	When setting limits, warns that he or she will let the parent know if the youth does not comply, and that there will be more serious consequences	Forcefully states that he or she is also the youth's parent and can set limits without consulting the parent; claims that his or her actions will be supported and not questioned

Section I

We have now given an overview of the importance of assessing the four pillar strengths and weaknesses of parents, stepparents, and adoptive parents to understand the reasons for their style of parenting and their ability to modify if needed. With this knowledge, the clinician will provide caregivers interventions tailored to the youth's needs. Here, we will review basic parenting principles to help youths with reasonably good strengths in their four pillars.

Parenting Principles

Having well-developed pillars is the basis of the knowledge and wisdom that parents and grandparents use to help their youths. Below, we provide age-specific principles that parents and caregivers can use to improve interactions and solve challenging situations.

Parenting Principles for Infants

Being Responsive to the Infant's Needs

During the preverbal years, infants begin to make sense of their world and recognize patterns in their environment that help them begin to predict what may occur. They implicitly learn that they can shape how their parents respond to them: smiling and laughing makes their parents happy, crying when they have a wet diaper leads parents to change it, crying when hungry brings food, etc. Due to the preverbal nature of the infant, the parents are surprised how good they are at being attuned to the infant's needs, thinking, and communications. This becomes evident when parents

Table 8.4 Parents' Tasks with Infants

Holding
Rocking
Touching
Singing
Using baby talk (mother/Fatherese)
Making demonstrative facial expressions
Feeding and changing diapers at appropriate times
Attending to changes in mood or eating patterns
Encouraging family visits
Making regular visits with primary care provider as indicated

have a second child and feel less anxious about holding, using baby talk, feeding, and changing their infant's diapers. In Table 8.4, we highlight the many positive and intuitive tasks parents successfully complete every day, stored in implicit nondeclarative memory as mental schemas, later known as insight or wisdom.

Sharing your Values and Understanding your Infant's Moral Development

How parents manage this phase influences their child's development of a moral compass, a precursor of understanding and incorporating social norms. The moral development in children is seen as they make choices while interacting with others, and as they manage difficult situations. A study by Barragan et al. [3] found that 19-month-old toddlers can altruistically share food with strangers. This type of behavior suggests that childrearing practices that emphasize connectedness with others convey to the infant/toddler that people tend to help others. For parents, the implications are clear: children astutely observe their parents' interactions with others, internalize their parents' social values, and inherit their parents' moral compasses.

Recognizing Concerning Development in your Infant

Importantly, the infant is busy early in his or her life. He or she stores volumes of visual and emotional information in nondeclarative memory. Although it is largely taken for granted, early temperamental difficulties and weaknesses in visual abilities in the infant can lead to early relational difficulties that parents may find stressful. Thus, attention to four pillars in the infant, although rudimentary, can lead to early prevention of later problems.

Parenting Principles for Preschoolers (2 to 5 Years of Age)

During the preschool years, children begin to understand words and practice using language to communicate their needs, wants, and dislikes (early arguing). Further, they make developmental leaps as they begin to talk, walk, draw, etc. In these early years, the child's four pillars, temperament, cognitive abilities, and attachment styles become apparent. At this age, children develop more sophisticated patterns in memory to predict what makes adults and peers happy and angry (cognitive flexibility; see Chap. 5). Due to the verbal and action-prone nature of children at this age, parents are happily surprised when things go as expected.

Terrible Twos

For decades, the "terrible twos" has been popularized as an inevitable stage that is fraught, because it represents a time of turmoil in the young child. This could not be further from the truth. The so-called terrible twos phase is a metaphor for the toddler's newly acquired abilities to use motor activity and language to experiment with issues of control. This stage is a very exciting time for parents, who begin to see their child voice opinions behaviorally (walking away or toward certain situations) and verbally, expressing likes and dislikes. At this age, the child's emotional regulation abilities are not yet fine-tuned, and they do not yet understand the impact their reaction will have on others. Most parents are surprised by the child's forceful and loud expression of discontent or dislike (e.g., I don't want to drink milk, I am not hungry, etc.). Parents with good four pillars who have children with good four pillars are often surprised by how short-lived (less than five minutes) difficult moments are.

Certainly, the parent's reaction to the child's discontent will influence how the child learns to self-regulate, as he or she becomes aware of the impact he or she can have on her parents. Additionally, young children's emotional regulation abilities are strongly influenced by their physical regulatory issues: nutrition, sleep, and environmental support.

Conversely, when parents approach these moments of independence with a dysregulated style, it will set the stage for "terrible twos" moments, and the child will learn to imitate the parent's maladaptive behavior. These episodes of poor self-regulation can range from mild to full-blown meltdowns. The main reason for difficult episodes is the presence of weaknesses of the child's and/or parent's four pillars. The child's behavior, also been described as a tantrum, can lead to throwing objects, hitting, kicking, or biting others.

Iris Goes to the Grocery Store

Iris, a two-year-old girl, goes to the grocery store with her mother to buy milk, eggs, and flour to make pancakes. Iris is excited about making the pancakes and asks her mother to get chocolate chips to put in the pancakes. Her mother, instead of redirecting Iris, says, "No, we are not getting chocolate chips." Iris escalates; instead of helping her calm down, her mother says, "If you don't stop getting upset, I will not make the pancakes." Iris escalates and begins to yell. Her mother begins to give consequences, which do not help Iris calm down ("You will be in time-out when we get home," and "If you don't stop acting this way, you won't be allowed to use your iPad at home"). This can be understood as Iris's mother having weaknesses in one or more of her four pillars. She attempts to redirect Iris, but since she uses a difficult/feisty temperament style, Iris escalates and will need help regulating her emotions. But her mother, who does not have the cognitive flexibility to intuitively know how Iris feels, does not recognize that Iris can be helped by modeling how to look forward to the activity of making pancakes later.

This situation is well-known to the reader, who has surely seen grocery-store tantrums in preschool children, mismanaged by parents. Unfortunately, these parents commonly feel shame when noticed by others, which reinforces their use of ineffective authoritarian approaches.

Iris Goes to the Grocery store with her Aunt

Iris goes to the grocery store with her aunt to buy milk, eggs, and flour to make pancakes. Iris is excited about making the pancakes and asks her aunt to get chocolate chips to put in the pancakes. Her aunt does not want to get chocolate chips, and thus playfully redirects Iris, saying, "Will you help me crack the eggs?" Iris smiles and agrees. Her aunt stays on topic as she walks toward the checkout counter, asking Iris, "Have you ever cracked eggs and seen how gooey they are?" Iris continues to smile and says she wants to go home to crack the eggs.

This situation is also well-known to the reader, who has no doubt gone to the grocery stores and seen preschool-aged children with good relationships with adults. This can be understood as both Iris and her aunt making use of the strengths of one or more of their four pillars.

Promoting Growth in Preschool Children

We review the parental tasks needed to promote the development of a child's internalized positive mental schemas to be used during their preschool school years.

Modeling Flexibility for Preschool Children

Modeling flexibility prepares children to develop social skills and tolerate a modicum of frustration; possessing flexibility will facilitate success in social interactions. However, this principle may conflict with the age-old guidance to maintain predictable schedules, which we find to be impractical for most parents. Having an adjustable schedule allows parents to model flexibility with attention to their child's four pillars. Children with an easy/flexible temperament may benefit from structure to help with predictability in their lives, for example, predictable wake-up and bedtimes, regular snack and mealtimes, enough time to get ready to visit grandparents or go to church services, etc. Children with a slow-to-warm-up temperament benefit from having time to transition to new activities or complete tasks; it will take them longer, for example, to wake up, go to bed, or finish their snack. Finally, a child with a difficult/feisty temperament will need parents to model how to regulate their emotions by encouraging play and using a calm, soft voice when asking their child to complete an activity or chore.

Introducing Preschool Children to their Parents' World

Introducing children to their parents' world not only helps them develop self-regulation and selective attention, but allows children a glimpse into their parents' day-to-day activities. In doing this, children observe their parents interacting with different settings and with others. In introducing the preschool child to his or her parents' world, he or she also learns about his or her parents' likes and dislikes. Running errands is one good way to do this. However, it is important to be mindful of timing. Parents should time errands according to their child's emotional state, and not the parents' convenience, as running errands at an inopportune time may negatively impact the child's regulating abilities. Also, parents should consider taking only one child at a time on errands, instead of all; it can be viewed as a treat the child can earn. At stores, plan to walk to the items needed and to avoid walking through aisles with tempting items; this will prevent meltdowns in stores.

Promoting Self-Regulation in Preschool Children

- Encourage hands-on active play daily; play provides the mental space children need to regulate their mood.
- Communicate the importance of each other (e.g., good morning, have a good day, I love you, etc.).
- Model and encourage positive social skills by greeting or offering to help other people.
- Avoid overstimulating children.
- Accept that children have different palates and preferences in food taste, scent, and texture. It is counterproductive to ask a child to eat something he or she does not like if it can be substituted for another nutritious item. Experienced parents know that the foods a child dislikes now will likely be enjoyed at a later age.
- Promote enjoyable collaboration: ask the child to help with simple fun tasks (e.g., decorate cookies, wash dishes, pick up toys, etc.) (Tables 8.5).

Table 8.5 Additional Guidance for Preschool Children in Special Circumstances

Limit the number of chores or tasks according to age to prevent children from feeling overwhelmed, which can lead to disruptive behaviors
Rehearse managing unusual activities (e.g., attending a wedding, graduation, receiving immunizations, going to the dentist or to a medical specialist). Playfully act out or draw what will happen several days before the activity
In the case of the death of a loved one, whether expected or not, the preschool child will not fully understand the permanency of the loss; this understanding occurs at age 4 to 5 years
A child's reaction can vary, and parents will need to pay attention to the child's emotional reaction when told of the death of the loved one
Help the child with his or her emotions; do not ask his or her to feel the same as others. If the child's reaction is to feel anxious or distraught, spend one-on-one time to reassure his or her and share happy memories about the loved one
Model how to manage the sad event by reflecting on the reasons the person that passed was important to the family
While some children may be overwhelmed and cry, others will ask questions or appear unaffected. Some children may ask parents or other adults near them to share the reasons for their sad feelings
If a parent is emotionally overwhelmed by the death of the loved one, the child should be reassured and supported by a different family member
Drawing or writing a story about the person that died has been helpful for many
The question of whether to bring children to funerals is a difficult one. As a general rule, it is best to avoid bringing preschoolers to funerals. Preschool children often continue to rely on fantasy and have limited understanding of the permanence of death; it may be overwhelming to see many distressed, crying, or emotional adults
Disruptive children should not attend funerals

Teaching Limit-Setting for Preschool Children

Difficult moments are part and parcel of any childhood. Difficult moments are times when young children become emotionally overwhelmed and struggle with self-regulation. They may display intense feelings of sadness or anger. We provide a few principles to make these ubiquitous moments less stressful.

- Create a safe and calming space in the home where the child can calm down and regain control when upset (a chair where stuffed animals sleep, favorite couch, etc.). Encourage him or her to use the safe space when sad or upset.
- Choosing battles and avoiding power struggles is not always possible. It is a misconception that young children intentionally make their parents mad. Rather, they make their parents mad when they do not know how to manage a stressful and difficult situation due to weakness in reasoning (because of either their young age or weaknesses in their four pillars). Therefore, it is important to avoid attributing negative intentions to the child and help them regulate by modeling how to manage difficult situations.
- Do not match the child's loud or angry tone of voice.
- Avoid applying negative labels to the child's behavior, as this will lower self-esteem and promote more disruptive behaviors. For example, phrases like "You are hyper/difficult/push me to get mad/a troublemaker," should be avoided.
- Teach the child special words they can use when they need help regulating their emotions and are unable to articulate this. The word or phrase can be something like "purple," "green eggs," or the name of a stuffed animal or family dog, etc. When the child uses the code word, the parent will provide a DEAR moment followed by a Wait, Watch, and Wonder approach (see below).
- Use clear, age-appropriate directions regarding limit-setting and consequences. We avoid the use of the word "discipline," as it implies punishment.

DEAR Moments

When a child sends nonverbal or verbal signals that he or she needs help with emotional regulation, we should consider DEAR moments. These moments occur when a parent or other adult Drops Everything And Relates to the child in a calm manner. The presence of a parent or adult, in the moment, is reassuring, particularly when the parent or adult abstains from commenting unless requested. While these moments may seem time-consuming, this approach will ultimately save time while also preventing the child's emotional upheaval from becoming unmanageable—a much more time-consuming outcome. Frequently, the Wait, Watch, and Wonder (WWW) approach can follow DEAR moments.

The Wait, Watch, and Wonder Approach

A parent's first inclination toward a distraught child is often to actively inquire (or even demand) that the child share what is bothering him or her. When parents implicitly convey an urgency for understanding what has driven the child's distress, albeit with the goal of helping their child feel better, the child cannot learn self-regulation and problem-solving abilities from the experience. Moreover, when the child notices the parent's anxiety or frustration, he or she may fear how the parent will react. As a result, the child may be more hesitant to share the reasons behind his or her distress.

Our Wait, Watch, and Wonder approach encourages parents to promote self-regulation and problem-solving skills. Our model asks parents to wait—and allow the child to share what troubles him or her when he or she is ready. While the parent waits, he or she will also be observing—or watching—how his or her child is managing the new challenging situation emotionally and behaviorally. Waiting gives the child time to settle and the parent time to "watch" before forming opinions or judgments about what may be causing their child distress, as well as what the child needs. Once the child has been able to calm himself or herself, the parent may now "wonder" aloud: "I wonder what I can do to help you? Are you feeling sad, angry, or overwhelmed?" The child's response is not as important as the process of teaching the child that asking for help in difficult moments is valuable. Parents' active listening implicitly provides the child a sense of competency. Some clinicians may note that Wait, Watch, and Wonder sounds similar to the dyadic infant-mother psychotherapy process: Watch, Wait, and Wonder, a child-led psychotherapeutic approach that requires parents to receive training in its use [10]. However, our approach represents an important difference, because it is an in-the-moment parenting approach that takes into account developmental milestones and can be used at all ages (Fig. 8.1).

Mark, a 5-Year-Old Boy, Becomes Frustrated and Angry when he Has Difficulties Tying his Shoes before Leaving for Church

The parent asks, "Anything wrong?"

Mark, feeling anxious, says, "Nothing!"

The parent waits and watches how Mark handles the situation.

Mark continues to feel frustrated.

The parent wonders, "Let me know if I can help you." [Modeling how to regulate].

Mark responds, "You'll be mad at me."

The parent calmly says, "I want to help you. I am not mad."

The parent, by waiting for Mark to feel safe, observing his reaction, and communicating to the child, "You can tell me what's bothering you when you are ready," allows Mark to feel emotionally and relationally secure, and therefore eager to

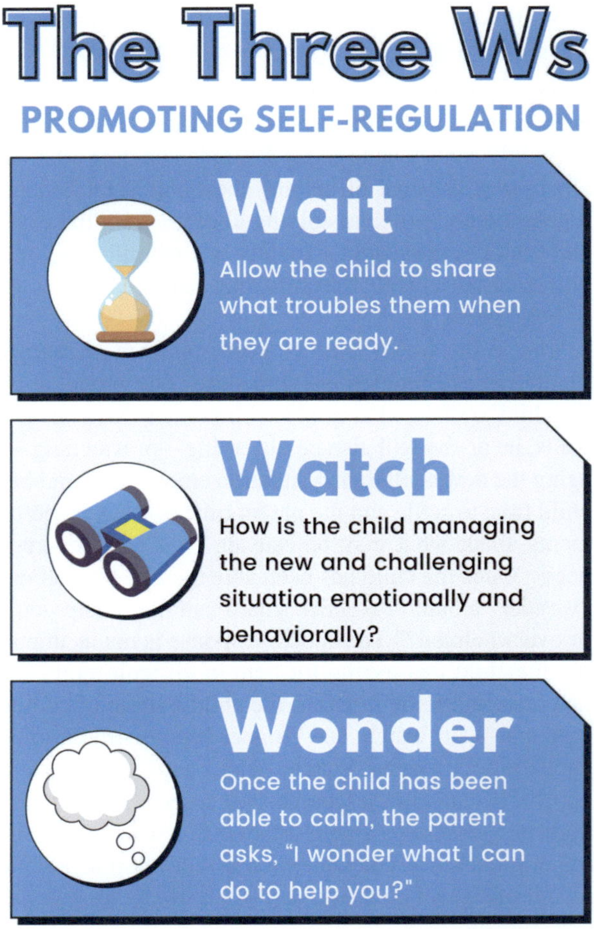

Fig. 8.1 A Wait, Watch, and Wonder moment. This original figure was created with Canva.com under a one design use license commercial agreement

communicate the whole story. Conflict is avoided, and the child internalizes the parent's active listening and pride in him.

Later…

Mark states, "I know you will be mad at me because I'm not smart. It's hard to tie my shoes." [Parent is aware that tying his shoes is a newly acquired task and that it is developmentally appropriate to struggle].

His father replies, "We have plenty of time before we need to go. Do you want to try again, and if you can't tie them, I'll help you?"

Mark replies, "Can you help me tie my shoes now and help me practice later?"

Mark shared that he was worried his parent would be critical of him for not being "smart" enough to tie his shoes. In reviewing Mark's difficulties, his responses will depend on his four pillars. In this case, Mark has good four pillars, and calmly (easy/flexible temperament) shares with his parent that tying his shoes is difficult (cognition: tying shoes is expected to be difficult at his age) and hopes to practice later that day with his parent's help (cognitive flexibility), within the context of a secure attachment style in his family.

In reviewing Mark's situation with developmental milestones in mind (**Appendix A**), at 5 years of age, children do not usually have the fine motor skills or coordination required to tie their shoelaces. Learning to tie shoelaces also requires patience and practice. By using the Wait, Watch, and Wonder approach, the parent learns what can be expected and develops realistic expectations (e.g., that tying shoes is not easy for all 5-year-old children).

Mark's Father Successfully Uses the Wait, Watch, and Wonder Approach
Wait: Recognizes Mark is frustrated and silently waits to see how he proceeds.
Watch: Observes how Mark expresses why he is frustrated: "You will be mad at me."
Wonder: Wonders what would help him to promote competency.
"I wonder if you want me to help you ties your shoelaces?"

With a Different, Less Successful Approach, Mark Feels Mistrust and Low Self-Esteem. Below is a Hypothetical Example of How Mark's Father Might have Reacted

With a sense of urgency, Mark's father demands, "What's wrong?"

Mark anxiously says, "Nothing!"

Mark's father becomes frustrated and forcefully states, "You need to tell me what's wrong if you want me to help you."

Mark responds, "You always get mad at me."

Frustrated, Mark's father says, "I am mad at you when you don't tell me what's wrong."

Mark replies, "Even if I tell you what's wrong, you get mad. It's too hard to tie my shoes."

Mark's father says, "You are smart, and you know how to ties your shoes. Hurry up."

In essence, Mark's father demands that he communicate; he fails to recognize that Mark feels badly about not being able to tie his shoes. Parents frequently assume that children should share their feelings, without recognizing a child may fear their parent's frustration and criticisms. This developmental and emotional mismatch sets the stage for relational difficulties between the child and his or her parents.

Lying, Defiance, and Oppositional Behavior in Preschool Children

During the preschool years, many youths respond to their parents' caring but firm limit-setting and develop adaptive patterns that allow them to get along with others. However, some preschool children occasionally lie and demonstrate defiant and oppositional behaviors. When these maladaptive behaviors are infrequent and emerge when the child feels misunderstood by others, they are healthy developmental steps that allow him or her to become independent and voice disagreement. These behaviors can be viewed as a rehearsal for disagreeing with adults when he or she feels safe and understood, and prevents the need to lie or become aggressive. However, when these maladaptive behaviors are frequent, the severity is largely related to the extent of the child's four pillar weaknesses. The preschool child with a difficulty/feisty temperament will lie about his or her contribution to problems when reprimanded. Further, young children with cognitive weaknesses become defiant and argumentative when they sense they have done something wrong, but, due to their weakness, do not grasp the extent of the problem. We can see this dynamic play out in daycare and preschool, where the need for adaptive social skills is increased.

Clinicians and parents often agree that a child's maladaptive behaviors fit the diagnostic categories of oppositional defiant disorder, disruptive behavior disorder, or impulse control disorders. Unfortunately, these diagnoses do not address the root of the maladaptive behaviors, and the clinician may suggest behavioral approaches that aim to interrupt a cycle of escalating negative behaviors by teaching parents to use clear limit-setting within an authoritative relationship. Ultimately, this exacerbates family conflict. Alternately, by understanding the causes of the maladaptive behaviors, the clinician can provide tailored and practical interventions for these young children (Chap. 7) that are informed by the child's weaknesses in the four pillars. This approach implicitly allows the parent to work around the child's four pillar weaknesses and enhance his or her strengths.

At times, clinicians refer patients for possible pharmacologic interventions to help youths with emotional regulation difficulties. For example, when oppositional behaviors in preschoolers are due to attention-deficit hyperactivity/disorder, early pharmacologic intervention leads to good outcomes. However, we emphasize that some difficult-to-treat preschool children may have both attention-deficit hyperactivity/disorder and weaknesses in their four pillars. However, in these youths, medication and traditional psychotherapeutic approaches may not be enough, or treatment could unmask the weaknesses in their four pillars.

Throughout this book, we posit that lying, defiance, and oppositional behaviors may also result from parenting styles that are themselves influenced by parental weaknesses in the four pillars. In fact, in some longitudinal studies of youths, harsh discipline in the first five years of life is associated with aggression in adolescence [4, 12, 33]. However, for parents with good four pillars, several evidence-based interventions can decrease these disruptive behaviors. Specifically, Parent-Child Interaction Therapy (PCIT) represents one approach for disruptive behavior problems in children aged 2 to 7) [6]. PCIT involves two phases, child-directed interaction (CDI) and parent-directed interaction (PDI), in which therapists instruct and coach parents in play therapy and operant conditioning skills. In PCIT, clinicians typically observe sessions through a one-way mirror, communicating with caregivers by a bug-in-the-ear system. The goals are to encourage warm, secure parent-child relationships, and to increase child compliance and decrease disruptive behaviors. The foundational skills include praise, verbal reflection, imitation, behavioral description, and enjoyment [21].

Unfortunately, when families have weaknesses in their four pillars and struggle with other external challenges, PCIT attrition rates may be high. These external challenges include internalizing problems in parents (e.g., depressive disorders, anxiety disorders, maladaptive personality characteristics, being a single parent, having less education, having had a child removed from the home, and a lack of resources). Also, parents who have more negative talk and behavior, are younger, and experience more distress (e.g., employment, housing, and transportation and childcare difficulties) tend to struggle more in PCIT [35].

Grandparents Think We Are Parenting Wrong

Whether sharing happy and humorous stories about their children with their grandchildren or simply spending time with them, grandparents' involvement in their grandchildren's lives enhances family closeness. Ideally, grandparents have joyful and special roles with their grandchildren, and emotionally support their adult children. Grandparents' involvement—taking the grandchildren to play at a park, taking them for ice cream, or helping with homework—often makes life easier for their children. However, at times, the generational gap in parenting styles presents challenges for parents. Conflict with close family members or grandparents regarding parenting approaches can be detrimental for the children, and the issue will need to be addressed by the parents.

A colleague, adept at intuiting the emotional needs of his 2- and 5-year-old children, shared his difficulties with his parents and in-laws, who were critical of his parenting style. They disapproved of his choice to not set limits on his children's clothing and food choices. The grandparents criticized his decision to allow children to help choose what to wear for church, and to make their own (reasonable) breakfast choices. "I would never do it that way," the grandparents said. "They should not have choices. They need to learn that you are in charge and eat what you give them." Finally, the grandparents argued, "It worked when you were little," implying their approach was correct.

The reader knows that we would be the first to say that a one-size-fits-all approach, in parenting, is not helpful. Each generation has had its own parenting approaches and beliefs, which have changed over the years. Today, children have healthier food choices, develop skills by using electronic devices that promote learning, and more.

Although it is common to suggest that parents let close family members or grandparents know when they have overstepped their boundaries, this may lead to more conflict. In certain situations, the well-known adage "I bit my tongue," is helpful to remember. Stepping back and looking at the bigger picture of the benefits of having family members and grandparents close to their (grand)children helps diffuse frustrations and anger. When conflict is infrequent, it is best to avoid the instinct to engage and to become overly critical of family members and grandparents. Talking through the reasons for parenting decisions and listening to the family members and grandparents' philosophies may not lead to a quick solution, but it promotes understanding and reduces discord.

Common Struggles for Parents of Preschool-Aged Children (Fig. 8.2)

My Child Can't Sleep

Children benefit from good sleeping patterns. Sleep promotes health and growth, self-regulation, and learning. However, sleep problems are common in children, with rates between 25% and 40%. Young children most commonly exhibit what is referred to as "bedtime problems and night awakenings"; these problems also occur in middle childhood (ages 4 to 12). Importantly, for many children, these problems persist. Insufficient sleep in children and adolescents worsens inattention and daytime fatigue, increases family stress, and decreases parental well-being [47]. Sleep can be disrupted by medical conditions, medications, and environmental factors (stressful situations or loud evening noises). Having a good understanding of the reasons for sleep disturbances in children and adolescents is a critical tool for parents and clinicians alike. While a review of the medical and neuropsychiatric causes of dysomnias is beyond the scope of this text and has been reviewed elsewhere [14, 34, 46], we will focus on sleep problems as they relate to the four pillars.

Youths with weaknesses in the four pillars can have difficulties judging time and may having problems falling asleep or staying asleep. Based on the child's understanding of their sleep difficulties, parents may enlist the help of primary care

Fig. 8.2 Sleep

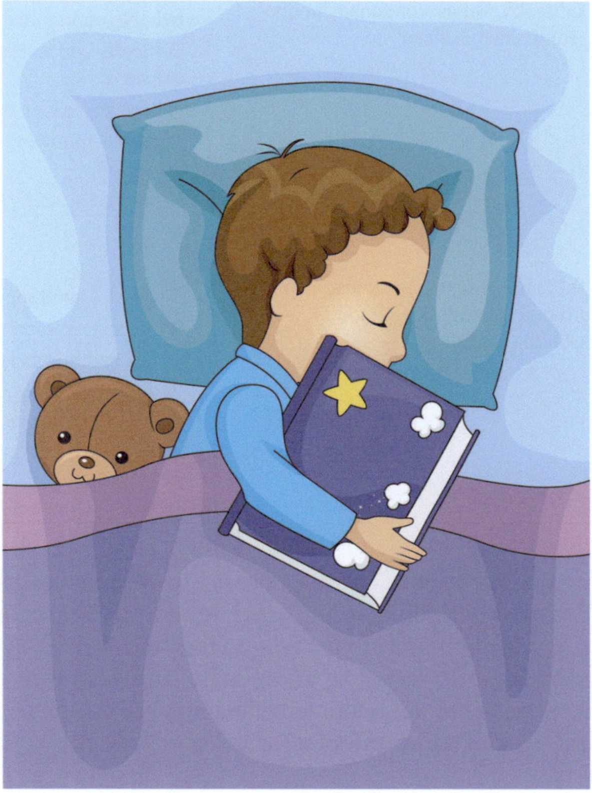

clinicians, complaining that "He can't fall asleep." Such complaints, in the clinical setting, may result in a request for a medication or a prescription for a soporific medication or melatonin. In our work in outpatient and inpatient settings, we have found that many times, parents have observed that their youth had slept well although the youth's experience was that of not having slept well. Our recommendation has been to assess a youth's sleep hygiene by asking the youth to use a method of communication they have mastered. This will allow for a better understanding and documentation of the problem (e.g., have the child write down or text his or her parents if he or she is awake after bedtime). Parents are often surprised their child slept most of the night.

The comparison between children's self-reports and parents' reports is useful to depict perceptions of children's sleep. Children with good cognitive abilities are, by the age of 8, mature enough to complete a 7-day self-report journal of their sleep. It is also important to analyze sleep patterns for school days separately from weekends [40]. An alternative option for younger children is for parents to check in every one or two hours after bedtime to see if their child is having trouble sleeping (Tables 8.6 and 8.7).

Table 8.6 Signs a child may not be getting enough sleep

Irritable or argumentative over minor issues
Difficulty concentrating at school or at home on certain days
Falls asleep easily throughout the day
Struggles following conversations and is often distracted
Experiences timing changes in their appetite

Table 8.7 Interventions that help promote healthy sleep (modify according to age)

Establish a soothing bedtime routine
Create a sleep-inducing environment (see below)
Read a bedtime story with child (less than 20 minutes)
Sing a calming song
Use a sticker chart as an incentive for good sleep behavior
Reduce conflict before bedtime

We reiterate that one size does not fit all. Some youths can fall asleep better with background noise from fish tanks, music, etc. Others find it helpful to read or play simple games for a limited time on their media devices while in bed. For others, the reduction of screen time after 9 p.m. correlated with earlier sleep-onset time and increased total sleep duration with improved daytime vigilance. These findings provide evidence that restricting screen use in the evening represents a valid and promising approach for improving sleep duration in adolescents, with potential implications for daytime functioning and health [48]. The reasons for this are poorly understood and seem to be related to their temperamental traits in rhythmicity, or the internal rhythm of the child [9]. Importantly, at bedtime, youths are at particular risk of social media misuse, including cyberbullying, "sexting," or overdisclosure. Parents should become familiar with websites that explain how to use parental controls on their youth's devices.

My Child Asks for One More (Glass of Water, Trip to the Bathroom, YouTube Episode) at Bedtime

Consistent with what we have shared, the reasons why children delay the going-to-bed process are multifactorial. Some youths fear falling asleep if they have had repetitive frightening dreams, while others may have obsessive anxiety: "I can't shut my mind off." These youths may hope that the last ritualized trip to the bathroom will help them go to sleep. Finally, some youths may fear going to bed if worried about a family member's health, school problems, or conflicts with peers. Therefore, it is best to understand the reasons and develop a realistic strategy to address the issue. An authoritarian approach at bedtime should be avoided, because it conveys frustration and will increase the youth's anxiety about not being loved and accordingly increase his or her struggle to fall asleep.

Can my Child Take Melatonin for Sleep Problems?

For healthy children with insomnia who practice good sleep hygiene, melatonin might be appropriate. Melatonin is the primary regulator of the sleep-wake cycle and may be the preferred initial pharmacotherapy for sleep-onset insomnia due to its ability to reset the body's normal circadian clock [7]. In clinical studies of children and adolescents, both immediate-release [31, 58] and extended-release melatonin [26] reduced sleep-onset latency and increased total sleep duration in youths. Further, melatonin appears to be well-tolerated. A two-year randomized trial of prolonged-release melatonin for insomnia in pediatric patients found no adverse effects with regard to growth, BMI, and pubertal development [37]. Additionally, significant improvements in sleep quality, sleep patterns, and caregiver satisfaction were maintained throughout the trial, and no withdrawal symptoms were observed upon discontinuation. However, while melatonin appears to be well-tolerated, it should be avoided in children with immune disorders or those using immunomodulating treatments [30].

My Child Has Nightmares

Nightmares are frightening or unpleasant dreams and may reverberate with typical fears in preschool-aged children, including the dark and separation. Having a night light in the room may help comfort a child and reduce his or her fear of the dark. When a child has nightmares, ask him or her to share (or draw) the nightmare and what it was about. This helps reassure the child that it is not real, and encourages him or her to use his or her imagination to create a problem-solving scenario.

Reasons for persistent nightmares are multifactorial. It is best to complete a psychiatric evaluation to identify the stressors that may be contributing to nightmares. Play or art therapy facilitates identifying themes the child may have problems sharing. Interventions can be tailored accordingly.

My Child Has Night Terrors

Night terrors (or sleep terrors) in children are considered parasomnias. These are characterized by episodes of screaming, intense fear, and flailing while still asleep and are often paired with sleepwalking. The reasons for night terrors are poorly understood, although it is commonly thought that they are due to stress, lack of sleep, or medications. Night terrors are not due to a serious psychological issue or medical problem, and they usually resolve with age.

Unlike with nightmares, children are not aware of a night terror as it is happening. Still, seeing a child have a night terror is challenging and unsettling. Although the child is not awake, he or she may scream in distress, sit up in bed, breathe heavily, and have tachycardia. Episodes usually last a few minutes, although some can last up to 45 minutes. Attempting to wake the child might cause him or her more distress. Efforts should be made to gently guide the child back to bed until he or she falls back asleep.

My Child Has Potty-Training struggles (Enuresis and Encopresis)

Enuresis is a physiological issue that occurs when young children struggle with bladder control at night. This usually occurs in children between 2 and 4 years of age; however, it can continue in school-aged children. Most children grow out of enuresis, although it can be distressing. Primary care providers can evaluate and help with pharmacologic approaches to help with self-esteem issues. Parents that were enuretic when they were young are more likely to have a child that is enuretic as well.

Importantly, parents should not punish children who struggle with enuresis. Some parents take punitive measures, telling their child in a critical manner that he or she is responsible for changing his or her wet bedsheets. This increases anxiety and lowers self-esteem. Education about enuresis should be provided to the parents so that they can take a collaborative approach with their child to address the problem, change the bedsheets, and seek help from their primary care provider.

Parents often ask at what age a child is expected to be toilet-trained. Most children are toilet-trained and can control their bowels by 4 years of age, although it is often hoped this will occur by age 2 because of social expectations or daycare requirements. Problems controlling bowel movements can cause soiling, which leads to frustration and anger for the child, parents, and teachers. In addition, this problem can lead to severe social difficulties—the child is often teased by friends and shamed by adults. When soiling is not caused by a physical illness or disability, it is called idiopathic constipation, a functional bowel disorder characterized by difficult, infrequent, and/or incomplete defecation.

Although most children with idiopathic constipation do not have a physical condition, they should first have a complete physical evaluation by their primary care provider. If no physical causes are found, we suggest the next step be a referral to a psychotherapist. This can prevent the use of invasive procedures if the problem with idiopathic constipation is due to a stressful change in the child's life, such as the birth of a sibling, separation/divorce of parents, family problems, or a move to a new home or school. Idiopathic constipation is more common in boys than in girls.

Idiopathic constipation can be treated with a combination of educational, psychological, and behavioral methods. However, the various treatment methods from these theoretical viewpoints have not been consistently effective [5]. Currently, there is limited literature reviewing and synthesizing functional defecation disorders, making it challenging to comprehensively characterize and delineate behaviors indicating a need for specific intervention. Most cases of encopresis are the result of chronic constipation. Approximately 1–2% of children younger than 10 years old have had encopresis, and it is more common in boys. Importantly, early treatment of constipation can attenuate the social and emotional impacts of encopresis.

A 5-Year-Old Girl Is Afraid to "Poop Because the Angels Could Get Mad"

A 5-year-old girl was referred to a child and adolescent psychiatrist by her pediatrician due to idiopathic constipation. A trial of laxatives, including mineral oil, was not only unsuccessful, but also made her feel embarrassed when the mineral oil leaked and failed to help her have a bowel movement [15]. Her family was well adjusted and had good four pillars. The only stressor identified was that her paternal grandfather had become ill from pneumonia and was hospitalized for three days prior to the onset of her constipation. Her parents did not think this was a major stressor since "her grandfather is fine now."

The child was very bright and charming, and related well to family and friends until her constipation began to interfere. She no longer wanted to play with friends due to the abdominal pain. She began to ask about how her grandfather was feeling and thought he was "not funny and silly anymore," which her parents shared was not accurate: "He is the same old funny grandpa." Prior to the onset of her symptoms, she was described as "the perfect child."

In consultation with her pediatrician, it was agreed that play therapy could be of help due to the many protective factors she had: easy/flexible temperament, superior intelligence, well-developed cognitive flexibility, and a secure attachment. She began play therapy.

Second Session

Child: Get in the trash can [*The psychiatrist stands in the empty trash can*] … now you know how it feels!

Psychiatrist: I feel stuck.

Child: You should be. You were bad. You were angry at God's angels for making your grandfather go to the hospital.

Psychiatrist: I didn't know why he was sick. I was scared.

Child: It was because he was old and old people die.

Psychiatrist: [*Steps out of the story.*] What should I say now?

Child: *[Laughs anxiously.]* Ha ha! I am happy you are stuck in the trash. Your poop is stuck, and angry feelings will fill the trash can. You are dirty.

Psychiatrist: Kids can have angry feelings. Let's keep playing and maybe you will feel better and not worry about letting your poop out.

Child: I get mad when my parents give me the poop medicine.

Psychiatrist: Maybe you're worried about being mad at God's angels about your grandfather and you don't poop … [*Makes connection of symptom and anxiety*]

Child: Yes, I'm afraid to poop, because the angels could get mad and take him to the hospital again!

The Following Session.

Child: [Looks happy.] Guess what? I pooped at McDonald's. It was a lot! I know it's okay to be angry with the angels.

Psychiatrist: Great! You're not worried about being mad at God's angels now.

We acknowledge that not all cases will have such a remarkable outcome as with this child. However, this case highlights the benefit in considering a psychotherapeutic process to explore possible psychosocial stressors as a source of anxiety before invasive studies are used.

My Child Displays "Nervous Habits," Including Nail-Biting and Skin-Picking

Parents of youths with transient or persistent tics (vocal or motor) or Tourette's syndrome struggle knowing how to best help their child with their tics. Often parents are frustrated at the sight of seeing their child display tics and want them to stop.

Parents typically say, "Please stop clearing your throat," or "Don't bite your lip," etc. Unfortunately, asking a youth to stop the behavior increases his or her anxiety, as he or she recognizes the parent's frustration and feels embarrassed, which exacerbates the tics.

Table 8.8 Redirection to help with mild tics or tic-like behavior

Tic or tic-like behavior	Redirection
Licks lips, bites lips, or grimaces Licking lips is more pronounced during winter because of dry lips	Give the youth something to have in his or her mouth (e.g., a lollipop, gum, hard candy, tootsie roll, etc.) Use lip balm for dry lips; help ensure it is not used excessively
Makes finger or arm movements	Ask him or her to play with a fidget toy or an electronic device
Picks insect bites or scabs	In addition to the use of a fidget toy or electronic device, applying clear nail polish over an insect bite can decrease the urge to pick at skin Prevent dry skin by using moisturizing lotion

Parents benefit from learning about the neurobiology of tics: it is not a conscious action; youths may not realize they are having tics; it can have seasonal waxing and waning in frequency, etc. An approach of reassurance and redirection is helpful. Additionally, sharing information about tics with people close to the youth can help them to be more understanding. In Table 8.8, we list a few comments that can help redirect youths and help with mild tics. If tics are severe and disruptive—such as causing pain or causing the youth to be teased by others—consider treatment with the use of medication or habit reversal therapy.

Parenting Principles for Elementary- and Middle-School-Aged Youths (6 to 13 Years of Age)

Parent Principles for Elementary School-Aged Youths

Youths typically begin elementary school (primary education) at 5 to 6 years of age, after kindergarten. Elementary school generally goes through the sixth grade, typically to 11 years of age. In elementary school, youths learn the basics of reading, math, science, and other subjects, upon which later learning will build. During the elementary school, the most salient developmental steps are competition in games, enjoyment of conversation in groups, increased interest in the opposite gender, and respect of parents (**Appendix A**). Socialization skills are an important aspect of this period. Granic and Patterson [25] eloquently state, “Parents and children are confronted with a variety of daily tasks (e.g., clean-up time, playing games, problem-solving when conflict arises, eating dinner together).” They further suggest that the extent to which parents can flexibly and appropriately respond, emotionally, cognitively, and behaviorally, to shifts in contexts, may tap a repertoire of alternative strategies that correspond to how children will adapt to future challenges. Thus, during this age, parents need to be reminded that a youth’s most effective way of communicating his or her affective states is through elaborate storytelling, play, and drawings. Parents benefit when given information about their youth’s developmental abilities in communicating their emotional states. As Krimendahl [32] states, "I do not view my role as finding ways to 'get' school age children to talk, for talking is not the most developmentally natural medium for children." Additionally, Schaefer [52] states that children use play to communicate when they do not have the words to share their needs, and look to adults to understand their language. Later, in preadolescent years—middle school—verbal communication takes hold.

Parenting Principles for Middle-School-Aged Youths

Middle-school-aged youths are those from ages 11 to 13. This period is also referred as prepuberty, preadolescence, or early adolescence. During this period, youths experience dramatic changes in physical development, encompassing height, weight, and sexual development. Although maturity rate during this period occurs at varied rates, generally in girls it occurs one and a half to two years earlier than in boys. Major cognitive changes occur during this period, with transitions from concrete thinking to abstract thinking. During this stage, youths experience mixed feelings about how they fit in society and may experiment with different roles until they achieve a sense of identity [41]. Further, they develop a better understanding of higher levels of humor, are inquisitive about adult roles, and may challenge authority. During this period, youths are psychologically curious and idealistic about the world and themselves.

Middle-school-aged youths start turning away from their parents and relying more on friends, teachers, and coaches. Social relationships and roles change dramatically as they join youth programs and become involved with peers and adults outside of their family. During this period, adolescents develop a sense of individuality by actively comparing themselves to their peers and seeking approval from them. This facilitates developing close friends their own age, which can provide the sense of "belonging" to a larger similar group. During this age, the child's cognitive abilities expand, and he or she is better able to problem-solve and hold two opposing viewpoints in mind. This allows for the vitality needed to remain engaged in peer group activities; difficulties in this area frequently reflect cognitive and relational difficulties (Table 8.9).

Helicopter Parents with Elementary- and Middle-School-Aged Youths

Parents have a natural inclination to solve youths' problems when seeing them in distress (e.g., crying, angry at themselves, etc.). This often fails to recognize that this can interfere in the youth's acquisition of skills that promote independence and

Table 8.9 Growth-promoting tasks for elementary- and middle-school-aged youths

"Catch them being good" is the most used and helpful phrase shared with parents to convey the important task they have during this stage, complimenting and supporting their youth's accomplishments
Parents can model and encourage positive social skills by inviting family friends and their children to dinner or evening activities
Occasionally, parents can model positive social skills by inviting adult friends without their children for dinner or weekend gatherings. This allows youths to learn how to give space to adults by engaging in an activity independently
Avoid overscheduling in after-school activities such as swimming lessons, soccer, gymnastics, dance lessons, baseball, etc
As with preschool children, accept that youths have different palates and preferences in food taste, scent, and texture. It is counterproductive to ask a youth to eat something he or she does not want
Demonstrate and talk about the importance of altruism. Encourage youths to spend time alongside parents helping people in need. Donate clothing, volunteer, or donate money to a charity with your child present
As with preschool children, with elementary-school-aged children, errands should be timed according to the youth's emotional state and not for parent convenience, as it may negatively impact the youth's self-regulating abilities
Mealtimes with family have been shown to have positive effects in family relationships. Encourage youths, without forcing them, to sit with the family at mealtime to share and hear stories about the day, even if they are not hungry
When a youth is unwilling to engage in activities with the family, consider it an opportunity to model how to communicate by asking him or her to share her logic. This may inform the parent of possible anxieties or weaknesses
Avoid solving their problems and offer to help (see wait, watch, and wonder approach above)
Help youths create and use one or two code words to signal when they're feeling overwhelmed or need help regulating their emotions. These words can be a specific color not often used (purple), the name of a family pet, etc. when the child uses the code word, the parent will provide a DEAR moment (drop everything and relate) with the youth (see section above) to help with emotional regulation. An alternative to code words is color-coded index cards or sticky notes
Choosing battles and avoiding power struggles is not always possible. When conflict occurs, the most important step is to avoid matching the youth's loud or angry tone of voice as this negatively models how to manage difficult situations
When setting limits, use clear, age-appropriate directions and give short, easy-to-complete consequences to promote adaptive behaviors
Avoid negatively labeling behaviors. This decreases self-esteem and promotes disruptive behaviors. Phrases to avoid include: "You are stubborn/ungrateful/selfish/push me to get mad." if negative behaviors occur often, clinicians should assess weaknesses in the youth's four pillars (and those of his parents), which may be at the root of the problem
With middle-school-aged youths, it is important to maintain trust. By spending a few minutes listening to what they like, the clinician can more easily engage, laugh, and discuss difficult subjects that are hard to address directly

self-sufficiency. Solving a youth's problem can prevent them from learning to tolerate a healthy degree of frustration and uncertainty that allows them to learn from the experience.

Jessica, An 11-Year-Old, Becomes Frustrated While Helping her 6-year-old Brother with a Spelling Assignment

Parent: *Jessica, you are really good at spelling. Can you please help your brother with his spelling assignment?*

Jessica: *Yes, I like to spell. [Begins to help her brother work on the assignment]*

Jessica: *[Yells at her parents] He doesn't care about spelling. [She crumples up her brother's assignment]. He doesn't want to learn; he doesn't pay attention to me.*

Parent: *Okay, you can leave him alone. I will help him.*

Although there may be many causes of the problems between Jessica and her brother, it is important for parents to learn not to solve these problems without understanding the origin of the distress. In this case, for practical purposes, let's assume that Jessica's brother had typical spelling difficulties for his age. However, Jessica was too young to be aware of his level of understanding, and may have thought he should have the same skills as her. This would have been an opportunity for the parents to compliment Jessica for helping her brother and to teach her about spelling skill acquisition at her brother's age. Jessica would feel validated and hopefully more willing to help her brother later. When her parents agreed to allow Jessica to leave and not help her brother, they prevented her from learning to tolerate a healthy degree of frustration that would have allowed her to learn that her brother had spelling skills below her level, which is why he needed help.

Jessica Becomes Frustrated with her Best Friend

Parent: *Jessica, what happened? You seem angry.*

Jessica: *Yes, I am. Kali doesn't want to be my friend anymore.*

Parent: *I am sure that is not true. Let me call her parent and see what happened and why she hurt your feelings.*

Jessica: *[Looks pleased at her mother's willingness to solve her problem.] She is my best friend; I need her to like me.*

Parent: *Okay, I will call now.*

The reasons for problems between 11-year-old friends can be many. In this situation, when Jessica's parent called to make things better, he or she prevented Jessica from learning to tolerate a healthy degree of frustration—and from learning from the experience. The long-term goal is for Jessica to learn to be flexible in her thinking and come up with what to suggest to her friend as a possible solution. In other words, youths benefit when they are allowed to figure things out on their own.

Transitions

Transitions are part of every youth's life, and some are easier than others to manage. We provide suggestions on how to manage the most common transitions youths face.

- If a family is planning to move to a new home and the child will be attending a new school, several things can be helpful.
  - Drive by (stopping to get out, if possible) to view and explore the new home or school when empty. After the visit, parents should take the youth to a comfortable setting (e.g., to have ice cream or a snack) and talk about the youth's impressions of the new place.
  - Initially, most youths will have negative or ambivalent feelings about the new home or school, because it is part of a significant loss and change from their prior home or school. Parents should use the Wait, Watch, and Wonder approach to help with the youth's ambivalence.
  - In preparation for leaving the youth's home or school, parents can help by asking the youth what photos he or she would like from important rooms or places for them (living room, bedroom, backyard, school building or classroom, etc.) and then capturing these photos. The photos can later be used to reflect on positive memories. Family and friends should be included in the photos when possible.
  - At times of distress, youths may ask to see the photos of their prior home or school to retrieve happy memories to cope with the sadness of leaving.
- In contrast to preschool children, in the case of the death of a loved one (in some cases, including pets), whether expected or not, elementary- and middle-school-aged youths are best helped when parents ask them to share their sad feelings and what the loved one meant to them. At this age, youths understand the permanency of the loss, and will have more memories and strong feelings about the person or animal that passed.
- Youths' reactions can vary. Some may be overwhelmed and cry, preferring comfort from close friends who are not as sad or overwhelmed as their parents. Others may intellectualize and ask many questions; these youths may appear unaffected but may be struggling internally. Therefore, it is best for parents to use the Wait, Watch, and Wonder approach to help youths as they experience their emotions and not to push them to feel what others experience.
- Parents may find it helpful to have one-on-one time with youths to look at pictures of their loved one together. If a parent is too overwhelmed, this task should be given to a different family member.

- Having a school-age youth attend a funeral may be appropriate for some, but not for all. Most have the capacity to understand the permanence of death, though, depending on their age, it may be overwhelming to see parents and trusted adults in an emotional state. A general rule that may be helpful is that school-age youths may attend funerals unless they request not to. Disruptive youths should not be taken to funerals.

Reactions to the Unexpected Death of An 8-Year-Old Girl

After the rapid, unexpected death of an 8-year-old girl from a malignant brain tumor, the parents of her close friends noted their children reacted differently to the tragic event. They wondered if this was normal. The parents asked a psychiatrist to meet with their daughters' close group of friends to help. The meeting began with one of the parents introducing the psychiatrist to the group; after that, parents were asked to leave the room. There were five girls and three boys, all 8 years old. After they shared their names, they were told that they could remain seated or move around the room if they felt doing so would help. The psychiatrist invited the group to share any thoughts or feelings they had about the loss of their close friend. Much occurred during the 40-minute meeting. Some of the children remained seated and began to cry, stating it wasn't fair their friend had to die so young. Others turned their backs to the group and began to play video games—avoiding the affect in the room. The children were emotionally responding to the loss of their close friend in many ways, some overwhelmed and others creating distance from the emotional upheaval. One girl came up to the psychiatrist with an article that she had printed from the internet, stating angrily, "It says right here that the type of brain tumor she had is very rare. So why did she get it?" She was intellectualizing her fear and anger at such a painful event. Others said they were too sad to talk about it and would pray for her later that night, while others felt safe and talked about how good a friend she was, saying that she would always be remembered. The psychiatrist listened empathically and gave suggestions on how to manage their emotions (e.g., crying, writing, talking to a parent, drawing, singing, praying, etc.).

The parents were later brought in and were told about the importance of not imposing their feelings or views on what they thought their youth should feel. The parents were then given an assignment: to check in with their child throughout the week by asking, "Anything I can do?" and to support their child's requests.

Six of the children continued to do well and were open with their parents during check-ins, while two of the children were seen in individual grief psychotherapy for a few months after the meeting, after which they resumed healthy developmental progress.

Days later, the psychiatrist was asked to return for a second meeting with the group. Surprisingly, the meeting was to thank him for helping parents allow their children to process the death of their close friend "our way."

When helping a youth with the death of a loved one, it is important to remember that reactions can vary. In this case, some were overwhelmed and cried, others intellectualized and asked many questions, and some isolated their affect by playing video games. These youths appeared unaffected but were likely struggling internally. Therefore, it is best for clinicians and parents to use the Wait, Watch, and Wonder approach to help youths with their emotions, rather than pushing them to "talk about [their] feelings."

Limit-Setting in Elementary- and Middle-School-Aged Children

Elementary- and middle-school-aged youths will have periods of healthy turmoil, with occasional intense displays of anger. Setting fair and reasonable limits to these behaviors is an important task of parenting. However, limit-setting and consequences do not always lead to positive changes. Youths benefit in knowing, at their developmental level, the reasons for the limits set and the consequences given. Developmentally, it is to be expected that elementary-and middle-school-aged youths will explore newly acquired abilities by challenging boundaries if they feel their parent, friend, or teacher is treating them unfairly. Although these youths may be upset with certain boundaries, it is part of their learning process, and, if reasonable, they will learn to incorporate these boundaries into their daily lives.

Firm limit-setting with clear consequences can be effective if used sporadically in the context of a parent-youth relationship with good four pillars. Youths are less angered and more willing to accept limits if they were involved in the process of setting them before they are needed; doing so gives youths some ownership of the rules and makes them more invested in following them to get along with their parents. Conversely, if an authoritarian approach is used frequently, the youth will create emotional distance from the parent because of fear and mistrust. The parental attitude of "I am in charge" usually reveals an underlying mismatch of four pillars that requires attention.

- Limit-setting for children and adolescents should be developmentally appropriate and fair.
- Children and adolescents should have input about rules and consequences in advance. This prevents intense negative reactions when they are enforced.
- Following through with consequences is easier when they are agreed upon. For example, if a youth is late to school, it is reasonable to ask him or her to help his or her young sibling with homework. A youth who is late for curfew may be asked to run errands, etc.
- The practice of "grounding" (including blocking phone/internet use for several weeks) for maladaptive behaviors is not helpful when done in a punitive manner, for example, yelling or in anger. Rather, setting limits on maladaptive behaviors if there are no known weaknesses in the four pillars (Chap. 7) is best accomplished by giving clear and concise reasons why the parent is upset, and providing

a short-term consequence that has been agreed upon before. The consequences should be brief—one or two days. More is not better nor more effective, and can lead to mistrust, ignoring of parents, worsening behaviors, and depressive feelings. Positive behavior will reinforce changes: "Great job! I know it was hard, but you managed to stay away from your phone/social media/friends for two days."

- When setting limits or giving consequences, parents should emphasize that they will not withdraw their love based on behavior. Keep criticism specific to the behavior, and avoid making derogatory statements. This will help youths know that even when they make mistakes, limit-setting and consequences represent the parents' efforts to prevent them from further distress.
- Perform good role-modeling by listening to the youth's point of view. Youths are more likely to comply when they understand a rule's purpose. Some youths may request an explanation for the parent's decisions regarding a consequence. This allows a youth to voice his or her opinion, which, surprisingly, can often improve the way the parent is handling the situation.
- Avoid setting rules that youths can't follow. For example, youths with weak visual-spatial abilities or those with attention-deficit/hyperactivity disorder will have trouble maintaining an organized bedroom (although they often surprise parents by knowing where things are in a messy room)! Designating one day a week in which the parent can help the youth organize his or her room improves trust and avoids conflicts that create distance between them.
- Avoid ultimatums. They create more conflict and prevent parents from considering what may be at the root of the youth's distress and contributing to his or her emotional dysregulation.

Lying, Defiance, and Oppositional Behavior in Elementary- and Middle-School-Aged Youths

During the elementary and middle school years, most youths respond well to parents' caring but firm limit-setting. Most youths learn to develop adaptive patterns to get along with others, and can appreciate the benefits in complying with social norms. However, some of these youths begin to openly lie, and may demonstrate defiant and oppositional behaviors. The severity of these behaviors is largely related to the extent of the four pillar weaknesses present. Youths with severe forms of difficult/feisty temperament will lie about their contribution to problems when reprimanded. They can become defiant, argumentative, and dismissive of social norms, as they often do not have the moral compass needed to understand their contribution to the problem. This can be exacerbated at family reunions or in school settings because of the increased social skills needed.

Why Do Elementary- and Middle-School-Aged Youths Lie? Why Are they, at Times, Defiant and Oppositional?

When youths have weaknesses in the four pillars and executive functions, they are at risk for emotional or behavioral problems: persistent patterns of lying, acting out, self-defeating behavior, academic failure, substance abuse, and promiscuity.

Youths who are unable to recognize emotions in others [20], assume hostile intent from family, peers, or teachers [17, 18], and/or have cognitive weaknesses that lead to poor social problem-solving [18] are at risk for later antisocial behavior. Hill et al. [28] found that a lack of parental involvement in school during the middle school years predicted a youth's later maladjustment. Verbal abilities, as assessed by intelligence tests, have also been found to predict later antisocial behavior [42].

Parents or teachers may be tempted to "hold back" children who have not met benchmarks, but it should be noted that kindergarten and early grade retention has long-term detrimental effects on behavior outcomes, despite temporary academic benefits [29]. Dodge et al. [17] found that the experience of social rejection by peers leads to growth in antisocial behavior across elementary school. Additionally, academic failure, indexed by grade retention, placement into special education, and failing test scores, represents another predictor of antisocial outcomes when due to cognitive weaknesses and living with family significant household conflict. Low levels of academic competence are associated with high levels of internalizing problems in middle childhood, and with high levels of externalizing problems during the transition from elementary school to middle school [44].

Parenting Principles for High-School-Aged Youths 14 to 18 Years of Age (Adolescence)

Adolescence is a developmental period that commences with the onset of puberty and artificially ends with adulthood and the ability to function independently within the context of one's environment and culture. The adolescent's primary developmental task is to successfully regulate shifts in the affective states of self and others in order to develop the capacity for intimate and stable interpersonal relationships (Fig. 8.3). During adolescence, healthy individuals develop increased capacity to attend selectively, to discern important information, and to control their behavior. This period of growth is marked by an increased ability to read social and emotional cues and an increased appreciation and dependence on interpersonal relationships [27].

Many think that adolescence is a period during which the quality of parent-adolescent interactions can be relatively stressed and conflictual. However, only approximately 5–15% of adolescents experience extremely conflictual relationships with their parents [11, 53, 54]. Thus, adolescence is not nearly as tumultuous as it may appear to be, with more that 80% of adolescents having high-quality

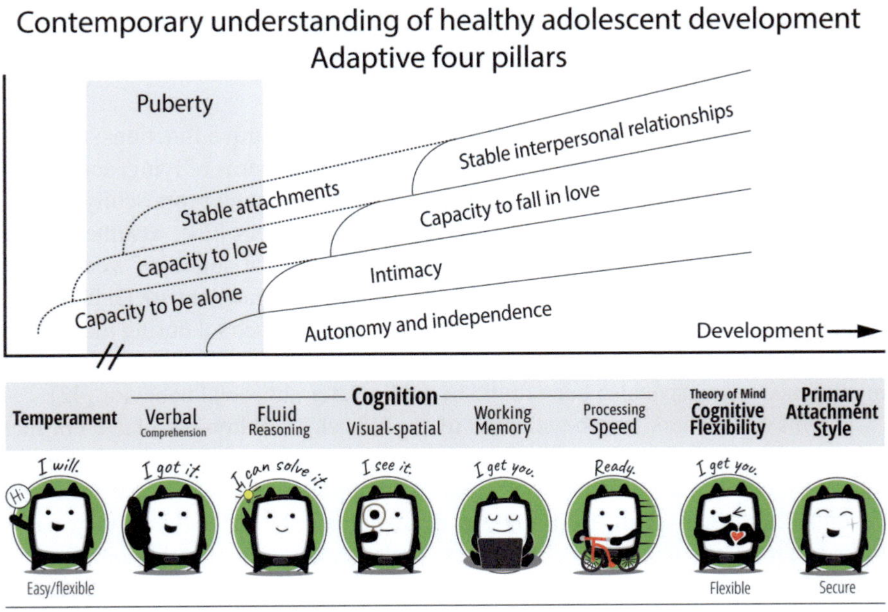

Fig. 8.3 Contemporary understanding of healthy adolescent development. (Adapted from [63])

socioemotional functioning [19]. Thus, the presence of 15% of adolescents with behavioral and emotional problems is consistent with the percentage of adolescents with four pillar temperamental and cognitive weaknesses [16]. Importantly, many adolescents with disease-based psychiatric diagnoses respond well to treatment interventions, and return to higher emotional and behavioral functioning unless they have weaknesses in their four pillars.

Research has suggested that cognitive development through the adolescent years is associated with progressively greater efficiency of executive control capacities, paralleled by increased activity within focal prefrontal regions [55]. Furthermore, with increasing age, prefrontal activity becomes more focal and specialized, while irrelevant and diffuse activity in this region is reduced. For example, imaging studies of adolescent brains confirm aspects of fluidity in decision-making and a number of other cognitive capacities [23, 24]. Gogtay explains that, during adolescence, the area of the brain responsible for organization, planning, and strategizing is not fully developed, as gray matter continues to thicken (Fig. 8.4). Additional imaging evidence in the affective domain suggests that the development of prefrontal modulation over emotional processing continues to develop throughout the adolescent years and into early adulthood [62] (Table 8.10).

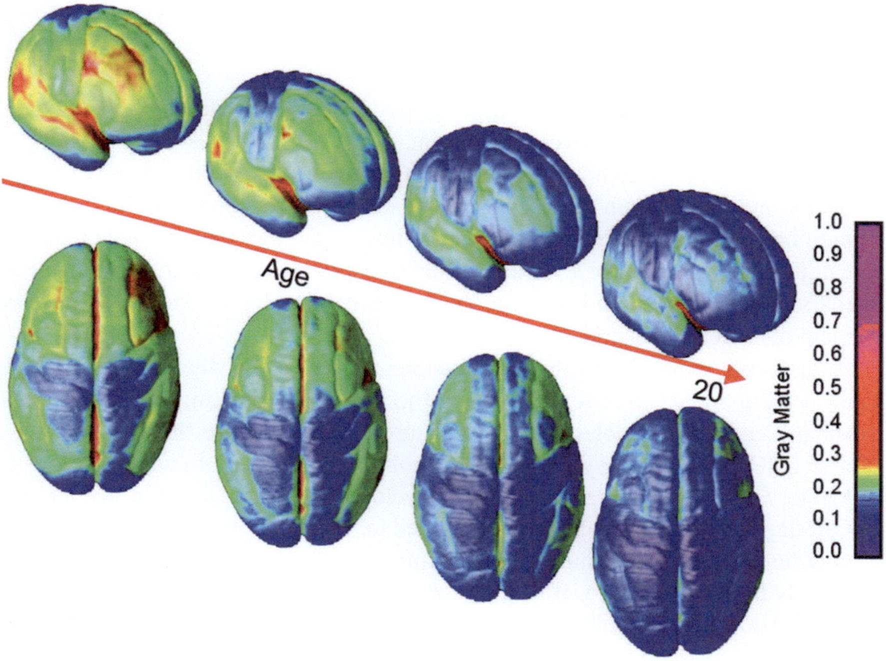

Fig. 8.4 Gray matter density significantly varies as a function of development, with latter maturation occurring in the prefrontal cortex in late adolescence [24]

How Can Parents Promote Independence?

Promoting independence in adolescents is essential to helping them establish their own identity, which changes over time. Parents may feel rejected by an adolescent's newfound independence, as he or she starts turning away from his or her parents and relying more and more on friends, teachers, and coaches.

- Parents should not step in and solve an adolescent's problems. Give him or her space to experience a wide range of emotions without feeling the urge to help him or her be happy. Rather, empathize with how hard it is to deal with what he or she is going through.
- Make time to listen to without interruptions.
- The phrase "Catch them being good" is also helpful with adolescents, who benefit from compliments and support of their accomplishments.
- When an adolescent demonstrates responsibility, he or she should be granted more freedom and privileges.
- Allow adolescents to have friends to their home and in a space that will allow for some privacy from parents. Plan, by age, how long they should be alone before checking in (providing food and/or beverages) as this provides an opportunity to learn about possible relational problems emerging with friends.

- There will be occasions when parents should compromise on preferences (e.g., clothing, hair style, music, foods, etc.) In general, this is best done regarding things that are not permanent.
- Encourage and help adolescents find employment, which teaches life skills, prevents boredom, and improves self-esteem.
- Adolescent eating habits are influenced by many factors: culture, family dietary habits, and more. When adolescents have eating problems due to difficulties with their body image, it is best to have their primary care physician provide the education necessary to make good dietary decisions. The primary care physician can reassure parents if these issues are due to normal developmental issues, or alert them of a need for treatment.
- Adolescents should know that their parents need to know where they are when away from home and have them call to check in during evening outings. Parents should remind their adolescent that they support them and that their safety comes first; a "Call us anytime you need help" policy is a good one to have.
- Mastery of driving is an important developmental task for this age group. Offering driving classes or having a trusted family member teach the adolescent may be more effective than parents taking on the task, because it prevents the anxiety both parties have. If that isn't possible, remember to allow for mistakes without devaluing or embarrassing him or her. Teach him or her to drive in heavy rain, snow, and ice in empty parking lots.
- Adolescents find it distressing when parents have long lists of questions: "How was the concert? How was the date? Who was there?" Rather, limit queries to one general question: "Anything you would like to share?"
- Parents should not strive to be their adolescent's friend. This is not a parent's job, and jeopardizes efficacy when the adolescent needs guidance or limit-setting.

Talking to adolescents about sexuality before they begin high school is important. Parents who find this difficult should ask another family member who is up to the task. Adolescents need accurate information, not value judgments. The conversation should review the risks involved in using drugs, sexual activity, risk-taking behaviors, and more. These conversations are important to adolescents even if they roll their eyes, seem uninterested or state they "already know." They are listening!

Table 8.10 Growth-Promoting Tasks for Adolescents 13 to 18 Years of Age

Role-modeling
Being a healthy role model is critical to helping adolescents maintain good moral character and healthy social norms
Parents should find enjoyable one-on-one or family time with their adolescent to share personal successes and failures during their own adolescence. This encourages communication and teaches adolescents that mistakes will be made and that the parent will understand
Consider occasionally working in the same space the adolescent uses (working on a project, reading a book, etc.) doing so may lead to a conversation about the adolescent's interests
Have meals as a family with the intent of sharing positive stories; doing so has been known to improve family relationships. At times, the adolescent may sit and participate, even if he or she has plans to eat with friends later
Preparing meals or getting things ready for upcoming activities together with adolescents is a great teaching tool and allows for openness in dialogue
When sharing important information of serious nature, share its purpose and ask for the adolescent's attention before you speak with him or her
When the adolescent wishes to share his or her thoughts and feelings, parents should be encouraged to model listening by providing a DEAR moment (described above) even if busy
Parents should not use a sarcastic, demeaning, or disrespectful tone directed at the adolescent
Do not embarrass the adolescent or instill a sense of shame (e.g., "your hair looks bad," "people are going to make fun of you for that," "I bet you are in love," etc.) as he or she will take a defensive position, creating distance and mistrust
Parents should not share personal problems that may negatively affect their youth
Adolescents have many life experiences, and the death of a loved one is not uncommon. Their reactions can vary. By this age, they are more articulate as to what they need from their parents and friends. Some adolescents will use denial to cope with death, while others may become involved in altruistic activities to honor the loved one. A general rule is to allow adolescents to attend funerals unless they request not to

Parenting the Adolescent as he or she Begins to Date

Dating in adolescence, or having a girlfriend or boyfriend, can boost the adolescent's confidence if the relationship is characterized by intimacy and good communication. Manning et al. [38] estimate adolescent dating to occur among 95 percent of that population. They conclude that adolescent dating and sexual relationships are fluid: having several sexual partners, or having a relationship that is not sexually exclusive. Moreover, youths value the support, trust, and closeness they experience in romantic relationships. Adolescents learn to confide in their partners about conflicts with their parents and peers. Adolescents use their romantic partner as a rehearsal for an adult intimate relationship and find value in spending time doing activities they both enjoy, in addition to discussing cultural and societal challenges, etc. While adolescent romantic relationships can support sexual development, not all do. Dating should not be confused with their sexual activity.

Another important aspect of dating during adolescence is the inevitable breakup. Developmentally, the breakup serves as a template for how to manage the loss of a loved one due to differences in beliefs and values. For youths, the breakup is a brief period of mourning, with some reflection on what may have been lost, with subsequent recovery and motivation to engage in another romantic relationship. Without a doubt, an adolescent's choice of romantic partner will be influenced by his or her four pillars.

As we stated in Chap. 6, youths with personality disorders will seek others who have similar beliefs and values, with the same high levels of instability (defying authority, demanding full attention from partner, etc.) Unfortunately, youths with deficits in cognitive flexibility form romantic relationships characterized by a lack of trust and constant conflict, which can ultimately lead to dating violence. Further, preteen dating often occurs in youths who come from families that are struggling and are at high risk for sexual trauma.

Setting Limits with Adolescents

Setting fair and reasonable limits is an important part of parenting adolescents. Limit-setting and consequences do not always lead to immediate positive changes although promotes change if youths benefit know, at the appropriate developmental level, a parent's reasoning behind limit-setting or consequences. Developmentally, it is normal for adolescents to challenge some limits in order to determine the boundaries. When they find a parent, friend, or teacher to be trustworthy, they will learn to incorporate these boundaries into their daily life.

- Limit-setting for adolescents should be fair.
- Adolescents should have input about rules and consequences in advance. This prevents intense negative reactions when they are enforced.
- Helping an adolescent follow through with agreed-upon consequences encourages him or her to know he or she can rely on his or her parents to help him or her from engaging in self-defeating actions. For example, restricting the use of a car after an adolescent breaks curfew can help him or her avoid telling peers that he or she does not feel comfortable with their increasing risk-taking behaviors.
- If an adolescent is late to school, ask him or her to help a younger sibling with homework; if late for curfew, asking him or her to run errands, etc.
- The practice of "grounding" adolescents for maladaptive behaviors is not helpful when done in a punitive manner (when accompanied by yelling or anger) nor is restricting smartphone use or socializing for several weeks. Rather, consequences should be brief—one or two days. More is not better nor more effective, and can lead to mistrust, ignoring of parents, increased acting-out behaviors, and depressive feelings.
- Reinforce positive behavior: "Great job! You managed to stay away from your phone/social media/friends/etc. for two days. I can imagine how difficult that must have been for you."
- When setting limits or giving consequences, parents must emphasize they will not withdraw love based on an adolescent's behavior. This will help him or her know that even when he or she makes mistakes, limit-setting and consequences represent the parent's efforts to prevent him or her from further distress.

- Perform good role-modeling by listening to a youth's point of view. Youths are more likely to comply if they understand the rules. Further, this allows a youth to voice his or her opinion, which, surprisingly, can often improve the way the parent handles the situation.
- Avoid setting rules that an adolescent cannot follow. Adolescents with weaknesses in verbal comprehension will be less likely to recall instructions given by parents (call your brother today, bring your clothes to the laundry room tomorrow, etc.) Sending information by text or having tasks in visual form in the home increases follow-through.

Lying, Defiance, and Oppositional Behavior in Adolescents

When adolescents routinely lie and become defiant, the severity of these behaviors is largely related to the extent of the four pillar weaknesses they may have. Like in younger age groups, adolescents with severe forms of difficult/feisty temperament or cognitive weaknesses will lie about their contribution to problems and can become defiant and argumentative when they are noted to violate social norms. This happens because they often do not possess the moral compass needed to understand the negative consequences of their maladaptive and risk-taking behaviors. This can be exacerbated by interpersonal conflict that results from a lack of adequate social skills.

Failure to supervise behavior and lack of engagement with an adolescent's schooling has been associated with antisocial outcomes [8]. Adolescents who reside in social areas of instability at risk for violence and become involved with peers that promote violating social norms are at higher risk for antisocial behaviors [28, 39, 50].

I Am a Good Parent, but this Week, I Am Exasperated with my Teenager!

We are all susceptible to fluctuations in our health (e.g., glucose, dietary, or sleep changes). These changes, as well as unexpected situations with family, school, or work, can tax us emotionally and lead to a disequilibrium on how we handle day-to-day matters. Youths and parents alike will have bad days that may lead to poor decisions or acting in a disruptive manner.

It is not surprising that when a youth has a bad, out-of-character day or week, it can disrupt the family system. Understandably, parents have difficulties when their youths unexpectedly become disruptive despite efforts to help them. It is important to help parents take a broad perspective to decipher if things are truly worrisome, or if the changes they're seeing are part and parcel of daily life in the developmental scaffolding of adolescence.

Occasionally, adolescents have bad days that lead to conflicts with their parents. Despite their desire to understand and solve things, parents need to be careful not to escalate their child's distress by asking questions in a rapid-fire way, hoping to gain insight. When an adolescent is frustrated, upset, or angry, the last thing he or she wants to hear is a barrage of comments or questions ("What is wrong?", "Why are you so mad?", "It looks like you are in a bad mood," etc.) Even though a parent may be asking out of concern and love, the *felt experience* by the youth is that of being pushed to talk about feelings, or being criticized. He or she might then resort to disruptive behaviors to create distance from the angry parent. Conversely, the parent feels dismissed for trying to help. Adolescents are not adults. They require parents to model how to manage and regulate their emotions when the *felt* experience is that the parent is being critical, confirming that they are defective and not lovable.

Under the best circumstances (good four pillars in both the youth and parent), with time and space, the family dynamic will return to its typical, healthy status, and both parties will be able to reflect about their experiences. The adolescent may say, "I know you were trying to help me." The parent may reflect, "I didn't give you time to adjust." From there, they can resume their normal healthy interactions.

Additionally, it is important that parents consider that out-of-character changes in a youth can be due to medication changes of his or her medical or psychiatric conditions. This information is crucial to share with the youth's physician.

The family dynamic may also be thrown off by a parent's behavior. Parents under stress from a work or family issue may become critical of their youth for minor issues. Often, a youth reacts to this out-of-character behavior by unknowingly becoming dysregulated due to the anxieties his or her unhappy or angry parent elicits.

Section II

Parenting Myths

This section provides a brief review of traditional parenting wisdom passed down through the generations, often viewed as bedrock. But just like the old adage that instructs us to avoid swimming after eating, many of these parenting "truths" are actually the opposite—myths. We posit that these myths need to be revised because (1) they do not capture the developmental complexities of youths and (2) and are based on unrealistic assumptions that can be detrimental to the emotional and behavioral success of children and adolescents.

You Must Obey Me Because I Am Your Parent

For decades, clinicians have suggested parents use limit-setting techniques outlined in popular books that mostly encourage reinforcing parental authority, or "a benign dictatorship," wherein parents are the judge and jury and have the final say [51].

Parents are surprised when, after diligently following the advice given by the clinician, this approach proves unsuccessful. They feel frustrated when their youth begins to mistrust them. "Why doesn't it work for my child?" they ask in dismay. "When my parents set limits, I obeyed them." Or, "I wouldn't have been allowed to do what my child is doing." These are all-too-familiar comments made by parents of difficult youths. Educating parents on how to develop effective parenting strategies to prevent maladaptive and oppositional behaviors in youths is a difficult endeavor.

Helping parents shift their parenting style from a paternalistic, authoritarian approach to a more supportive and growth-promoting approach can be difficult and counterintuitive. However, avoiding in-the-moment "I am in charge; you must obey" conflicts, which are the norm for most families, can greatly improve a youth's relationships with his or her parents. Ultimately, the goal is to teach youths to learn self-regulating and growth-promoting, adaptive skills while not losing trust in their parents' support and concern.

To improve parenting, the clinician must assess the underlying four pillar weaknesses in youth and parents to develop a course of action tailored to their strengths, with attention to their deficits.

We contrast parents with two different styles as they manage two different scenarios (Tables 8.11 and 8.12).

These cases are often familiar to clinicians. The authoritarian style can have significant negative consequences when youths with weaknesses in their four pillars are unable to meet the parent's expectations. This will increase their sense of being a failure and place them at risk for emotional or behavioral problems: persistent patterns of lying, acting out, self-defeating behavior, academic failure, substance abuse, and promiscuity.

Table 8.11 Parents with two different styles managing an 8-year-old boy with incomplete school assignments

Authoritarian style	Flexible style
You need to be responsible. You will be grounded to your room for two weeks without access to a TV, computer, or phone	What consequences do you think are reasonable for missing two assignments? [or] your consequence is to unload the dishwasher every day this week

Table 8.12 Parents with two different styles help a 15-year-old girl remember to take her morning medication

Authoritarian style	Flexible style
You are an adolescent, and I want you to take responsibility for taking your ADHD medication every morning and after school. I will not be checking, so if you forget the medication, you will have to face the consequences	You are an adolescent and I want you to learn why it is important to take your ADHD medication every morning and after school. I will be checking the pill holder; if you forget, I will let you know. If you take the medication regularly without reminders, you will earn more free time on weekends

My Parents Used Time-Outs, so they Must Work

We encourage the reader to help parents develop useful interventions to help children self-regulate. We encourage them to avoid approaching the child with a demanding and anxiety-producing limit-setting attitude. We teach parents that the goal of a time-out is for the child to be successful in self-regulating. A time-out should not be intended as punishment, which implicitly leads to further battles down the road. During a time-out, the child needs help from the parent to self-regulate, which seldom happens. We are sure the reader has read or heard of time-outs being extended—by adding 5,10,15, or more minutes—when the child is unable to calm down and self-regulate (AAP 2018; [51]). When a time-out is not completed and both parties become upset, the conflict that ensues reinforces its futility. The parent subjectively feels the need to win the "battle" and uses an angry tone of voice that reinforces their parental authority, which unfortunately models to the child what to do at a later time when he or she is angry at his or her parents.

We have found that brief (30–45 second) time-outs work best, to help the child learn how to settle and calm down. Upon completion of the time-out, the parent will benefit from saying "good job." At the end of the time-out, both child and parent will have stored in their memory how to self-regulate. Regardless of the youth's age, parents should keep in mind that not all youths will be able to settle down, depending on deficits in their four pillars, and may want to consider helping him or her learn how to regulate when distressed (Fig. 8.5).

As an example, a colleague recently shared with us that, after uncharacteristically cursing while driving and being visibly upset, her 3.5-year-old daughter said, "Mommy needs a time-out." The young child had stored in memory what was helpful to self-regulate and conveyed it in a playful manner to her mother.

Children with high levels of maladaptive behaviors due to deficits in their four pillars may remain unaffected by time-outs and other forms of appropriate limit-setting. They lack the skills to suspend reward-driven behavior and may respond with escalating anger and revenge. Suggested interventions for this population are reviewed in detail in Chap. 7.

If You Tell the Truth, You Will Not be in Trouble

Parents have an important role in helping children learn to be honest. Parents model a good moral compass that is internalized by the child. Many parents reinforce this by telling their children that by telling the truth they will be rewarded; or, if they broke a rule, they will be in less trouble than if they do not tell the truth. The problem with this approach is that parents, mostly unknowingly, fail to understand that children notice that parents themselves do not always tell the truth.

Some examples of when parents do not tell the truth.

- A parent tells an older youth not to tell her younger brother about the new goldfish or pet replacing the one that the child does not know has died.

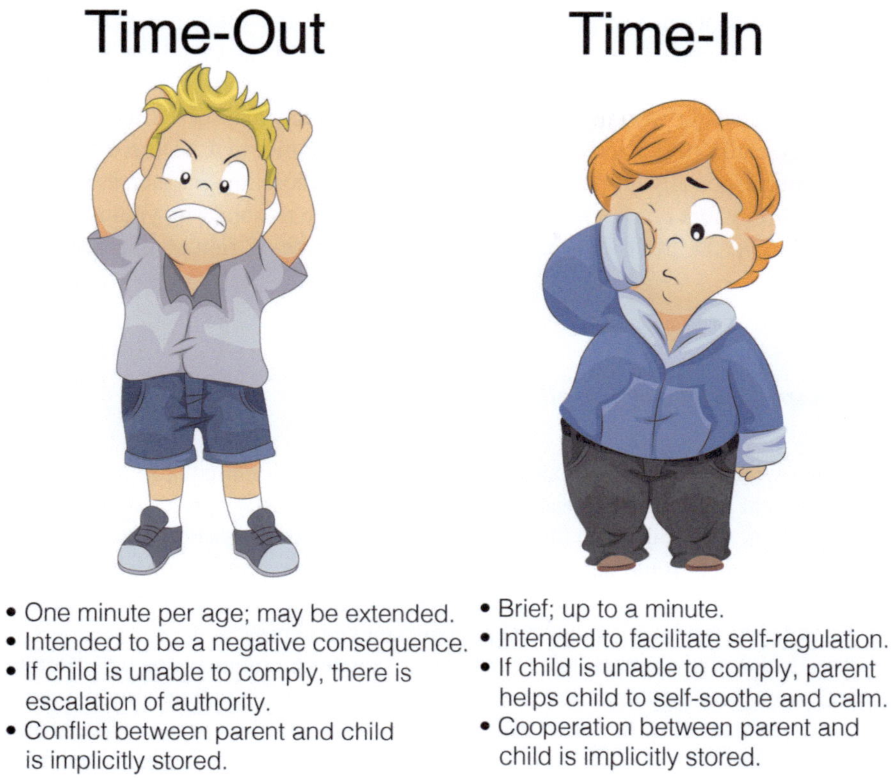
Time-Out
Time-In
• One minute per age; may be extended.
• Intended to be a negative consequence.
• If child is unable to comply, there is escalation of authority.
• Conflict between parent and child is implicitly stored.
• Brief; up to a minute.
• Intended to facilitate self-regulation.
• If child is unable to comply, parent helps child to self-soothe and calm.
• Cooperation between parent and child is implicitly stored.

Fig. 8.5 Time-out. This original figure was created with Canva.com under a one design use license commercial agreement

- A parent asks a child to say the parent is not home or available in order to avoid someone at the door or on the phone.
- Parents ask children to quietly follow them and skip ahead of a long line in an amusement park.
- A parent shares openly with the family that he or she is calling in sick from work to participate in an activity with friends.

Occasionally, there are times when youths choose to not tell the truth for altruistic reasons learned from parents and friends [61]. We are not adding judgment; rather, we aim to give a reminder regarding the importance understanding the context of social situations.

Some examples of when youths do not tell the truth for altruistic reasons.

- A youth lies to peers to protect a child that is frequently bullied, saying, “He or she is my friend; leave him or her alone.”
- An adolescent says he or she is not hungry, knowing about her grandmother’s financial struggles and limited food availability.
- A youth tells his or her uncle that he or she very much likes his birthday present, even though it may be for a younger child, knowing about the hardships his or her uncle is experiencing.
- A youth confides to his parents about a surprise party for his or her sister.

It is different when a youth repeatedly engage in lies that affect others in a negative way, for example, stealing something and saying he or she found the item in the street; calling and telling parents he or she is in a different place, etc. Further, youths with weaknesses in working memory or fluid reasoning may be telling the truth when they claim to not remember the details of a conflict that occurred hours or days earlier, especially if they found the incident overwhelming. Further, as we have outlined throughout this book, equally important are the reasons why youths may be afraid to share the truth with parents (e.g., a fear of being ridiculed, shamed, or devalued).

The Same Rules Go for all Siblings

Received wisdom states that parents love all of their children equally and use the same parental approach with each child. Although we mostly agree with this common wisdom, we remind the clinician that parental successes and frustrations are dependent on their youth being able to respond to the parenting approach used. We would add that "loving children equally" means understanding each child's unique biological, psychological, and social strengths and weaknesses.

A colleague had a first child who was very easy during infancy; she was often in a good mood, was easy to soothe, and slept well. When their daughter turned 3 years old, she had met all of her developmental milestones and was very well-behaved, which they believed was due to their good parenting style. Our colleague initially believed that most children could do as well if they were raised by good parents. Knowing we would disagree with this all-encompassing belief, our colleague suggested that our approaches were perhaps flawed: "Your approach has parents giving in to their child's tantrums too easily." As life would have it, our colleague had a second daughter with difficulties with mood regulation, who was difficult to soothe and struggled sleeping. By age 2, she had begun to have difficulties getting along with her sister, which made her sister feel bad. She had also begun to hit her parents when told "no." Initially, our colleague felt she and her husband had become too lax in their parenting, but quickly realized they had not changed their approach. They were able to appreciate that their approach with their first child was not a "good fit" for their second child. Our colleague has learned how temperamental differences in children can influence the parents' approach toward them (and no, we did not say "We told you so.").

Although many parents intuitively and seamlessly shift their parenting style to the specific needs of each child, other parents find this shift "too complicated; I can't always remember to parent in different ways." This reaction should alert clinicians to the possibility of a parent's four pillar weaknesses in temperament and perhaps working memory, or executive function deficits. Herein, the interventions suggested by the clinician will need to be understood and rehearsed by the parent during the appointment, so that they can be stored in the parent's implicit memory and later used at home. Occasionally, a psychiatrist will need to refer a family to an experienced family therapist to address parenting issues and work collaboratively.

Parenting children and adolescents must be based on the children's unique characteristics. In helping parents understand the need for different approaches with different children, we, at times, use an example of a family with three children. The parents have a 4-year-old boy and a 12-year-old girl who are thoughtful, compliant, and "easy to parent." These children complete their homework and chores without needing to be reminded. Their middle child, a 7-year-old boy with diabetes mellitus type 1 and attention-deficit/hyperactivity disorder (ADHD), predominantly hyperactive presentation, can be impulsive, careless, and demanding. When his glucose is stable and he has been taking his ADHD medication, he frequently completes his homework and chores mostly without reminders. If his glucose levels are not well-managed or his ADHD medication has worn off, he doesn't seem to care about earning rewards for good behavior and requires frequent redirection to remain focused on tasks.

This example allows clinicians to illustrate how the needs of one child can significantly differ from another—even within the same family. In the case of the 7-year-old boy visiting other family members, the visits need to be carefully monitored, with attention paid to his glucose as well as the "wearing-off" of his ADHD medication, which may cause or affect conflicts with others. Additionally, helping the family involves explaining to the other siblings why the parents' approach might seem discrepant. The biologic underpinnings of a youth influences his or her emotional and self-regulating abilities; these abilities are often different among siblings.

Appointment with a Parent with Good Four Pillars

Clinician: Can you please let Mary [*slow-to-warm-up child*] know she can play with the toys any time she feels ready? [*Toys are openly available in the office.*]

Parent: Sure. Mary, take your time; play with the toy you like when you are ready.

Clinician: Jeff (older child) prefers to talk with adults, although likes to play with his friends. You probably need to be firm in asking him to leave the adults alone and play with his friends. Mary probably gets nervous when you are firm with her because she is anxious playing with friends, and then worries you are mad at her. [*Mary smiles and nods in agreement.*]

Parent: So true. They are different. I guess that explains why Mary cries when I am in a rush and firmly pressure her to quickly get ready. She thinks I'm mad at her. Jeff would get ready just because he wants to talk my head off.

Clinician: I'm glad you appreciate that Mary needs a bit more time than Jeff. Even if you remember this three out five times, you are helping your children [*Supportive comment*].

Parent: Got it. I can't be the perfect parent all the time [*Accepts the suggestion and engages with humor*].

Appointment with a Parent with Weaknesses in his or her Four Pillars

Clinician: Can you please let Mary (slow-to-warm-up child) know she can play with the toys any time she feels ready? [*Toys are openly available in the office.*]

Parent: Why? She needs to learn that if she wants something, she needs to speak up. I do not want to baby her. Mary, go ahead and play with the toys.

Clinician: Is there anyone in your family that is shy and nervous like Mary?

Parent: No.

Clinician: Children that are shy and nervous like Mary usually have a genetic predisposition for this. Just like children who are genetically very good at sports. Parents can help them by adjusting their parenting style to the child's personality. Do you have any siblings?

Parent: Yes, the three of us all are different, and our parents raised us the same way. We turned out okay, except for my sister. She doesn't get along with anybody, but that was her fault; she was always difficult.

Clinician: I understand. It must be difficult to know that Mary is different from her brother and that they need you to parent them with different styles. It would be like parenting one child with diabetes that needs more help understanding how to use the medication, and another child without diabetes that is more independent. Does that make sense? [*Mary smiles and nods in agreement.*]

Parent: I disagree. Children need to be treated the same way so they can learn from the consequences if they do not obey me. We came here to see if you can prescribe medication to help her stop being so quiet and nervous.

Clinicians working with parents with weaknesses in the four pillars may find themselves understanding how the child feels around their parent. Mary's parent is not able to adapt to her needs. In these situations, by identifying the weaknesses in the parents as contributors to distress in the child, the clinician can modify the approach so that it can be useful to the parent.

It is important that clinicians consider that a youth's anxiety may be due to his or her parents' weaknesses, and to suggest family therapy, as a youth with this form of anxiety may not benefit from medication.

Parents Must Provide Structure at Home

The concept of providing structure for children and adolescents at home erroneously assumes that because structure at school helps a youth, a lack of sufficient structure at home explains why they are not doing well at home. Youths with good four pillars, who have the ability to incorporate informal parental and family structure in their daily routine, greatly benefit from it. However, for youths with weaknesses in the four pillars, attempts to enforce structure can be detrimental. Youths with cognitive weaknesses may perform better at school not necessarily because of the school structure alone; rather, it is because they learn to follow other students who follow the school structure. In teaching our colleagues, we share that youths with four pillar weaknesses rely on others to know what to do. As with a school of fish, youths learn by watching other students do (e.g., what book is needed for class, when to turn in assignments, when class is over). As a result, when these youths arrive home, many are not able to follow "home structure," since they do not have others to guide them on sequencing actions. This is particularly evident in youths with weaknesses in visual-spatial, fluid reasoning, and working memory. They may become argumentative and defy structures imposed because they do not have the ability to recall the reasons for it, nor the benefits of following it. As described in Chap. 7, youths with cognitive weaknesses require tailored interventions according to their needs in order to help them be successful.

Chelsea

Chelsea, a 12-year-old-girl, began to have problems with anxiety. A trial of selective serotonin reuptake inhibitor (SSRI) at therapeutic doses was minimally helpful. Her parents shared, "At home, she gets overwhelmed with anxiety, and doesn't get anything done." The psychiatrist inquired about what happened before Chelsea became overwhelmed. Her mother responded, "After school, we ask her to complete her homework, then play for 40 minutes, and then clean her room, because it is always messy. We find spoons, socks, and books shoved under her bed all the time." Her parents implemented a token system for Chelsea to earn rewards if she completed her chores. Chelsea, however, was not willing to follow the token system. The reason behind her refusal, we learned, was that she had trouble understanding the delayed rewards of the token system as a result of very low fluid reasoning. This surprised her parents. Chelsea's brother, who had attention-deficit/hyperactivity disorder, predominately hyperactive, did very well with the token system and structure. They added, "Chelsea does better than her brother at school. Why can't she follow the structure at home? If she spills a drink, she doesn't know what to do … she just walks away. She can't use her anxiety to hide from the world."

Chelsea's WISC-V revealed very low fluid reasoning and processing speed, with low average working memory. These weaknesses help us to understand the reason her struggles had increased with age, as the tasks required of her became more complex. In short, following home structure was difficult for Chelsea. Her psychiatrist suggested interventions for Chelsea from Chap. 7 that helped her understand that she would have more freedom and privileges by completing tasks, and that she could ask for help from her parents if she felt overwhelmed.

That's Not True; You Don't Feel That Way

Children learn early on that their parents are the best source to seek help from when a physical or emotional obstacle occurs in their life. In these situations, youths are open about why they feel overwhelmed, and are asking for help. Parents, however, struggle seeing their child in distress, and at times unknowingly interfere with their child's ability to learn how to cope with difficult experiences by "fixing" their youth's problem. Further, a parent can unwittingly fail to validate his or her youth's feelings by denying them: "That is not true. You are not a failure; you are smart." Or parents may state that the youth is not feeling the way she says she is: "No, you don't feel/depressed/mad/angry/ disappointed/etc." This response does not allow the youth to feel that her distress is important (Table 8.13).

Listening to the reasons for a youth's feelings and validating those feelings is important in helping a youth to implicitly acquire adaptive skills for future mishaps. Parents are often surprised at the many (often very reasonable) solutions that youths can develop if listened to and given time.

Table 8.13 "You Don't Feel That Way"

Youth obstacle and comment	Parents want to "fix" the problem	Using a Wait, Watch, and Wonder approach
His best friend says they are no longer friends Youth says, "nobody likes me"	"That is not true." [implying the youth is lying] "I am sure he or she still likes you. I am going to talk to his or her parents to help you"	Wait a few minutes and watch the youth's reaction; then, wonder aloud with the child how to help him or her Listen to his or her ideas about possible solutions
A youth is not chosen by his or her team coach to be a starting player "The coach thinks I am a terrible player"	"That is not true." [implying the youth is lying] "I know you are a very good player." [without knowing his or her abilities in the context of other team players]	Use a wait, watch, and wonder approach. Wonder what his or her thoughts are about not being a starting player He or she may need reassurance if his or her expectation is not commensurate with his or her abilities and experience
A youth gets a low grade on a school exam. "I am a stupid student"	"You are not stupid; you are a very smart student"	There are many reasons for a low grade. It is important to assess whether it is an isolated event, or whether the youth has true difficulties in understanding the subject material It is not helpful to tell the child that he or she is smart, as it may create unrealistic expectations. It may be better to compliment her dedication and work ethics

You're Intentionally Making Me Mad

When weaknesses in their four pillars prevent youths from managing stressful and difficult situations, they may react angrily toward others even as they implicitly hope for guidance. This represents a frequent misunderstanding between youths and their parents. For decades, difficult youths were erroneously credited for knowing how to push their parents' buttons. Comments such as "They know what they're doing" and "They're attention seeking" were frequently used to describe youths in these situations.

Moreover, popular parent media sources negatively portray youths with difficulties following social norms. In these media, it is assumed that youths use negative behaviors to intentionally manipulate parents (e.g., their lies become more sophisticated, they emotionally blackmail their parents, etc.). Further, the interventions suggested to parents in these sources often rely on one-size-fits-all approaches, asserting that a nonnegotiable, authoritarian approach will lead to improvement. This is unfortunate, because youths who resort to these behaviors ultimately prevent them from being able to get what they are hoping for or need (see "The Demanding Youth" and "Storm Chaser," Chap. 4).

In contrast, youths with good four pillars can often get what they want by mostly avoiding conflict with others, and actually enjoy seeing their parents be happy with them.

The Helicopter (DRONE) Parent (Fig. 8.6)

All parents have moments of intense vigilance. We intervened to retrieve our child's toy from another toddler who snatched it away, hovered over our child the first time they climbed a slide, waited for the school bus every first day of school, gave safety tips ad nauseam the first time they drove alone, lectured them before prom, etc.

The parent becomes a hypervigilant helicopter/drone parent when this behavior is persistent and detrimental to the youth's psychological and social development. Parents can be warm and loving and simultaneously overinvolved, intrusive, enmeshed, controlling; in these cases, they interfere in their youth's emotional and psychological autonomy [36, 60]. Helicopter/drone parents have strict expectations about their youth's behaviors, which prevent youths from establishing healthy boundaries with their parents. Accumulating evidence indicates that helicopter/drone parenting has detrimental effects for youths [43, 49]. Teaching youths independence is helpful in allowing them to develop healthy problem-solving skills and mastering self-regulation (Table 8.14).

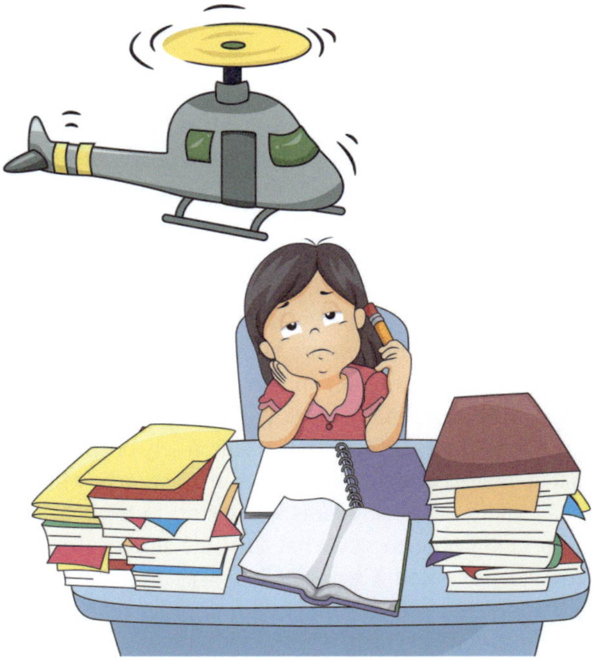

Fig. 8.6 Helicopter parent hovers over youth. This original figure was created with Canva.com under a one design use license commercial agreement

Table 8.14 Examples of helicopter/drone parent

Activity	Helicopter/Drone parent
Dressing	Chooses the child's clothes during preschool and elementary school years Helps child put on clothes when not needing help
Chores	Avoids giving their child chores; keeps their youth's room clean and tidy
Relationships with friends	Does not allow child to visit friends or play outdoors, for fear he will be hurt
	Solves child's minor arguments with friends by calling the friend's parents to work out the problem
	Sends frequent check-in texts when child is playing at a friend's home
Homework	Helps complete homework; takes over projects or tasks because they "need to be done right"
Extracurricular activities	Enrolls child in extracurricular activities and directs teachers or coaches on how their child should be treated

When Is Looking over a Youth's Shoulder Helpful?

The answer is "it depends." It is not helpful when a parent stifles a youth's psychological and social development. However, if a parent looks over a youth's shoulder to support him or her in a case of cognitive or language deficits and limited cognitive flexibility, it may be exactly what the youth needs. This sort of support should not be overbearing.

Special Situation: COVID-19

During the COVID-19 pandemic, many parents became hypervigilant because their youth had emotional and social needs beyond the safety precautions of wearing masks, frequent hand-washing, physical distancing, and limited access to older family members. Parents had to create new and complex virtual learning environments; many struggled to facilitate their children's learning and to monitor isolation, sadness, and relationships with peers. Further, limited social interaction with same age peers during the pandemic had negative effects, including increased anxiety and stress, boredom, low self-esteem, and more [1, 13].

Many parents did provide adequate support for their youth, although some—who were overly intrusive prior to the pandemic—had even more negative impacts on their children during the pandemic. For some of these youths, attending school in person prior to the pandemic created distance from their helicopter/drone parents. However, during the pandemic, some youths reported greater stress as parents sat beside them during virtual classes, continuously checked in on their assignments, interrupted classes by asking the teacher questions, and more. It will be important for clinicians to consider asking youths that experienced the COVID-19 pandemic about their educational experience, as this may reflect family dynamics that are directly related to a youth's emotional problems.

It Won't Hurt/You Will be Fine/There Is Nothing to be Afraid of

A common parental misconception is that it is best to tell youths they will not feel some discomfort, pain, or anxiety during a stressful and unusual life event such as a medical or dental procedure. Further, when they see their youth expressing pain, some parents attempt to minimize their pain, saying, "It doesn't hurt that much"; "You will be fine"; Toughen up"; etc. As explained in Chap. 3, youths' temperament style will influence their perception of and reaction to stressful life events.

For decades, the predisposition for pain tolerance in youths was underestimated because of the wide range of pain tolerance, family culture, and race that affect pain perception [22, 56]. The anxiety and pain one youth experiences when having sutures or casting for a fracture can be manageable, while another youth may be overwhelmed with anxiety and pain by a vaccination.

Parents quickly learn that a one-size-fits-all approach to helping their youth with pain or anxiety-provoking experiences can lead to more distress [57]. Parents will also learn that their tolerance for pain or anxiety-provoking situations can be very different from their youth's. Clearly, youths need reassurance that their pain or anxiety will end.

A youth's distressing experience should not be ignored or ridiculed.

Our colleague, an advanced-practice nurse, experiences vasovagal reactions when dilating eye drops are administered for routine ophthalmologic examinations.

"Don't tell me it's going to be fine," she says. "I always faint and end up on the floor." Some individuals need support and reassurance; teasing them will increase anxiety and can lead to mistrust of reassurance from others.

Therefore, it is best to allow youths to express their feelings. Using a developmentally appropriate pain scale according to a youth's age can be helpful in gauging the severity of their pain (e.g., use of illustrated faces for younger youths, and numbers for adolescents). The Wait, Watch, and Wonder approach is also helpful.

Helpful Comments for Youths Who Experience Pain

- It might hurt. Please let me know if it does. We will get something to eat or go for a walk to help the pain stop.
- If it hurts for more than 30 minutes, the doctor said we can give you medication to help.
- It is okay to be afraid [depending on the situation, provide possible solutions]. I am also afraid of needles, but I am happy when it stops hurting.

If you Sign up for an Extracurricular Activity, you Must Finish it

Parents often enroll youths in extracurricular activities that they believe will benefit their child's self-esteem. Most youths choose sport, arts, or musical activities that they like and correspond to their developmental skills. However, at times, youths choose activities that they are able to master, or have unrealistic expectations about how they will perform. To a parent's surprise, some youths may no longer like their choice of activity after attending a few sessions. Conflict may ensue because the parent expects the youth to complete the course or season of the activity. Parents should not assume that a youth's dislike or refusal to continue is due to stubbornness or defiance. Some youths need encouragement to continue. For others, the activity may be a poor fit for their abilities, or may be too difficult for a youth with cognitive weaknesses (Table 8.15).

They Need to Learn to Live in the "Real World"

The "real world" is subjective. One person may be a high achiever, graduate from high school, attend college and graduate school, and later become a professor. Others may drop out of high school and become world-renowned artists (Kristen Wiig, Chris Rock, Whoopi Goldberg, Eddie Van Halen, and many more are

Table 8.15 When extracurricular activities are a poor fit

Extracurricular activity	Weakness emerges	Recommendation
Playing musical instruments	Youths with visual-spatial and working memory weaknesses struggle to memorize basic elements needed to advance to higher levels These youths may find it frustrating to practice	Encourage the youth to participate in activities that have routines If a youth insists on playing an instrument, having an older youth give classes at home can be less anxiety-provoking and more supportive
Sports	Youth with weaknesses in verbal comprehension, working memory, visual spatial abilities, or nonverbal learning disorder may struggle to follow the flow of the team's verbal and nonverbal communications These individuals may struggle to consistently grasp the rules of the sport They may be clumsy and feel embarrassed	Encourage participation in activities that have routines If a youth insists on playing a sport, allow him or her to experience success playing noncompetitive sports Invite the youth camping, fishing, boating, and swimming for recreational exercise
Elite sports	If a youth is talented in a sport but has problems with cognitive flexibility, the competitive nature of the activity may lead to conflicts with coaches and teammates regarding fairness	Although a youth may excel in an elite sport, to prevent relational conflicts, limit time with peers after games
Other extracurricular activities: Chess, choir, swimming, debate, etc	A youth may initially perform well but gradually loses interest due to the amount of extra mental effort needed to enjoy the activity. This is especially likely if weaknesses in fluid reasoning, working memory, and processing speed are present. These youths find the extra time it takes to practice frustrating and may get upset because practice takes time away from friends	Promote activities in which the youth can be successful

examples). All are examples of real-world people. It's common for learning disorders to go undiagnosed until adulthood. As an example, the comedian, Chris Rock, described his struggles with taking things too literally and thinking in all-or-nothing terms. "Those things are really great for writing jokes," he said, "they're just not great for one-on-one relationships." Rock had cognitive testing and was diagnosed with nonverbal learning disorder (NVLD).

As we have seen throughout the book, an individual's four pillars shape the "real world" he or she seeks to fit into. Youths with difficult/feisty temperament seek others with high energy and, depending on the other three pillars, will excel in competitive, high-energy activities or live in constant conflict and use maladaptive behaviors that become their norm.

Our goal is to help parents ensure their children's emotional and behavioral success in their own real four pillar world. Here is a real-world personal example from one of our authors to his trainees and parents.

An Adolescent's "Real World"

A 15-year-old adolescent had struggled academically since middle school, and by high school, learning was substantially more difficult. As a sophomore, he was struggling to keep up with reading assignments in his language arts class, spent hours attempting to memorize vocabulary words, and "just couldn't get" geometry. He increasingly felt anxious and demoralized. He began supportive psychotherapy and was prescribed a selective serotonin reuptake inhibitor (SSRI) for generalized anxiety disorder (GAD). Psychological testing revealed dyslexia, which contributed to his anxiety at school. At that time, medication was discontinued by his clinician. However, his school did not recognize dyslexia as an "official" learning disability diagnosis that would allow him to receive accommodations. He eventually dropped out of high school and began working for a local newspaper drawing cartoons, as he had considerable artistic talent. His self-esteem improved, and he decided he no longer needed psychotherapy. In his last session, he gave his psychiatrist a goodbye cartoon in which both the patient and psychiatrist were laughing. Years later, in the middle of an overflowing sink at a party, a plumber was urgently called. When the plumber, who was the psychiatrist's former patient, arrived, the plumber immediately recognized his former psychiatrist with a bright, warm smile. The plumber now owned a successful plumbing business and, capitalizing on his graphic design skills, had even designed the company logo (which was striking). As they say, the rest is real world history.

Final Thoughts

Although both rewarding and challenging, successful parenting compels us to move beyond one-size-fits-all approaches. Successful parenting demands that we consider a child's unique weaknesses and strengths in his or her four pillars. Parenting approaches informed by the four pillars compel us to reevaluate inherent problems with bedrock parenting myths that have been passed down through the generations. Ultimately, revising these myths is crucial to address and temper unrealistic assumptions that undermine the emotional and behavioral success of youths.

References

1. Almaiah MA, Al-Khasawneh A, Althunibat A. Exploring the critical challenges and factors influencing the E-learning system usage during COVID-19 pandemic. Educ Inf Technol. 2020;25:5261–80. https://doi.org/10.1007/s10639-020-10219-y.
2. American Academy of Pediatrics. What's the best way to discipline my child? 2018. HealthyChildren.org. Available at: https://www.healthychildren.org/English/family-life/family-dynamics/communication-discipline/Pages/Disciplining-Your-Child.aspx. Accessed 29 Aug, 2019.
3. Barragan RC, Brooks R, Meltzoff AN. Altruistic food sharing behavior by human infants after a hunger manipulation. Sci Rep. 2020;10:1785. https://doi.org/10.1038/s41598-020-58645-9.
4. Bender HL, Allen JP, McElhaney KB, et al. Use of harsh physical discipline and developmental outcomes in adolescence. Dev Psychopathol. 2007;19(1):227–42. https://doi.org/10.1017/S0954579407070125.
5. Beaudry-Bellefeuille I, Booth D, Lane SJ. Defecation-specific behavior in children with functional defecation issues: a systematic review. Perm J. 2017;21:17–047. https://doi.org/10.7812/TPP/17-047.
6. Bjørseth Å, Wichstrøm L. Effectiveness of parent-child interaction therapy (PCIT) in the treatment of young Children's behavior problems. A randomized controlled study. PLoS One. 2016;11(9):e0159845. https://doi.org/10.1371/journal.pone.0159845.
7. Bruni O, Alonso-Alconada D, Besag F, et al. Current role of melatonin in pediatric neurology: clinical recommendations. Eur J Paediatr Neurol. 2015;
8. Calkins SD, Keane SP. Developmental origins of early antisocial behavior. Dev Psychopathol. 2009;21(4):1095–109. https://doi.org/10.1017/S095457940999006X.
9. Ciccone A. Rôle de la rythmicité dans le développement du bébé [Role of rhythmicity in infant development]. Encéphale. 2015;41(4 Suppl 1):S15–21. https://doi.org/10.1016/S0013-7006(15)30002-6.
10. Cohen N, Lojkasek M, Muir E (2006). Watch, wait and wonder: an infant-led approach to infant-parent psychotherapy. The signal. 14.
11. Collins WA, Laursen B. Parent–adolescent relationships and influences. In: Lerner R, Steinberg L, editors. Handbook of adolescent psychology, 2. New York: Wiley; 2004. p. 331–61.
12. Dadds MR, Salmon K. Punishment insensitivity and parenting: temperament and learning as interacting risks for antisocial behavior. Clin Child Fam Psychol Rev. 2003;6:69–86. https://doi.org/10.1023/A:1023762009877.
13. Daniel SJ. Education and the COVID-19 pandemic. Prospects. 2020;49:91–6. https://doi.org/10.1007/s11125-020-09464-3.
14. de Zambotti M, Goldstone A, Colrain IM, Baker FC. Insomnia disorder in adolescence: diagnosis, impact, and treatment. Sleep Med Rev. 2018;39:12.
15. Delgado SV. Psychotherapy rounds. Psychodynamic psychotherapy for children and adolescents: an old friend revisited. Psychiatry. 2008;5(5):67–72.
16. Delgado SV, Strawn JR, Pedapati EV. Contemporary psychodynamic psychotherapy for children and adolescents: integrating Intersubjectivity and neuroscience. Springer; 2015.
17. Dodge KA, Greenberg MT, Malone PS Conduct Problems Prevention Research Group. Testing an idealized dynamic cascade model of the development of serious violence in adolescence. Child Dev. 2008;79(6):1907–27. https://doi.org/10.1111/j.1467-8624.2008.01233.x. PMID: 19037957; PMCID: PMC2597335.
18. Dodge KA, Lansford JE, Burks VS, et al. Peer rejection and social information-processing factors in the development of aggressive behavior problems in children. Child Dev. 2003;74:374–93. [PubMed: 12705561].
19. Eisenberg N, Hofer C, Spinrad TL, et al. Understanding mother-adolescent conflict discussions: concurrent and across-time prediction from youths' dispositions and parenting. Monogr Soc Res Child Dev. 2008;73(2):vii–viii, 1–160. https://doi.org/10.1111/j.1540-5834.2008.00470.x. PMID: 18702792; PMCID: PMC2553724.

20. Eisenberg N, Spinrad TL, Fabes RA, et al. The relations of effortful control and impulsivity to children's resiliency and adjustment. Child Dev. 2004;75:1–22. [PubMed: 15015672].
21. Eyberg SM, Funderburk B. Parent-child interaction therapy protocol. Gainesville, FL: PCIT International; 2011.
22. Fein JA, Zempsky WT, Cravero JP. Committee on pediatric emergency medicine and section on anesthesiology and pain medicine; American Academy of Pediatrics. Relief of pain and anxiety in pediatric patients in emergency medical systems. Pediatrics. 2012;130(5):e1391–405. https://doi.org/10.1542/peds.2012-2536. Epub 2012 Oct 29. PMID: 23109683.
23. Giedd JN. The digital revolution and adolescent brain evolution. The Journal of Adolescent Health: Official Publication of the Society For Adolescent Medicine. 2012;51:101–5. https://doi.org/10.1016/j.jadohealth.2012.06.002. PMID 22824439.
24. Gogtay N, Giedd JN, Lusk L, et al. Dynamic mapping of human cortical development during childhood through early adulthood. Proceedings of the National Academy of Sciences of the United States of America. 2004;101:8174–9. PMID 15148381. https://doi.org/10.1073/pnas.0402680101.
25. Granic I, Patterson GR. Toward a comprehensive model of antisocial development: a dynamic systems approach. Psychol Rev. 2006;113(1):101–31.
26. Gringras P, Nir T, Breddy J, et al. Efficacy and safety of pediatric prolonged-release melatonin for insomnia in children with autism spectrum disorder. J Am Acad Child Adolesc Psychiatry. 2017;56(11):948–57.e4. https://doi.org/10.1016/j.jaac.2017.09.414. Epub 2017 Sep 19. PMID: 29096777.
27. Herba C, Phillips M. Annotation: development of facial expression recognition from childhood to adolescence: behavioural and neurological perspectives. J Child Psychol Psychiatry. 2004;45(7):1185–98. https://doi.org/10.1111/j.1469-7610.2004.00316.x. PMID: 15335339.
28. Hill NE, Castellino DR, Lansford JE, et al. Parent-academic involvement as related to school behavior, achievement, and aspirations: demographic variations across adolescence. Child Dev. 2004;75(5):1491–509. [PubMed: 15369527].
29. Holmes CT. Grade level retention effects: a meta-analysis of research studies. In: Shepard LA, Smith ML, editors. Flunking grades: research and policies on retention. Philadelphia: Falmer Press p; 1989. p. 16–33.
30. Janjua I, Goldman RD. Sleep-related melatonin use in healthy children. Can Fam Physician. 2016;62(4):315–7.
31. Jain SV, Horn PS, Simakajornboon N, et al. Melatonin improves sleep in children with epilepsy: a randomized, double-blind, crossover study. Sleep Med. 2015;16(5):637–44. https://doi.org/10.1016/j.sleep.2015.01.005. Epub 2015 Jan 21. PMID: 25862116; PMCID: PMC4425994.
32. Krimendahl E. "Did you see that?": a relational perspective on children who cheat in analysis. J Infant Child Adolesc Psychoth. 2000;1(2):43–58.
33. Lansford JE, Dodge KA, Pettit GS, et al. A 12-year prospective study of the long-term effects of early child physical maltreatment on psychological, behavioral, and academic problems in adolescence. Arch Pediat Adolesc Med. 2002;156:824–30.
34. Lewin DS, Wolfson AR, Bixler EO, Carskadon MA. Duration isn't everything. Healthy sleep in children and teens: duration, individual need and timing. J Clin Sleep Med. 2016;12(11):1439–41. https://doi.org/10.5664/jcsm.6260.
35. Lineman CC, Brabson LA, Highlander A, et al. Parent-child interaction therapy: current perspectives. Psychol Res Behav Manag. 2017;10:239–56. https://doi.org/10.2147/PRBM.S91200.
36. Locke J, Campbell M, Kavanagh D. Can a parent do too much for their child? An examination by parenting professionals of the concept of Overparenting. Aust J Guid Couns. 2012;22(2):249–65. https://doi.org/10.1017/jgc.2012.29.
37. Malow BA, Findling RL, Schroder CM, et al. Sleep, growth, and puberty after 2 years of prolonged-release melatonin in children with autism Spectrum disorder. J Am Acad Child Adolesc Psychiatry. 2021;60(2):252–61.e3. https://doi.org/10.1016/j.jaac.2019.12.007.

38. Manning WD, Longmore MA, Copp J, Giordano PC. The complexities of adolescent dating and sexual relationships: fluidity, meaning(s), and implications for young adults' Well-being. New Dir Child Adolesc Dev. 2014;144:53–69. https://doi.org/10.1002/cad.20060.
39. Mazerolle L, Bennett S, Antrobus E, et al. Disrupting the pathway from truancy to delinquency: a randomized field trial test of the longitudinal impact of a school engagement program. J Quant Criminol. 2019;35:663–89. https://doi.org/10.1007/s10940-018-9395-8.
40. Mazza S, Bastuji H, Rey AE. Objective and subjective assessments of sleep in children: comparison of Actigraphy, sleep diary completed by children and Parents' estimation. Front Psych. 2020;11:495. https://doi.org/10.3389/fpsyt.2020.00495.
41. McDevitt TM, Ormrod JE. Child development and education. 4th ed. Upper Saddle River, NJ: Pearson Education; 2010.
42. Moffitt TE, Caspi A. Childhood predictors differentiate life-course persistent and adolescence-limited antisocial pathways among males and females. Dev Psychopathol. 2001;13:135–51.
43. Moilanen KL, Manuel ML. Helicopter Parenting and Adjustment Outcomes in Young Adulthood: A Consideration of the Mediating Roles of Mastery and Self-Regulation Journal of Child and Family Studies. 2019;28:2145–58.
44. Moilanen KL, Shaw DS, Maxwell KL. Developmental cascades: externalizing, internalizing, and academic competence from middle childhood to early adolescence. Dev Psychopathol. 2010;22(03):635–53. https://doi.org/10.1017/S0954579410000337.
45. Morris AS, Silk JS, Steinberg L, et al. The role of the family context in the development of emotion regulation. Soc Dev. 2007;16(2):361–88. https://doi.org/10.1111/j.1467-9507.2007.00389.x.
46. Newton AT, Honaker SM, Reid GJ. Risk and protective factors and processes for behavioral sleep problems among preschool and early school-aged children: a systematic review. Sleep Med Rev. 2020;52:101303.
47. Owens JA, Babcock D, Weiss M. Evaluation and treatment of children and adolescents with excessive daytime sleepiness. Clin Pediatr. 2020;59(4–5):340–51. https://doi.org/10.1177/0009922820903434.
48. Perrault AA, Bayer L, Peuvrier M, et al. Reducing the use of screen electronic devices in the evening is associated with improved sleep and daytime vigilance in adolescents. Sleep. 2019;2019:42(9).
49. Perry NB, Dollar JM, Calkins SD, et al. Childhood self-regulation as a mechanism through which early overcontrolling parenting is associated with adjustment in preadolescence. Dev Psychol. 2018;54(8):1542–54. https://doi.org/10.1037/dev0000536.
50. Pettit GS, Bates JE, Dodge KA, Meece DW. The impact of after-school peer contact on early adolescent externalizing problems is moderated by parental monitoring, neighborhood safety, and prior adjustment. Child Dev. 1999;70:768–78. [PubMed: 10368921].
51. Phelan TW. 1–2-3 magic: effective discipline for children 2–12. 5th ed. Glen Ellyn, IL: ParentMagic; 2014.
52. Schaefer CE. Foundations of play therapy. 2nd ed. NJ: Wiley; 2011.
53. Smetana JG, Campione-Barr N, Daddis C. Longitudinal development of family decision making: defining healthy behavioral autonomy for middle-class African American adolescents. Child Dev. 2004;75:1418–34.
54. Smetana JG, Campione-Barr N, Metzger. Adolescent development in interpersonal and societal contexts. Annu Rev Psychol. 2006;57:255–84.
55. Tamm L, Menon V, Reiss AL. Maturation of brain function associated with response inhibition. J Am Acad Child Adolescent Psychiat. 2002;41:1231–8.
56. Thrane SE, Wanless S, Cohen SM, Danford CA. The assessment and non-pharmacologic treatment of procedural pain from infancy to school age through a developmental lens: a synthesis of evidence with recommendations. J Pediatr Nurs. 2016;31(1):e23–32. https://doi.org/10.1016/j.pedn.2015.09.002.
57. Trottier ED, Doré-Bergeron MJ, Chauvin-Kimoff L, Baerg K, Ali S, et al. Managing pain and distress in children undergoing brief diagnostic and therapeutic procedures. Paediatr Child Health. 2019;24(8):509–35. https://doi.org/10.1093/pch/pxz026.

58. van Geijlswijk IM, van der Heijden KB, Egberts AC, et al. Dose finding of melatonin for chronic idiopathic childhood sleep onset insomnia: an RCT. Psychopharmacology (Berl). 2010;212(3):379–91. https://doi.org/10.1007/s00213-010-1962-0. Epub 2010 Jul 29. PMID: 20668840; PMCID: PMC2952772.
59. Wallerstein JS, Blakeslee S. Second chances: men, women, and children a decade after divorce. New York: Ticknor and Fields; 1989.
60. Walkup JT, Friedland SJ, Peris TS, Strawn JR. Dysregulation, catastrophic reactions, and the anxiety disorders. Child Adolesc Psychiatr Clin N Am. 2021;30(2):431–44.
61. Yin L, Hu Y, Dynowski D, Li J, et al. The good lies: altruistic goals modulate processing of deception in the anterior insula. Hum Brain Mapp. 2017;38(7):3675–90. https://doi.org/10.1002/hbm.23623.
62. Yurgelun-Todd D. Emotional and cognitive changes during adolescence. Curr Opin Neurobiol. 2007;17(2):251–7. https://doi.org/10.1016/j.conb.2007.03.009. Epub 2007 Mar 26. PMID: 17383865.
63. Delgado and Strawn. Psychodynamic understandings. In: Levesque RJ, editor. Encyclopedia of adolescence. Springer International Publishing Switzerland; 2016.

Correction to: Intelligence: "Why Don't You Behave?"

Correction to: Chapter 4 in: S. V. Delgado et al.,
***Promoting the Emotional and Behavioral Success of Youths*,**
https://doi.org/10.1007/978-3-030-88075-0_4

Owing to the oversight on the part of the Author, figure 4 in this chapter was initially published with an error.

In the figure (labels are in the chapter), "Michael" should be over the red figure and "Noah" should be over the green figure. It was opposite in the original. This has now been updated and the correct presentation is given below:

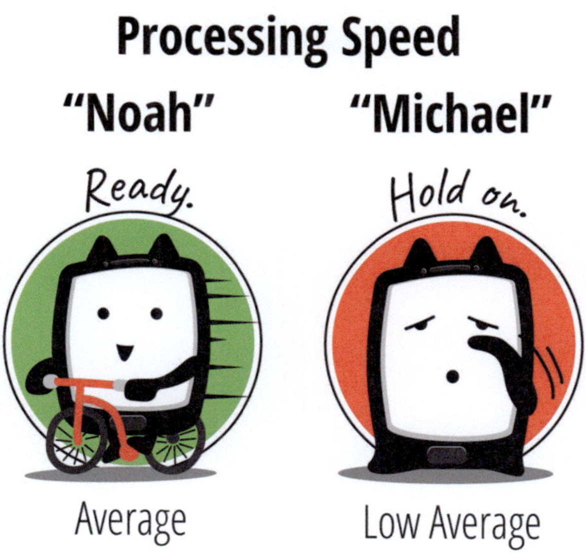

The updated original version of the chapter can be found at https://doi.org/10.1007/978-3-030-88075-0_4

S. V. Delgado et al., *Promoting the Emotional and Behavioral Success of Youths*, https://doi.org/10.1007/978-3-030-88075-0_9

Appendix A

S. V. Delgado et al., *Promoting the Emotional and Behavioral Success of Youths*,
https://doi.org/10.1007/978-3-030-88075-0

Developmental milestones: 2- to 3-year-old toddlers

Developmental Domain	Proficient	Concerning
Social/Emotional	At 2 years old, plays mainly beside other children, does not like sharing, and may grab and push. At 3 years old, shows affection for friends without prompting, takes turns in games, shows concern for a crying friend, and has a wide range of emotions.	Poor affection for friends. Aggressive forms of play. Poor self-regulation while playing. Does not know how to make use of toys or enjoy play. Little interest in taking turns in games.
Language/Communication	At 2 years old, average vocabulary should be 50 to 300 words. By 3 years old, should have a vocabulary of 1,000 words and be able to carry a conversation using two- to three-word sentences using plurals and pronouns.	Limited amount of words used. Use of offensive words, likely heard from adults. Loud use of infantile voice.
Cognition	At 2 years old, completes phrases of two to three words and communicates needs (hunger, thirst, pain, etc.). At 3 years old, plays make-believe with dolls, animals, and people, completes puzzles with three or four pieces.	Play is simple or disorganized. Poor ability to play make-believe and speaks of negative view of others. Concrete play without story line.
Behavior/Motor	At 2 years old, begins to run and kicks a ball, builds a tower of six to seven cubes. At 3 years old, runs easily and climbs well, has control of bowel and bladder during the day.	Impulsive with poor self-regulation. Repetitive behaviors or actions. Often aggressive actions.
Parental "Milestones"	Creates a stimulating and colorful environment. Reads to the child. Displays consistent and predictable discipline and routines. Attunes to child's needs even during episodes of angry feelings.	Unpredictable routines. Abrupt and inconsistent discipline. Poor recollection of feeding and sleep schedules. Unaware of child's distress during conflict between parents. Bothered by child's needs and yells at child rather than attunes.

Adapted from: Division of Birth Defects, National Center on Birth Defects and Developmental Disabilities, Centers for Disease Control and Prevention; Shelvov SP, Hannemann RE, Trubo R (2004) The American Academy of Pediatrics: Complete and Authoritative Guide for Caring for Your Baby and Young Child. Bantam Books

Developmental milestones: 4- to 6-year-old children

Developmental Domain	Proficient	Concerning
Social/Emotional	Enjoys exploring and is curious about toys and games. Increasing creativity with make-believe play. Wants to please and agrees to rules, although may change rules often. Increasingly cooperates and plays with other children over playing alone. Likes to sing, dance, and act. By 5 years old, can tell the difference between pretend and real and is aware of gender. May be very demanding at times, and very compliant at other times.	Restricted range of emotions. Ignores other children. Argues with persons outside of the family. Shows extreme behavior, usually aggressive or sad. Limited repertoire of games and activities. No interest in make-believe or interactive games.
Language/Communication	Sings a song or recites poem from memory. Tells stories with full sentences. Can say first and last name. Increasingly uses future tense. Uses basic rules of grammar. By 5 years old, recites the alphabet and counts to 10. By 6 years old, average expressive vocabulary should be 2,500 words, and receptive vocabulary should be 20,000 words.	Speaks unclearly and is difficult to understand. Cannot retell a favorite story or video. Frequent errors with pronouns. Unable to comment on daily activities or experiences. Limited and repetitive vocabulary. Poor use of grammar, especially plurals and past tense. Imitates words of others and uses out of context.
Cognition	By 6 years old, identifies many colors and numbers. Can draw a person and geometric shapes with increasing complexity. Can count 10 or more things. Developing idea of “same” and “different.”	Has trouble scribbling. Resists dressing self and toilet training. Difficulty staying focused on a single activity for more than three minutes. Difficulty distinguishing between pretend and real. Cannot follow three-part commands.

	Remembers parts of stories and tells you what may happen next in a story. Developing an understanding of time. Knows about things used every day, like money and food. Can draw a circle or triangle.	Speaks in infantile manner. No depth to their stories or play.
Behavior/Motor	Can print some letters or numbers. Stands on one foot for 10 seconds or longer. Hops and eventually skips. Uses a fork and spoon and sometimes can use a knife to spread. Can use the toilet on his or her own. Swings and climbs. Can dress independently; may need help with laces and buttons.	Unable to jump in place. Unable to brush teeth, wash and dry hands, or get undressed without help. Draws pictures in very simple form. Restlessness, over-activity, and abrupt behavior/motors.
Parental "Milestones"	Reads stories and attunes to the child's reactions to the story line. Is consistent, repeats instructions with tone of voice and gestures reflecting care and firmness. Is warm and affectionate when child expresses angry feelings. Has predictable routine in parenting and playful activities.	Frequently involves children in conflict between parents. Consistently displays affect in harsh manner. Inconsistent and abrupt discipline. Frequently shouts when the child needs attention. Unrealistic expectations of the child. Use of corporal punishment.

Adapted from: Division of Birth Defects, National Center on Birth Defects and Developmental Disabilities, Centers for Disease Control and Prevention; Shelvov SP, Hannemann RE, Trubo R (2004) The American Academy of Pediatrics: Complete and Authoritative Guide for Caring for Your Baby and Young Child. Bantam Books

Developmental milestones: 7- to 9-year-old children

Developmental Domain	Proficient	Concerning
Social/Emotional	Fears of monsters, kidnappers, and large animals. Play includes use of fantasy and imagination. May have imaginary friends. Develops a sense of humor, expresses simple jokes and rhymes. Initially desires to play with parents, but gradually shifts toward friends. Can play in organized sports and follows rules. Develops a greater sense of empathy with same-sex peers, but still mostly self-focused.	Intense sadness or despair. Only smiles or laughs at the expense of making fun of peer or adult. Problems making and keeping friends, demanding of their loyalty. Displays anger, aggression, or temper tantrums. Demands privileges of older siblings. Does not fear being alone in public places.
Language/Communication	Can describe with some detail a favorite activity, video, or book. Uses correct grammar and sentence structure most of the time. Recognizes and reads simple words. Able to thank others for help.	May steal or lie with a poor understanding of the consequences. Poor comprehension of age-appropriate books and videos. Self-injurious behavior such as head banging, scratching, or biting when angry. Frequently uses foul language.
Cognition	Develops the skills to process more abstract concepts and complex ideas. Is able to focus on the past and future as well as the present. Can draw a figure with a head, body, arms, and legs. Identifies right and left easily.	Learning becomes increasingly difficulty; avoids doing homework. Frequent disruptive behavior at school. Continues to communicate with simple sentences. Does not pick up on humor. Difficulty with changes in routine or transitions. Speaks in infantile manner. Seems younger than age.
Behavior/Motor	Usually has good balance and enjoys running, jumping, skipping, and other forms of physical play.	Frequently falls during simple activities.

	Able to hold a pencil and clearly write letters. Can copy triangles and diamonds. Can ride a bicycle and tie shoes. Increasing height and weight.	Inability to hold and use writing instruments. Repetitive behavior/motors such as hand flapping or rocking. Frequent physical pains such as stomachaches, headaches, or vomiting. Frequent aggressive behaviors toward siblings and peers.
Parental "Milestones"	Is involved in child's extracurricular activities. Delegates age-appropriate responsibilities within the home. Works to reduce changes in child's life, shields children from parental conflict.	Often asks the child to take sides between parents when in conflict. Frequent complaints of other persons in the presence of the child. Usually is harsh; inconsistent discipline may include corporal punishment. Always expresses anger verbally by yelling. Relies on child to listen to adult problems or loneliness.

Adapted from: Division of Birth Defects, National Center on Birth Defects and Developmental Disabilities, Centers for Disease Control and Prevention; Shelvov SP, Hannemann RE, Trubo R (2004) The American Academy of Pediatrics: Complete and Authoritative Guide for Caring for Your Baby and Young Child. Bantam Books

Developmental milestones: 10- to 12-year-old adolescents

Developmental Domain	Proficient	Concerning
Social/Emotional	Close friendships to same-sex peers. Becomes critical of adults. Has intense interest in belonging to a team and enjoys organized competitive games. Anger is common, resents being told what to do, and rebels at routines. Reacts emotionally rather than logically. Experiences many fears and worries about physical changes and appearance.	Doesn't smile or laugh, prefers to argue or demand. Problems making and keeping friends. Angry and aggressive comments or behaviors, temper tantrums. Dislike of organized games.
Language/Communication	Begins to be interested in world and community events. Has strong urge to conform to peer-group morals. Good abstract reasoning, with meaningful conversations with peers.	Does not see the consequences of stealing or lying. Prefers to view age-inappropriate books and videos, which can include violence and sex. Self-injurious behaviors such as head banging, scratching, or biting, when stressed. Use of foul language.
Cognition	Challenges adult knowledge. Increased ability to use logic. May have interest in earning money. Has interest in having privacy.	Frequent negative behavior at school. Declining grades with increased difficulty. Difficulty with small changes in routine or transitions. Avoids schoolwork, and it does not bring pleasure.
Behavior/Motor	Rapid growth if in puberty and is increasingly aware of body changes (e.g., voice, body odor). Girls begin to show secondary sex characteristics. Increased coordination and strength. Enjoys sports and video games	Impulsivity is common. Aggression is aimed at hurting others. Bullies other children who are not as strong. Frequent use of physical aggression. Begins to resort to self-harming activities when angry or unhappy.

	with peers, both organized or in community. Shift in sleep patterns.	
Parental "Milestones"	Is able to anticipate and discuss pubertal changes. Is understanding and supportive. Helps child set the rules and decide own responsibilities. Gives child opportunity to make decisions. Provides for organized activities in sports or clubs.	Undermines other parent. Gives the child adultified role in caring for younger siblings. Unable to perceive academic or social struggles in child. Makes fun of child if child makes mistakes. Increases use of negative comments and blames the child often.

Adapted from: Division of Birth Defects, National Center on Birth Defects and Developmental Disabilities, Centers for Disease Control and Prevention; Shelvov SP, Hannemann RE, Trubo R (2004) The American Academy of Pediatrics: Complete and Authoritative Guide for Caring for Your Baby and Young Child. Bantam Books

Developmental milestones: 13- to 15-year-old adolescents

Developmental Domain	Proficient	Concerning
Social/Emotional	Withdraws from parents, who are invariably called "too old." Needs less family companionship. Worries about grades, appearance, and popularity. Identifies with peer group. Ambivalent about sexual relationships. Body image and dieting patterns begin to have prominence. Age-specific moodiness.	Irritability, mood swings. Expects to fail and blames parents. Bullies other children. Blames parents for unhappiness. Enjoys teasing others. Engages in self-defeating, aggressive, antisocial, or impulsive behavior; may withdraw or isolate. Does not respect others' property. Body image avoids mainstream peers' image.
Language/Communication	Enjoys reading or being involved in school projects Thrives on arguments and discussions by using logical thinking.	Unable to enjoy being with peers unless involved in negative behaviors. Argues with adults using foul language.
Cognition	Increasingly able to memorize. Thinks logically and hypothetically about concepts. Engages in introspection and probing into own thinking. Has realistic plans for the future.	Concrete thinking. Behaves as if societal rules do not apply. Difficulties at school lead to disruptive behavior. Use of nicotine, alcohol, and drugs.
Behavior/Motor	Experiences sudden and rapid increases in height, weight, and strength with the onset of adolescence. Enjoys competitive sports and video games, both organized or in community. Participates in outdoor chores with parents.	Aggression is aimed at hurting others. No inhibitions of sexual or substance abuse activity. Bullies other children who are not as strong. Frequent use of physical aggression.
Parental "Milestones"	Decision making is done as a parental unit, even when divorced. Assists in navigating through pubertal changes. Models emotional and behavioral regulation during arguments. Engages in consistent support and limit setting. Models by engaging in altruistic activities	Undermines other parent. Unable to perceive struggles in peers. Makes fun of other's mistakes with foul language. Engages in unilateral authoritarian parenting with limited collaboration. Overly identifies with adolescent, has poor limit setting, and is too permissive Allows the adolescent to have an adult role when needed for selfish reasons

Adapted from: Division of Birth Defects, National Center on Birth Defects and Developmental Disabilities, Centers for Disease Control and Prevention; Shelvov SP, Hannemann RE, Trubo R (2004) The American Academy of Pediatrics: Complete and Authoritative Guide for Caring for Your Baby and Young Child. Bantam Books

Developmental milestones: 16- to 19-year-old adolescents

Developmental Domain	Proficient	Concerning Similar to deficits in 13- to 15-year-olds, although in more extreme form.
Social/Emotional	Usually has many friends and a few in whom they confide. May be strongly invested in a single romantic relationship; may begin to become sexually active. Worries about failure. Has conflicting feelings about dependence/independence. Age-specific moodiness.	Irritability, mood swings. Bullies peers and adults. Blames parents for any mishap. Begins to speak of physical actions toward others, self-harm, and suicide if demands to be liked or loved are not met. Difficulties trusting.
Language/Communication	Able to fluidly shift between different contexts, including ages and peer groups. Able to use more complex communication to express ideas, including nonverbal and abstract ideas. Establishment of ethical and moral values.	Enjoys being with peers only if they use the same foul language. Involved in negative behaviors with more planning. Argues and threatens adults and uses foul language without concern for hurting others. Unable to form or maintain satisfactory relationships with peers.
Cognition	Beginning to integrate knowledge leading to decisions about future. Makes steps toward intimacy. Conscious choices about which adults to trust. Respects honesty and straightforwardness from adults.	Concrete thinking is common Critical of parents and believes societal rules do not apply. Difficulties at school lead to disruptive behavior. Use of nicotine, alcohol, and illegal drugs.
Behavior/Motor	Has essentially completed physical maturation; physical features are shaped and defined. Probability of acting on sexual desires increases.	Aggression is aimed at hurting others. No inhibitions of sexual activity. Takes pleasure in bullying peers. Frequent use of physical aggression.

	May become sexually active or experiment with drugs.	
Parental "Milestones"	Discusses appropriate clothing in context of changes in physical maturity. Is available to talk and to listen. Avoids ridicule of inconsistent behaviors. Provides accurate information on consequences of sexual activity. Gives limited supervision roles in household of siblings. Engages in promoting college or other adult roles.	Unable to understand or dismisses the adolescent's struggles. Makes fun of adolescent if adolescent makes mistakes. Demands respect in angry and hostile manner. Unaware of adolescent's whereabouts. Failure to be aware of adolescent's developmental needs. Expects adolescent to be overly involved in parent role of younger siblings, although demands respect at other times.

Adapted from: Division of Birth Defects, National Center on Birth Defects and Developmental Disabilities, Centers for Disease Control and Prevention; Shelvov SP, Hannemann RE, Trubo R (2004) The American Academy of Pediatrics: Complete and Authoritative Guide for Caring for Your Baby and Young Child. Bantam Books

Index

S. V. Delgado et al., *Promoting the Emotional and Behavioral Success of Youths*,
https://doi.org/10.1007/978-3-030-88075-0

D

MIX
Papier aus verantwortungsvollen Quellen
Paper from responsible sources
FSC® C105338

If you have any concerns about our products,
you can contact us on
ProductSafety@springernature.com

In case Publisher is established outside the EU,
the EU authorized representative is:
Springer Nature Customer Service Center GmbH
Europaplatz 3, 69115 Heidelberg, Germany

Printed by Libri Plureos GmbH
in Hamburg, Germany